Ultrasound for the Ge

Ultrasound for the Generalist

A Guide to Point-of-Care Imaging

Edited by

Dr Sarb Clare
Consultant Acute Medicine, Deputy Medical Director, Sandwell and West Birmingham Hospitals
NHS Trust, United Kingdom.

Dr Chris Duncan
Specialist Registrar in Intensive Care Medicine, London, United Kingdom.

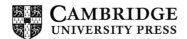
CAMBRIDGE
UNIVERSITY PRESS

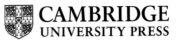

Shaftesbury Road, Cambridge CB2 8EA, United Kingdom

One Liberty Plaza, 20th Floor, New York, NY 10006, USA

477 Williamstown Road, Port Melbourne, VIC 3207, Australia

314–321, 3rd Floor, Plot 3, Splendor Forum, Jasola District Centre,
New Delhi – 110025, India

103 Penang Road, #05–06/07, Visioncrest Commercial, Singapore 238467

Cambridge University Press & Assessment is a department of the
University of Cambridge.

We share the University's mission to contribute to society through the pursuit of
education, learning and research at the highest international levels of excellence.

www.cambridge.org
Information on this title: www.cambridge.org/9781108850483
DOI: 10.1017/9781108850476

First published 2022
Reprinted 2022

Printed in Great Britain by CPI Group (UK) Ltd, Croydon CR0 4YY

A catalogue record for this publication is available from the British Library.

Library of Congress Cataloging-in-Publication Data
Names: Clare, Sarb, Dr., editor. | Duncan, Chris, Dr., editor.
Title: Ultrasound for the generalist : a guide to point of care imaging /
  edited by Sarb Clare, Chris Duncan.
Description: Cambridge, United Kingdom : New York, NY : Cambridge
  University Press, 2022. | Includes bibliographical references and index.
Identifiers: LCCN 2021019839 (print) | LCCN 2021019840 (ebook) |
  ISBN 9781108850476 (epub) | ISBN 9781108797078 (paperback)
Subjects: | MESH: Ultrasonography–instrumentation | Ultrasonography–
  methods | Point-of-Care Systems
Classification: LCC RC78.7.U4 (ebook) | LCC RC78.7.U4 (print) |
  NLM WN 208 | DDC 616.07/543–dc23
LC record available at https://lccn.loc.gov/2021019839

ISBN 978-1-108-79707-8 Paperback
ISBN 978-1-108-85047-6 Cambridge Core
ISBN 978-1-108-85048-3 Print/Online bundle

. . . .

Contents

Foreword   vi
Preface   vii
Abbreviations   viii
Editors and Contributing Authors   xii

Introduction   1

1   **Basic Physics, Knobology and Artefacts**   4

2   **Echocardiography**   26

3   **Thoracic Ultrasound**   68

4   **Abdominal Ultrasound**   97

5   **Vascular Ultrasound**   127

6   **Soft Tissue and Musculoskeletal Ultrasound**   140

7   **Ultrasound for Neurology**   168

8   **Gynaecology and Early Pregnancy Ultrasound**   180

9   **Hospital at Home**   190

10   **Palliative Care and End of Life Care**   195

11   **Ultrasound in Prehospital, Remote and Austere Environments**   200

12   **COVID-19 – A World Stage**   217

13   **Governance and Quality Assurance**   231

14   **Training and Accreditation**   236

Meet the Authors   245
Index   247

Digital media accompanying book can be accessed online via the code printed on the inside of the cover

Foreword

It is a pleasure and a privilege to write a foreword and contribute to this unique ultrasound field book. From the clinician just starting out on their point-of-care ultrasound (POCUS) journey to those who are already established and well advanced, this book will prove to be an invaluable companion. The increasingly recognised value of POCUS for all clinical decision-making means that this book will appeal to General Practitioners, Family Medicine Physicians, Emergency, Acute and Critical Care Physicians, Paramedics and Prehospital Practitioners, Physiotherapists, Podiatrists and Advanced Nurse Practitioners.

Ultrasound for the Generalist – A Guide to Point-of-Care Imaging provides you with the knowledge and skills to learn the basics and progress to develop more advanced skills. You will understand how ultrasound images are created, how to acquire and interpret them for each organ and to apply them in your daily work. You will learn what is normal and what is abnormal in the context of real cases and appreciate the importance of quality assurance, limitations and accreditation. The combination of digital media and case descriptions brings this book alive and will inspire you to reach for the scanner. This is an ideal book to take out with you in your field of clinical work as a real-time reference guide.

Ultrasound for the Generalist definitely addresses the needs of the generalist as it covers a wide range of organ systems where POCUS informs management decisions. Chapters range from thoracic ultrasound and echocardiography through to gynaecological and musculoskeletal ultrasound and considers new care settings where even experienced POCUS users may not have seen ultrasound at the bedside. The coverage of remote and austere medicine, including prehospital, military and humanitarian medicine, highlights the essential diagnostic role of POCUS in resource-limited settings.

As a senior clinician, POCUS has enabled me to deliver and practice the best clinical medicine of my career. It has empowered me with a skill that provides prompt and accurate information to make decisions wherever I see patients – in the home, care home or in the hospital. It has been a complete 'game changer' in my day-to-day practice as I have been able to deliver more acute care within community settings. This has been critical for the development of Acute Hospital at Home so that patients and families have a more credible choice over where they would like to be treated during an acute illness. POCUS is now a routine part of my assessment of patients.

I have worked alongside the authors Dr Sarb Clare and Dr Chris Duncan for a number of years and am really proud to have them as my colleagues. Their dedication, clinical expertise and passion for POCUS is inspirational and contagious. All clinical cases within this book are original and display the extensive experience of the authors and contributors.

I highly recommend this very special book for all generalists. It is beautifully written for the learner and easy to follow with fantastic illustrations, scans, photos and digital media. This indispensable text will allow you to acquire and apply this increasingly critical skill to provide the highest quality of care to all patients you see and in whatever setting you see them.

Professor Dan Lasserson
MA MD MRCGP FRCP Edin
Professor of Acute Ambulatory Care, Warwick University
Clinical Lead, Hospital at Home, Oxford University Hospitals NHS Foundation Trust, UK
Twitter @DanLasserson
2021

Preface

Point-of-care ultrasound (POCUS) has become an essential tool within acute specialties to enhance bedside diagnostics, facilitate safe interventional procedures and guide referral to specialist services. It is vital for this tool to be expanded to community and prehospital settings where access to definitive investigations is limited. With the evolution of technology, ultrasound is becoming increasingly available due to reducing costs, machine size and remote image review for quality assurance purposes. This skill is invaluable for clinicians at all levels of training from medical school through to consultancy and allied healthcare professionals in any discipline.

With extensive experience using POCUS and seeing the uncountable benefits from swift diagnoses, streamlining the patient journey, carrying out safe procedures and ultimately saving lives, we are both hugely passionate about sharing this skill with all generalist colleagues. We were inspired to write *Ultrasound for the Generalist – A Guide to Point-of-Care Imaging* to provide a field handbook with the fundamentals and foundation of knowledge for clinicians to apply to whatever their normal practice may be.

It is only once you start using ultrasound in day-to-day practice that you will see and appreciate its true utility. US is a simple skill to acquire and yet it confers huge benefits for patients. It will enhance your clinical decision-making and identify pathology you would previously wait days or weeks to confirm. We are very keen to hear from you when you scan the cardinal case where ultrasound makes the difference!

This book will teach you how to use the machine, acquire images, recognise key anatomical landmarks and the appearance of pathology. You will learn to scan all systems and how to achieve competency and accreditation. It starts with the basics and progresses beyond conventional POCUS accreditation pathways. We have complemented the chapters with examples from our extensive library of real-life patient cases.

Key areas of inclusion are the application of US within 'Hospital at Home', Palliative Care, Soft tissue and Musculoskeletal, COVID-19 and Remote, Austere, Military and Humanitarian medicine. US does not 'belong' to any one specialty and clinicians should identify and incorporate the techniques applicable to their daily practice.

We would like to thank all our mentors and the POCUS enthusiasts championing this skill. A massive thanks to our contributing authors and the publishers at Cambridge University Press, in particular Catherine Barnes and Kim Ingram, for believing in us and our vision. Final thanks to our family and friends for their relentless support!

Enjoy the read and please spread the Power of POCUS!

Dr Sarb Clare and Dr Chris Duncan
2021
www.GeneralistUltrasound.com

This book provides access to an online version on Cambridge Core, which can be accessed via the code printed on the inside of the cover.

Abbreviations

A2C apical two-chamber view

A3C apical three-chamber view

A4C apical four-chamber view

A5C apical five-chamber view

AAA abdominal aortic aneurysm

ACA anterior cerebral artery

AF atrial fibrillation

AFB acid fast bacilli

AIM acute internal medicine

ALI acute lung injury

AMVL anterior mitral valve leaflet

Ao aorta

AP anterior-posterior

AMS acute mountain sickness

AR aortic regurgitation

ARDS acute respiratory distress syndrome

ARVC arrhythmogenic right ventricular cardiomyopathy

AS aortic stenosis

ASD atrial septal defect

ASE American Society of Echocardiography

ATT anti tubercular treatment

AV aortic valve

AXR abdominal X-ray

BLUE basic lung ultrasound examination

BP blood pressure

BSE British Society Of Echocardiography

CAP community-acquired pneumonia

CBD common bile duct

CFM colour flow mode

CKD chronic kidney disease

CO cardiac output

COPD chronic pulmonary obstructive disease

CPAP continuous positive airway pressure

CPD continual professional development

CPR cardiopulmonary resuscitation

CRP C-reactive protein

CRL crown rump length

CT computed tomography

CTPA computed tomography pulmonary angiogram

CW continuous wave

CWD continuous wave Doppler

CXR chest X-ray

dBs decibels

DC direct current

DCM dilated cardiomyopathy

DCS decompression stress

DICOM digital imaging and communications in medicine

DVT deep vein thrombosis

EBV Epstein–Barr virus

ECG electrocardiogram

Echo echocardiogram

ECMO extracorporeal membrane oxygenation

ED emergency department

EF ejection fraction

EM emergency medicine

ESR erythrocyte sedimentation rate

EtCO2 end tidal carbon dioxide

ETT endotracheal tube

FAC fractional area change

FASH focused assessment sonography HIV-associated tuberculosis

FAST focused assessment with sonography in trauma

e-FAST extended focused assessment with sonography in trauma

FB foreign body

FH frank hypovolaemia

FUSIC focused intensive care echocardiography

GB gallbladder

GCA giant cell arteritis

GCS Glasgow Coma Scale

GP general practitioner

HACE high altitude cerebral oedema

HAPE high altitude pulmonary oedema

HAPH high altitude pulmonary hypertension

HCG human chorionic gonadotropin

HCM hypertrophic obstructive cardiomyopathy

HIV human immunodeficiency virus

HPB hepatobiliary

HRCT high resolution computed tomography

HTN hypertension

Hz Hertz

IAS interatrial septum

ICD intercostal drain

ICP intracranial pressure

ICU intensive care unit

IIH idiopathic intracranial hypertension

ITU intensive therapy unit

IVC inferior vena cava

IV intravenous

IVDU intravenous drug user

IVS interventricular septum

IUD intrauterine device

IUP intrauterine pregnancy

IVF in vitro fertilisation

IVSd interventricular septum diastole

JVP jugular venous pressure

KHz Kilohertz

LA left atrium

LBBB left bundle branch block

LP lumbar puncture

LUQ left upper quadrant

LUS lung ultrasound

LV left ventricle

LVAS left ventricular assist system

LVEDP left ventricular end diastolic pressure

LVIDd left ventricle internal diameter in diastole

LVIDs left ventricle internal diameter in systole

LVH left ventricular hypertrophy

LVNCC left ventricular non compaction cardiomyopathy

LVOT left ventricular outflow tract

LVOTO left ventricular outflow tract obstruction

LVPWd left ventricle posterior wall in diastole

m/s metres per second

MAPSE mitral annular plane systolic excursion

MCA middle cerebral artery

MDR TB multi drug resistant tuberculosis

MERT medical emergency response team

MHz Megahertz

MI myocardial infarction

M-Mode motion mode

MPA main pulmonary artery

MR mitral regurgitation

MRI magnetic resonance imaging

MS mitral stenosis

MSK musculoskeletal

MSKUS musculoskeletal ultrasound

MSSA methicillin susceptible staphylococcus aureus

MV mitral valve

NF necrotising fasciitis

NHS National Health Service

NICE National Institute of Clinical Excellence

NSTEMI non ST elevation myocardial infarction

NYHA New York Health Association

ON optic nerve

ONSD optic nerve sheath diameter

PA pulmonary artery

PACS picture archive and communication systems

PCA posterior cerebral artery

PCI percutaneous coronary intervention

PD power Doppler

PE pulmonary embolism

PEA pulseless electrical activity

PEEP positive end expiratory pressure

PG porcelain gallbladder

PHEM prehospital emergency medicine

PHT pulmonary hypertension

PHUS prehospital ultrasound

PIMS paediatric multisystem inflammatory syndrome

PLAPS posterolateral alveolar and/or pleural syndrome

PLAX parasternal long-axis view

PMVL posterior mitral valve leaflet

POCUS point-of-care ultrasound

POD Pouch of Douglas

PSAX parasternal short-axis view

PSS Paget-Schroetter syndrome

PV pulmonary valve

PW pulse wave

PWD pulse wave Doppler

QA quality assurance

RA right atrium

RBBB right bundle branch block

RCEM Royal College of Emergency Medicine

RCR Royal College of Radiologists

REBOA resuscitative endovascular balloon occlusion of the aorta

RHD rheumatic heart disease

ROSC return of spontaneous circulation

RUQ right upper quadrant

RV right ventricle

RVESA right ventricular end systolic area

RVID right ventricular internal dimension

RVOT right ventricular outflow tract

RWMA regional wall abnormalities

SAH subarachnoid haemorrhage

SAM systolic anterior motion

SBE subacute bacterial endocarditis

SC subcostal view

SFJ saphenofemoral junction

SLE systemic lupus erythematosus

SMA superior mesenteric artery

SOB shortness of breath

SS suprasternal view

STIs sexually transmitted infections

STEMI ST elevation myocardial infarction

SV stroke volume

TAB temporal artery biopsy

TAP transversus abdominis plane

TAPSE tricuspid annular plane systolic excursion

TAUS temporal artery ultrasound

TB tuberculosis

TCD transcranial Doppler

TDI tissue Doppler imaging

THI tissue harmonic imaging

TGC time gain compensation

TOE transoesophageal echocardiography

TR tricuspid regurgitation

TTE transthoracic echocardiography

TV tricuspid valve

TVUS transvaginal ultrasound

UGRA ultrasound guided regional anaesthesia

US ultrasound

USS ultrasound scan

UTI urinary tract infection

VATS video assisted thoracoscopic surgery

VEXUS venous excess ultrasound

VGE venous gas emboli

V/Q ventilation and perfusion

VSD ventricular septum defect

VTE venous thromboembolism

VTI velocity time integral

VUJ vesicoureteric junction

WES wall echo shadow

WHO World Health Organization

Editors and Contributing Authors

Editors and Lead Authors

Dr Sarb Clare MBE
Consultant Acute Medicine, Deputy Medical
Director, Sandwell and West Birmingham Hospitals
NHS Trust, United Kingdom.

Dr Chris Duncan
Specialist Registrar in Intensive Care Medicine,
London, United Kingdom.

All ultrasound images and online videos are originals
of Authors and Contributors unless otherwise stated.

Graphic design and image annotation by **Dr Chris
Duncan**.

Contributors

Front cover artwork by **Miss Samantha Allwood**.

Mr Carl Bellamy
Medical Photographer, Sandwell and West
Birmingham NHS Trust, United Kingdom.

Dr Jonathan Benham
Consultant Radiologist, Sandwell and West
Birmingham NHS Trust, United Kingdom.

Miss Alice Corbett
Specialist Musculoskeletal Podiatrist, London,
United Kingdom.

Dr Paramjeet Singh Deol
Consultant in Emergency Medicine and General
Practitioner, Urgent Care General Practice Lead,
Chelsea and Westminster Hospital, United Kingdom.

Dr Alex Hackney
Foundation Year Doctor, West Midlands,
United Kingdom.

Dr Vesna Homar MD
General Practitioner and Consultant in
Emergency Medicine, Ljubljana, Slovenia. Assistant
Lecturer, Faculty of Medicine, University
of Ljubljana.

Dr Sam Hutchings OBE
Surgeon Commander Royal Navy, Consultant in
Intensive Care Medicine, Department of Military
Anaesthesia and Critical Care, Royal Centre for
Defence Medicine and King's College
Hospital London.

Professor Daniel Lasserson
Professor of Ambulatory Care. University of
Warwick, United Kingdom
Clinical Lead, Hospital At Home, Oxford University
Hospital NHS Foundation Trust, United Kingdom.

Dr Catherine Lester
Consultant in Sports and Exercise Medicine, London,
United Kingdom.

Dr Gaynor Prince
Consultant Emergency Physician, FACEM, DDU,
Committee Member Emergency Medicine
Ultrasound Group (EMUGs) New Zealand, ACEM
and EMUGs Collaboration Working Group. World
Extreme Medicine Faculty.

Mr Naveed Saeed
Consultant Echocardiographer, Sandwell and
West Birmingham Hospitals NHS Trust, United
Kingdom

Dr Maheshwari Srinivasan
Consultant Obstetrician and Gynaecologist, Sandwell
and West Birmingham Hospitals NHS Trust,
United Kingdom.

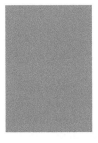

Introduction

About Point of Care Ultrasound

Point of care ultrasound (POCUS) is the use of limited ultrasound (US) protocols performed at the patient's bedside to assess a wide range of clinical conditions. This is distinctly different to the sonographer and radiologist delivered departmental studies which require many years of training and experience to provide a systematic structured assessment.

The purpose of POCUS is to answer key clinical questions that have been guided by the conventional history, physical examination and preliminary investigations (blood tests, X-rays). It is an invaluable tool in the arsenal of general clinicians and can avoid unnecessary delay in the confirmation and identification of pathology.

Point of care ultrasound has grown exponentially over the past 15 years in hospital settings and the COVID-19 pandemic has been a catalyst to accelerate training of this vital skill.

Point of care ultrasound has been facilitated by technological advances which have created more portable, handheld devices at significantly lower costs. Although bedside US is established within certain specialities, particularly Emergency Medicine, Intensive Care Medicine and Acute Medicine, it is becoming more accessible to all healthcare providers including Internists, General Practitioners, Family Physicians, Paramedics, Physiotherapists and Advanced Nursing groups. With the advent of portable US machines, clinicians can now apply the same principles and techniques in any location ranging from Critical Care to the more extreme, austere environments and low resource populations.

How Point of Care Ultrasound Can Help

- Empowers you as a clinician.
- Puts you on the right pathway by improving diagnostic accuracy.
- Gives you confidence in referral and non-referral to specialists.
- Aids decision-making with ceilings of care and withdrawal of medical intervention.
- Identifies reversible pathology within the peri-arrest and arrest scenarios.
- Enhances safety and accuracy of procedural intervention.
- Reduces time to diagnosis leading to reduced length of stay in select cases.
- Gives you confidence in discharging patients.
- Improves the patient-doctor relationship and the patient journey.

What Is the Evidence?

Unlike physical examination of palpation, percussion and auscultation, US allows clinicians to directly visualise what is going on inside the patient's body. It should be seen as an extension of your conventional clinical history and physical examination. There is a wealth of developing evidence suggesting POCUS is superior to physical examination and reduces time to diagnosis, augments the doctor-patient relationship and improves overall patient satisfaction. POCUS has been suggested to improve diagnostic accuracy and deliver these diagnoses at a lower overall cost.

Numerous studies have demonstrated that thoracic US outperforms auscultation and chest radiographs in diagnosing common causes of acute respiratory failure such as pneumonia, heart failure, asthma, COPD and pulmonary embolism.

One of the pioneering works was published by Lichtenstein and Meziere in 2008. They demonstrated excellent diagnostic accuracy of thoracic US in acute respiratory failure within a rapid, protocolised and reproducible framework – the *BLUE Protocol*. They reported an overall diagnostic accuracy of 90.5% which is significantly greater than auscultation and chest radiography combined. This protocol is described in more detail in Chapter 3 – 'Thoracic Ultrasound'.

In view of the growing popularity and evidence base for POCUS, there are published recommendations for the use of focused cardiac ultrasound in shocked patients which have been endorsed by the American Society of Echocardiography (ASE) and the British Society of Echocardiography (BSE).

Point of Care Ultrasound Is Simple to Learn …

Physicians at different levels of training and experience appear to greatly improve their diagnostic ability beyond history and physical examination after brief training in POCUS. A study of first-year medical students who had received 18 hours of US training were able to detect pathology in 75% of cases in comparison to only 49% of certified cardiologists using a stethoscope.

Point of care ultrasound training is becoming widely implemented within the undergraduate curriculum within select medical schools across the world. Multiple postgraduate specialist training pathways endorse and mandate US training prior to completion of training. This is described in detail in Chapter 14 – 'Training and Accreditation'.

It is clear this skill can be learned quickly with effective outcomes no matter where you are in your training journey. The technological advances producing low-cost hand-held devices are making POCUS increasingly accessible and training should develop to reflect this change. Figure I.1 is an example of an 'all-in-one' hand-held US device.

The Momentum Is Growing

Emergency Care across the world has led the POCUS momentum by mandating accreditation before qualification. It is now gaining popularity in other acute specialties with established training pathways such as Acute Medicine and Intensive Care Medicine. Europe, USA, Canada and Australia have pathways and curricula for family physicians and this book aims to carry the principles learned from acute settings and apply them to patient care in any environment by any healthcare provider. We anticipate the greatest diagnostic gains will be seen within lower resource settings, including general practice, where accessibility to definitive investigation is limited and POCUS may rapidly exclude key pathology in a timely manner.

A Mandatory Skill for all Generalists

As experienced clinicians within POCUS we believe this core skill should be mandated for all generalists. Not only is there mounting evidence of its benefits but it is becoming increasingly cost effective. Throughout medical school we continue to teach the same clinical examination skills we used centuries ago. Whilst there is rationale behind teaching the principles and processes of a detailed examination there are many skills, such as tactile vocal fremitus and whispering pectoriloquy, that are rarely performed in day-to-day clinical practice. There are many examples of technological advances improving patient care and superseding historic clinical standards. US in the hands of general clinicians is one of these advances.

With significantly increased time pressure and volume of patients we need to work efficiently to

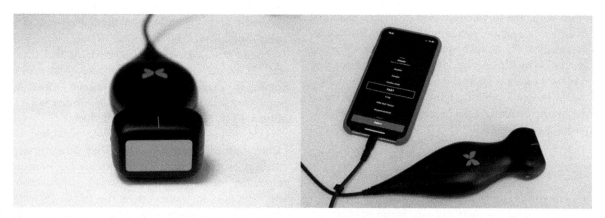

Figure I.1 **The Butterfly iQ is an example of an 'all-in-one' ultrasound probe that plugs directly into a phone or tablet.** Other examples of portable all-in-one probes include the Philips Lumify, EchoNous Kosmos, GE Vscan, Sonosite iViz, Clarius C3 and the Healcerion Sonon.

ensure patients receive high quality care in a timely manner. Ensuring we get the diagnosis correct first time is key to streamlining the patient journey and POCUS vastly enhances the diagnostic capability of frontline and generalist clinicians.

Mandating POCUS as a core skill at undergraduate level will aid the understanding of anatomy and pathology by seeing it in real life rather than simply reading about in books. This will lead to competence and consolidation of knowledge and aid a seamless transition from theory to clinical practice.

It is key to emphasise that POCUS will never replace conventional history and basic examination. These core steps of patient assessment guide the indications for US which vastly enhances the pre-test probability for POCUS. Users should understand the limitations of the training pathways they are accredited within and not attempt to diagnose beyond their expertise.

We promote the mantra of history, examination, observation, palpation, percussion, auscultation and guided sonography as compulsory elements of clinical assessment of all patients.

Summary

- Point of care ultrasound is designed to answer key questions at the bedside and is becoming more accessible for all clinicians with the advent of smaller, portable hand-held devices.
- There is an increasing evidence base for POCUS highlighting that it is superior to physical examination and traditional diagnostics and may be delivered in a time-efficient manner.
- Across the world there is an increasing momentum of training and accreditation within undergraduate and postgraduate training programmes.
- Ultrasound for the Generalist is a critical mandatory skill within the medical field and, alongside history and physical examination, will become an indispensable tool for modern clinical practice.

Basic Physics, Knobology and Artefacts

Ultrasound physics is a dreaded and frequently neglected topic by many POCUS enthusiasts. However, a basic understanding of the principles behind how US generates images will aid the clinician with interpretation, optimisation and troubleshooting unexpected findings. Many signs, particularly in lung ultrasound (LUS), rely solely on the interpretation of artefact patterns, making it an essential element to diagnosis.

This chapter will discuss the basic physics of US, common artefacts and top tips the user needs to know when learning to scan. Understanding the machine and controls ('knobology') is a critical step in acquiring the best possible image.

Physics

Introduction to Ultrasound

Sound travels as longitudinal mechanical waves through mediums such as air, water or solid substances. It therefore cannot be transmitted through a vacuum. Each soundwave is characterised by its frequency and intensity. US describes soundwaves with a frequency higher than the threshold of human hearing.

Ultrasound probes contain a grid of crystals known as **piezoelectric crystals** which deform when a charge is applied to them. Using an alternating current, they will oscillate (rapidly expand and contract), which leads to generation of US. The transformation of electrical oscillations into mechanical oscillation (sound) is known as the **piezoelectric effect.**

These same crystals are able to act as receivers. The transducer will emit a burst of US for a few microseconds and then wait for a returning signal for the same period of time. The time taken for a signal to return and the intensity of that signal is used to construct an US image. Key elements to the US transducer are shown in Figure 1.1.

Frequency describes the number of oscillations per second and is measured in Hertz (Hz). Audible sound is roughly 20–20,000 Hz (20 KHz). US is characterised by frequencies over 20,000 Hz (20 KHz). As the frequency increases, common order of magnitude prefixes may be used such as kilohertz (KHz, 1000 Hz) and megahertz (MHz, 1,000,000 Hz). Medical US typically uses frequencies between 1 and 20 MHz. Figure 1.2 shows the spectrum of sound frequency.

When sound travels through a medium there are regions of higher density and pressure where particles have been pushed closer together known as *compression*. Other particles are subsequently under less pressure and density and therefore spread further apart. This is *rarefaction*.

This longitudinal wave may be plotted on a graph with *distance* on the x-axis and *time* on the y-axis creating a graph that is analogous to a normal sinusoidal waveform. The time taken for one complete cycle of moving from resting pressure, to compression, rarefaction and back to resting pressure equates to the **wavelength** (see Figure 1.3).

If this graph were to plot *pressure* (y-axis) against *time* (x-axis) describing the single point in space going through a complete cycle of compression, rarefaction and back to resting pressure, this is known as the **period** (Figure 1.3).

Amplitude describes the *strength* of a sound wave measured as the difference between the peak pressure and average pressure in decibels (dBs). This is a logarithmic scale with a change of 6 dBs representing a doubling of amplitude.

Propagation velocity is the speed at which the sound wave travels through a particular medium. This relates to the speed upon which the US wave travels through the patient and back to the probe. Propagation velocity is variable depending on the *medium* through which it is travelling (Table 1.1). The US machine takes the average propagation velocity and assumes the beam is travelling at a constant velocity of 1,540 m/s.

Table 1.1 Propagation velocity through different mediums

Tissue	Air	Water	Muscle	Fat	Liver	Spleen	Kidney	Bone
Velocity (m/s)	331	1496	1568	1476	1570	1565	1560	3360

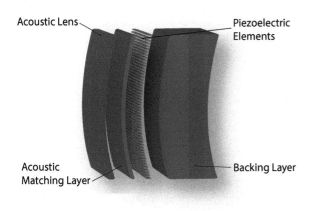

Figure 1.1 Key elements of the ultrasound transducer.

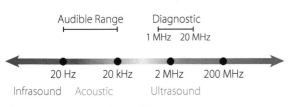

Figure 1.2 Spectrum of sound frequency.

The equations that describe the relationships between these parameters are listed below:

$$Frequency\ (Hz)\ -\ 1\ /\ Period\ (s)$$
$$Velocity\ (m/s)\ =\ Frequency\ (Hz) \times Wavelength\ (m)$$
$$Wavelength\ (m) = Velocity\ (m/s)\ /\ Frequency\ (Hz)$$

These equations demonstrate that frequency is *inversely related* to wavelength. This is a key principle to understand for clinical US.

Wavelength is one of the key determinants for *axial resolution* – the ability to distinguish between structures along the axis of the US beam. Our ability to visualise a structure relies on it being larger than the wavelength of the US beam. As the frequency falls, the wavelength will increase. This describes how better *resolution* may be achieved by using a *higher frequency* transducer.

Ultrasound in the Body

Clinical US relies on the generated kinetic energy being reflected back towards the probe to be processed into an image. Tissues have a different degree of **acoustic impedance** which is closely related to the density – higher density tissues have a higher acoustic impedance.

Structures with a low acoustic impedance will allow US to pass readily through them leading to less reflection and a darker image to be generated. Liquid allows

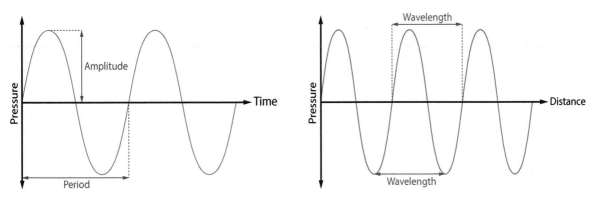

Figure 1.3 Sound waves plotted as graphs showing pressure on the y-axis and either time or distance on the x-axis. Note the annotations describing amplitude, period and wavelength.

5

easy transmission of US with minimal reflection and therefore appears black on the screen. This is described as *anechoic* (see Figure 1.4). This explains the dark appearance of structures such as blood vessels, heart chambers, effusions, ascites and the bladder.

By contrast, solid structures with a high acoustic impedance, such as bone, cause a higher degree of reflection leading to a much brighter image. This is described as *hyperechoic*. As minimal US will be transmitted beyond the bright reflective surface an *acoustic shadow* develops beyond the hyperechoic structure. This is commonly seen with bone, stones (e.g. gallstones, renal calculi) and foreign bodies (see Figure 1.5).

Remaining structures in the body will have an *echogenicity* that is between these two extremes. The brightness may be described in relation to one another. *Isoechoic* describes structures that appear to have the *same brightness* whereas *hypoechoic* will describe an object that is *darker* than surrounding structures.

An example of a structure with variable echogenicityis the kidney where the medullary pyramids are more hypoechoic than the renal cortex. Figure 1.6 shows a normal kidney.

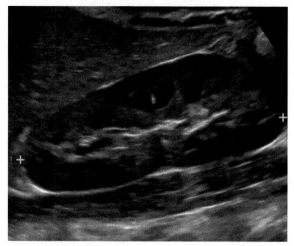

Figure 1.6 **The kidney is an example of a structure with variable echogenicity. Note the hyperechoic pelvis compared with the hypoechoic medulla.**

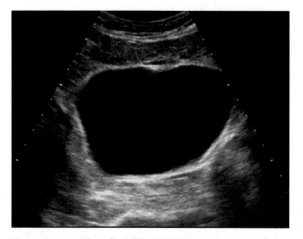

Figure 1.4 **Anechoic fluid-filled bladder.** Note the bright area deep to the bladder. This is due to acoustic enhancement.

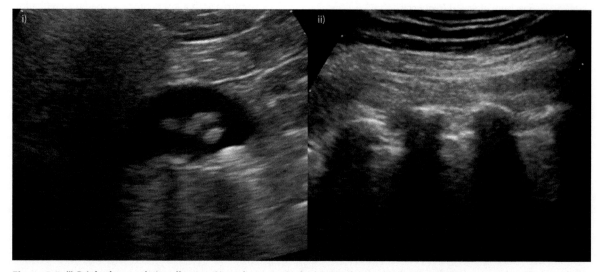

Figure 1.5 **(i) Bright, hyperechoic gallstones. Note the acoustic shadowing deep to the stones. (ii) Ribs are hyperechoic structures that cause a very prominent acoustic shadow.**

Table 1.2 Acoustic impedance of different mediums'

Medium	Impedance Z (10^6 Ns/m^3)	Velocity (m/s)	Density (10^3 kg/m^3)
Air	0.00041	331	0.0012
Fat	1.47	1476	0.928
Water	1.49	1496	0.997
Kidney	1.61	1560	1.032
Liver	1.65	1570	1.051
Muscle	1.66	1568	1.058
Spleen	1.66	1565	1.061
Bone	6.2	3360	1.85

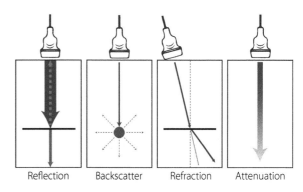

Figure 1.7 **Key ultrasound principles.**

As US crosses the boundary between two tissues with very different acoustic impedance, such as air and soft tissue, a higher proportion will be reflected back towards the probe. The use of US gel limits the acoustic impedance between the air and skin which would result in much of the US reflecting before it even reached the body. Table 1.2 shows the various acoustic impedance for different mediums.

Most US imaging arises from scattering of transmitted waves from small structures within tissues which are too small to resolve. This results in interference and produces a speckled appearance due to the various intensities of echoes received by the transducer causing irregularities in the greyscale of the image. To the untrained eye this looks like a snowstorm, but with experience it may be sufficiently characteristic to assist in tissue differentiation. Modern ultrasound systems use image post-processing to smooth the image and reduce the specular appearance to varying degrees depending on the settings and user preference.

Specular reflection and backscatter are two simplified concepts of reflection depending upon the size of the reflective structure and the wavelength (Figure 1.7):

- **Specular reflection** – this is a 'mirror-like' reflection that occurs at a reflector that is relatively large – at least two wavelengths in size. The degree of reflection is highly dependent on the *angle of incidence* of the beam. The greatest degree of reflection occurs when the probe is *perpendicular* to the reflective surface. As the angle of incidence moves further away from 90 degrees, less of the reflected energy will return to the probe, resulting in the image appearing less bright.

- **Backscatter** – this occurs with small structures that are smaller than the wavelength. When the US beam hits these structures, it is reflected in many different directions independent of the angle of incidence. The strength of the returning signal is many times weaker than with specular reflection.

Attenuation is the final principle to consider. As US passes through tissue it will gradually lose energy. This is through several mechanisms:

- **Absorption** – energy will be converted to heat due to absorption by the tissues it passes through. This is responsible for the largest proportion of attenuation.

- **Reflection** – energy is lost to specular reflection and backscatter. Whilst some energy is reflected back to the probe, much is reflected away from the probe and therefore lost.

Attenuation is directly related to the **frequency** of the US wave. Waves with a higher frequency are associated with a greater degree of attenuation meaning they are unable to reach deep structures. This explains the trade-off between using a *high frequency* transducer to achieve **good resolution** but at the expense of limited tissue **penetration**. A *low frequency* transducer will allow visualisation of **deeper** structures but with poorer **resolution**.

Higher frequency → Smaller wavelength → Better resolution at superficial structures

Lower frequency → Longer wavelength → Better visualisation of deeper structures

Understanding these concepts will allow the user to select the optimal transducer to achieve the best possible resolution for each scan.

Beginning to Scan

There are six fundamental steps to consider when beginning to scan:

Step 1 – Know your machine.

Step 2 – Choose the correct probe and preset.

Step 3 – Understanding orientation.

Step 4 – Acquiring your images.

Step 5 – Image optimisation.

Step 6 – Saving your images.

Step 1 – Know Your Machine

The US machine may appear intimidating to novice users due to the perceived complexity. Figure 1.8 is a typical portable US machine. For POCUS, only a few essential features are required and most users can ignore many of the remaining buttons. Understanding the knobs on the machine is the art of *knobology* and critical in acquiring the highest quality images possible.

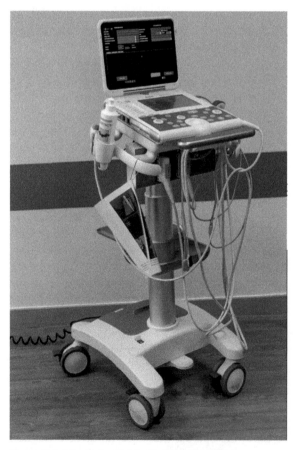

Figure 1.8 A typical portable ultrasound machine.

Getting to know your machine will also increase the speed of image acquisition and user confidence which is key for busy general clinicians. All machines will have the same basic settings and their use will become second nature with practice.

Power Button

Turning on the machine is clearly an essential initial step! When the machine is not in use it should be switched off and placed on charge. The battery life of machines tends to reduce rapidly and many do not function without mains connection after several years of use. Remember to plug into mains when performing scans to avoid loss of images.

Patient Details

Including patient demographics when saving images is important for governance and quality assurance. This should include name, date of birth, hospital number (patient identifier) and the person completing the scan (Figure 1.9). In an emergency setting this may not be possible but the users should enter details retrospectively or clearly document an emergency scan number.

Ultrasound Basic Controls and Functions

All machines will have the same basic controls. Figure 1.10 shows an example of a layout with annotations. Understanding the machine control panel will allow rapid image optimisation and seamless freezing, saving and switching between imaging modes.

All machines will have a central control wheel and adjacent buttons. This should be considered as the 'computer mouse' of the ultrasound machine and

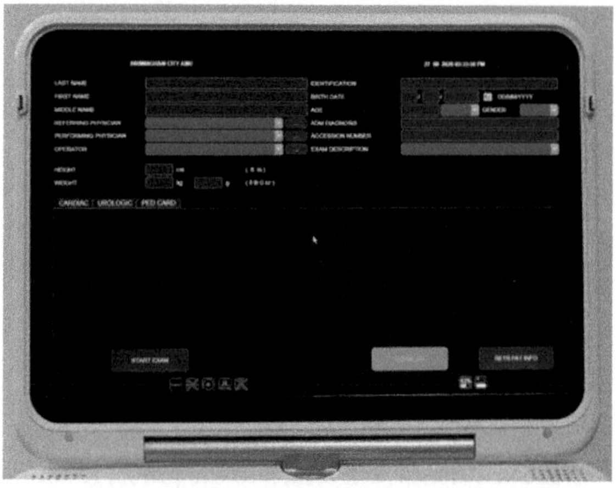

Figure 1.9 Data entry screen for patient demographics.

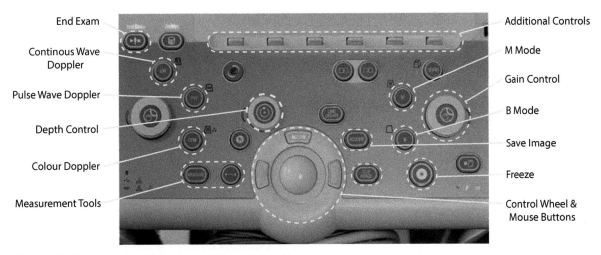

End Exam
Continous Wave Doppler
Pulse Wave Doppler
Depth Control
Colour Doppler
Measurement Tools

Additional Controls
M Mode
Gain Control
B Mode
Save Image
Freeze
Control Wheel & Mouse Buttons

Figure 1.10 Basic controls available on any ultrasound machine.

enables direction of the screen cursor, sizing of colour boxes and directing of spectral doppler pathways.

Step 2 – Choose the Correct Probe and Preset
The Probes

Correct probe selection is essential to acquiring an interpretable image based on the indication.

Before you start scanning ask yourself the following questions:

– What part of the body am I scanning?
– How deep are the structures?
– Is the footprint big or small?
– Am I doing a procedure?

All probes consist of the head, wire and the connector. The transducers may be detached from the machine to allow it to be interchangeable. Some machines will allow multiple probes to be connected simultaneously and selected using the probe button or icon on the screen.

Footprint and Field of View

The skin area that needs to be contacted by the probe to produce an image is called the *footprint* of the probe. This is dictated by the size of the piezoelectric array and can easily be appreciated by the size of the probe tip.

Larger footprints provide a more expansive scanning field but will struggle to image through small acoustic windows. For example, the curvilinear probe and phased array probe have very similar imaging frequencies and both allow visualisation of deep structures. The phased array transducer is far more

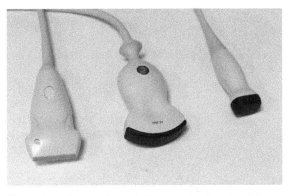

Figure 1.11 Commonly used ultrasound probes. From left to right: high frequency linear probe; curvilinear probe; phased array probe.

suited to cardiac imaging due to the smaller footprint allowing imaging through the rib spaces. A larger footprint is particularly suited for scanning large structures close to the surface of the body such as in abdominal ultrasound. The field of view is also an important characteristic for deciding which probe to use. The curvilinear and phased array probes generate a 'wedge shaped' field of view due to the beam fanning outwards from the probe. The distance between these structures on the screen may appear greater if they are situated deeper in the imaging field. Modern machines aim to compensate for this by beam steering or image reconstruction. Linear probes, by default, will create a 'rectangular' field of view using a higher resolution. This makes them ideally suited for US-guided procedures as they provide a more reliable location of needles as they are advanced. Figure 1.11 shows the commonly used US probes.

9

A guide to the common imaging modalities used with different probes is listed in Table 1.3.

Curvilinear Probe (Figure 1.12)

- Low frequency 2–5 MHz.
- Allows for visualisation of deep structures at the expense of resolution.
- Large footprint so not ideal for small acoustic windows.

Table 1.3 Types of probe, imaging frequency and common applications

Probe	Frequency (MHz)	Applications
Curvilinear	2–5	Abdominal Thoracic Bladder Focused assessment with sonography in trauma (FAST) Aorta Spinal
Linear	5–18	Thoracic – particularly for pleural abnormalities e.g. pneumothorax/pleural line irregularities Vascular access DVT MSK and soft tissue Optic nerve sheath
Phased Array	1–5	Cardiac Abdominal Inferior vena cava (IVC) Transcranial Doppler

- Generates a wedge-shaped field of view.
- Generally used for abdominal and pelvic examination. Thoracic imaging when deeper imaging required e.g. diaphragm or effusion assessment. Use for cardiac imaging limited by its large footprint providing poor visualisation through rib spaces.

Linear Probe (Figure 1.13)

- High frequency 5–18 MHz.
- High resolution of superficial structures at the cost of penetration. Reliable to 6–8 cm.
- Large footprint.
- Generates rectangular field of view which makes it suited for US-guided procedures.
- Should be used for imaging of any superficial structure where a small footprint is not required.

Phased Array Probe (Figure 1.14)

- Low frequency probe 1–5 MHz.
- Designed to provide a small footprint to enable penetration through rib spaces for cardiac imaging.
- Array of piezoelectric elements that are steered electronically to fan backwards and forwards across an image.
- Better focusing capability than other probes.
- May be used for other 'low frequency applications' such as abdominal US but will tend to provide poorer resolution.
- Probe marker will default to the *right* side of the screen when selected as this is the automatic setting for cardiac imaging presets.

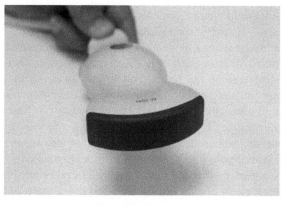

Figure 1.12 The curvilinear probe.

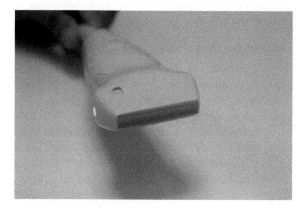

Figure 1.13 The linear probe.

All-in-One Handheld Probes

Handheld devices are now available that connect directly to a tablet or smartphone and can simulate multiple different probe types with computer algorithms. The Butterfly iQ is an example of this (Figure 1.15). The footprint is larger than a phased array probe and the weight is heavier due to the battery and processor being housed within the probe. Although these machines cannot match the image quality of their larger counterparts, they are a fraction of the price and unrivalled in their portability enabling diagnostic US in more resource-limited environments.

Presets

All US machines have system-based presets that automatically select the optimal frequency, depth, gain, penetration and measurement package for the selected application. This is of particular importance when performing echocardiography as the probe

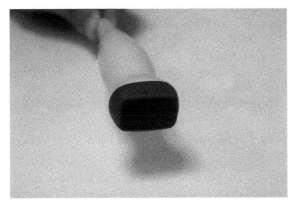

Figure 1.14 The phased array probe.

marker should default to the *right* of the screen rather than the *left* as is used with other modalities. The presets are an excellent 'starting point' to gain good picture quality and can be fine-tuned with other settings based on the images obtained.

Probe and Display Marker

Every probe will have a *marker* which may be a ridge, notch, mark or light. The aim of this marker is to aid with orientation of the patient's anatomy with the images on the screen. Each imaging application will have a *dot* or *marker* on the US display that should correlate with the direction of the probe marker.

For almost all applications this display marker should be located on the *left* of the screen. If imaging in the transverse plane the transducer should then be held with the probe marker pointing to the *patient's right-hand side*. This will mean that when the user moves the probe to *their left* it will correlate with a movement to the left-hand side on the US display. When performing longitudinal imaging the probe marker should be pointing towards the patient's head with the more cephalad structures located on the *left-hand side* of the screen (Figure 1.16).

The display marker for cardiac imaging is placed on the *right* of the screen. This is purely due to convention and differs from country to country. The probe marker in echocardiography changes orientation depending on the particular view. This will be covered in more detail in the echocardiography chapter.

The top of the screen represents the part of the body closest to the probe – in POCUS this is usually the skin. If performing transoesophageal echocardiography (TOE) this would be the oesophagus. The

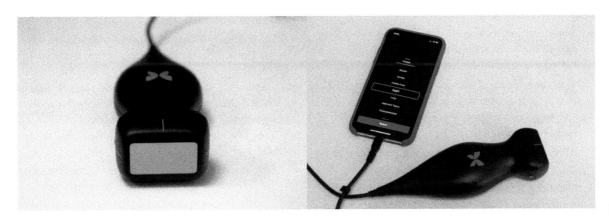

Figure 1.15 The Butterfly iQ is an example of an 'all-in-one' ultrasound probe that plugs directly into a phone or tablet. Other examples of portable all-in-one probes include the Philips Lumify, EchoNous Kosmos, GE Vscan, Sonosite iViz, Clarius C3 and the Healcerion Sonon.

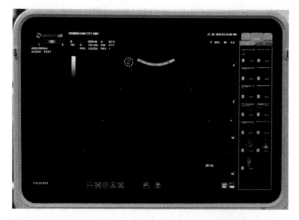

Figure 1.16 Orientation of the probe marker with the display marker (circled) is a key initial step when performing ultrasound.

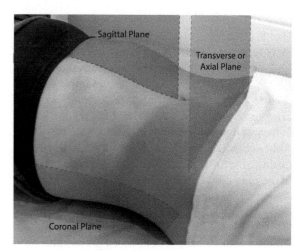

Figure 1.17 Normal imaging planes.

lower down the screen the structure becomes then the further away it is from the probe and therefore is visualised with poorer resolution.

The display area at the top of the screen is referred to as the '*near-field*' and the bottom of the screen is the '*far-field*'.

Step 3 – Understanding Orientation

In the previous section we have discussed orientation of the probe marker compared with the display marker. Being disciplined with orientation will ensure the user understands the structures displayed on the monitor and how to adjust the probe to optimise the image.

Imaging Planes

The imaging planes used for US are the same as for all other modalities. The body is divided into three distinct planes (see Figure 1.17).

- *Sagittal* or *longitudinal plane* – parallel to the long axis of the body acting as an imaginary line between the right and left sides of the body.
- *Transverse or axial plane* – perpendicular to the long axis and separates the top of the body (cephalad or superior) from the bottom of the body (caudad or inferior).
- *Coronal plane* – separates the long axis of the body from front (anterior) to back (posterior).
- *Oblique* refers to any imaging modality that uses a combination of these planes. These planes would be used to gain a particular anatomical view or to acquire a window through a structure, e.g. ribs.

Long axis and *short axis* are also commonly used terms and relate to the orientation of a particular anatomical structure. Long axis refers to a plane that is parallel to the maximal length of the structure. Short axis, by comparison, is perpendicular to this plane and usually achieved by rotating the probe 90 degrees from the long axis. The most common usage for this is cardiac imaging and this will be discussed further in Chapter 2 – 'Echocardiography'.

Step 4 – Acquiring Your Images
Gel

Ultrasound gel will provide a conductive medium between the transducer and skin reducing the impedance. Novice sonographers should be liberal with the use of gel to aid image acquisition.

Image Generation and Modes

We have already discussed how the piezoelectric crystals in the probe are capable of both transmitting and receiving signals. After transmitting, the crystals stop and wait for returning kinetic energy signals which are then passed into the ultrasound machine to be analysed and converted into an image.

The machine will receive information related to the:

- *Amplitude* of the received signal – determined by the amount of energy reflected by a structure.
- Amplitude is converted to a *brightness* value on a greyscale with dark shades representing low amplitude and bright shades the high amplitude.

– The *time taken* for a signal to return is used to calculate the *distance* of a structure from the transducer.

This information is the basis for the numerous modes available on an US machine. More advanced Doppler modes will be discussed later in the chapter.

A Mode

A mode is the simplest form of US and stands for *Amplitude Mode*. A single imaging line scans through the body with the amplitude of returning signals and depth plotted as lines. Larger lines represent a stronger returning signal. This is no longer used in clinical practice.

B Mode

B mode, or *Brightness Mode*, is the conversion of amplitude into the greyscale image. This will generate a more familiar US image based upon the returning signals.

2D Mode

Modern machines will generate many single B mode imaging lines that fan out from the transducer. The gaps between these lines are then *filled in* by the machine with an averaging process to generate a 2D image. This is the most commonly used mode in clinical practice and is important to be familiar with.

Many machines will refer to 2D mode as B mode. If you accidentally end up in a different mode or become lost on the US machine, then pressing the B-mode button should return back to the standard imaging mode.

A key consideration with this mode is the *frame rate* it generates. Frame rate is the number of frames per second and is described in *Hertz* (*Hz*). A higher frame rate is advantageous for imaging moving structures because it will more accurately track the changes over time. The more information an US machine has to process, for example a deeper image, larger sector width or use of spectral Doppler, the lower the frame rate will be.

M Mode

M mode, or *Motion Mode*, will take a single B mode line and display it graphically as changes over time. Changes in depth will be plotted on the y-axis against time on the x-axis. M-mode produces images with an excellent frame rate as the US machine is only having to process one imaging slice. This makes it perfectly suited to analysis of fast-moving structures such as heart valves or for displaying the changes in structure calibre over time e.g. blood vessels or cardiac chambers. M-Mode is discussed in more detail in Chapter 2 – 'Echocardiography'.

Ultrasound Probe Movements and Manipulation

It is important to be confident when handling the transducer and understand how certain deliberate movements may alter the image. Firstly, it is essential to handle the probe at the base in as comfortable a way as possible. Holding the transducer like a pen will allow the user to create a stable platform to prevent unnecessary movement artefact.

The four basic movements to be familiar with when scanning are *sliding, rotating, tilting* and *rocking*. Appreciating these movements will allow the mentor to verbally direct a novice sonographer to improve image quality. Another technique is compression that is commonly used in vascular US. This will be discussed in further detail in Chapter 5 – 'Vascular Ultrasound'. Each of these are considered in turn with a video demonstrating the movement.

Sliding

Sliding (see Figure 1.18) involves moving the entire probe in a specific direction to change the imaging window, move to a different area of the body or follow a specific structure such as a blood vessel. It is the only movement that requires the user to change the location of the transducer footprint.

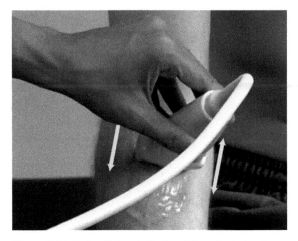

Figure 1.18 **Probe sliding.** *A video is available to view in the online video library.*

Rotating

Rotation (see Figure 1.19) of the probe clockwise or anticlockwise will allow the user to change between the long axis and short axis images of a structure such as the heart, kidney and blood vessels.

Tilting

Tilting (see Figure 1.20) the probe describes elevating or lowering the tail of the probe along its short axis. The transducer footprint should remain in the same location. This will allow the user to visualise multiple cross-sections of a single image by 'fanning' through an image. This is commonly used in cardiac and renal imaging.

Rocking

Rocking motion (see Figure 1.21) will move the tail of the probe to the left or the right along the long axis of the probe. Again, the transducer footprint should remain in the same location. This movement will cause structures to *swing* on the screen. An example is rocking to centralise the septum when imaging the apical four-chamber view of the heart.

Compression

Applying downward pressure onto the skin will assess the compressibility of a structure. This is typically used when differentiating between blood vessels or for diagnosing deep vein thromboses.

Advanced Imaging Modes

Certain imaging modes utilise the Doppler principle to gain further information about flow and movement characteristics. These modes include colour Doppler (CFM), power Doppler (PD), pulse wave (PW) Doppler and continuous wave (CW) Doppler. These are less commonly used in POCUS but are available for the more advanced user to assess blood flow characteristics and tissue or muscle motion.

The Doppler principle describes the change frequency of a soundwave if the source is moving relative to the probe. When US is reflected from moving fluid, the frequency is increased if the fluid is moving towards the probe and decreased if it is moving away. This is analogous to the change in pitch of an ambulance siren as it moves towards and away from a static individual (Figure 1.22).

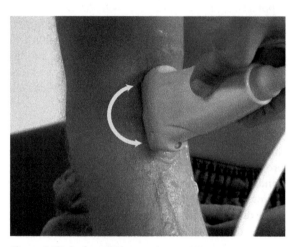

Figure 1.19 Probe rotation. *A video is available to view in the online video library.*

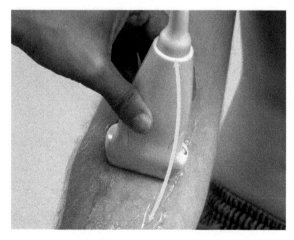

Figure 1.20 Probe tilting. *A video is available to view in the online video library.*

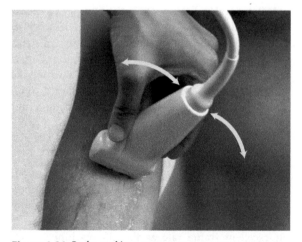

Figure 1.21 Probe rocking. *A video is available to view in the online video library.*

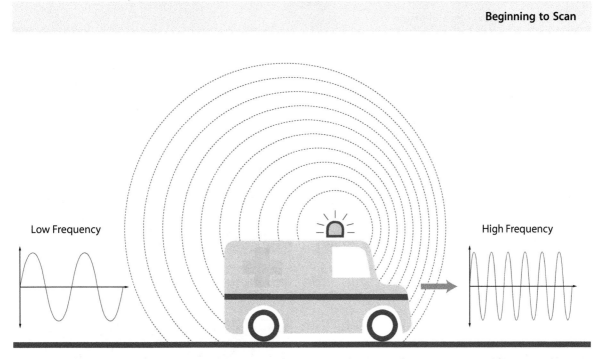

Figure 1.22 **The Doppler Effect describes the change in frequency when the source of waves is moving relative to an observer.**

The change in frequency between the transmitted and received signals is termed the *Doppler shift*. *Velocity* may be calculated from the Doppler shift by using the *Doppler equation*:

$$V = \frac{c \times f_d}{2 \times f_t \times \cos \theta}$$

The amplitude of the returning signal is dependent upon the alignment of the ultrasound beam with the direction of flow. Optimal alignment for accurate velocity estimation is for the beam to be parallel to the blood flow. The larger the angle between the beam and direction of flow, the more the velocity will be *underestimated*. The suggested threshold above which measurements should no longer be taken is 20 degrees from parallel. As the probe is moved to a 90 degree angle there will be no change in direction *relative* to the probe and therefore no flow will be detected. Electronic steering of the ultrasound beam is possible to achieve better alignment in circumstances where probe manipulation is insufficient or not possible.

Colour Doppler

This is the most commonly used mode of Doppler imaging. It provides a visual representation of the direction of blood flow by applying a blue or red colour within a region of interest. Blue flow is directed away from the probe and red is towards the

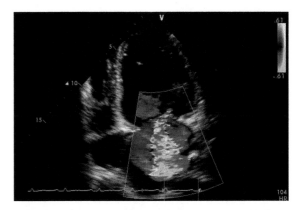

Figure 1.23 **Colour Doppler demonstrating severe mitral regurgitation in a patient with post-partum cardiomyopathy.**

probe. This may be remembered with the *BART* mnemonic: Blue Away Red Towards.

Larger colour boxes require the US machine to use more processing power causing a reduction in frame rate. It is therefore important to resize the box to only include the region of interest (Figure 1.23).

Power Doppler

Power Doppler is a modality integral to musculoskeletal US. It follows the same principles of colour Doppler but generates a signal that is independent to the velocity and direction of flow (Figure 1.24). This makes it more sensitive for detecting low velocity signals when compared with colour Doppler. It is

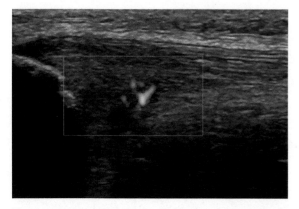

Figure 1.24 **Power Doppler signal showing neovascularity in the proximal patella tendon.**

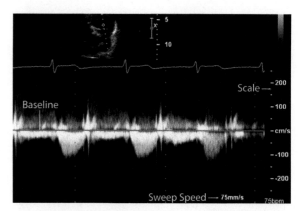

Figure 1.25 **Spectral Doppler trace with annotations of the commonly adjustable parameters.**

particularly useful for diagnosing neovascularity in tendon pathology. PD will be discussed in more detail in Chapter 6 – 'Soft Tissue and Musculoskeletal Ultrasound'.

Spectral Doppler

Spectral Doppler incorporates the pulse wave and continuous wave Doppler modalities. These are far more complex modes and will not be used by inexperienced sonographers. Flow is detected towards or away from the probe using analysis of Doppler shift and flow velocity is plotted upon a graph called a *spectral Doppler display*.

A positive deflection on the graph will reflect movement towards the transducer and a negative deflection is away from the transducer. This graph plots velocity on the y-axis against time on the x-axis. The *baseline*, *velocity scale* and *gain* may be adjusted to optimise the appearance of the graph (Figure 1.25).

Pulse Wave Doppler

Pulse wave Doppler is predominantly used to measure the velocity of blood flow at a single point. You may specify the exact location using a sample gate that usually appears as two horizontal lines along the cursor.

Pulse wave Doppler cannot be used for high velocity applications, e.g. very high blood flow or stenotic valves, due to a concept called aliasing. PW relies on the probe transmitting an US signal and then sampling only the signals received from the point of interest which is calculated by time (Figure 1.26). The further away from the transducer the sampling point is, the longer the transducer must wait for the signal

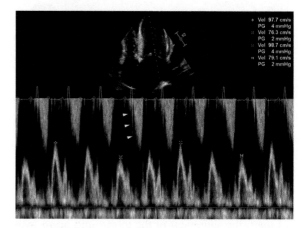

Figure 1.26 **Pulse wave Doppler of the mitral inflow.** Note the negative deflection from the baseline (blood flowing away from the probe) that wraps around the spectral trace (labelled). This is aliasing.

leading to a longer *round-trip time* between pulses. The time between pulses is called the *pulse repetition frequency*.

There is a limit on the maximum velocity that may be detected using PW Doppler which is termed the *Nyquist Limit*. Any velocity that exceeds this will *alias*. Practically speaking this means flow that wraps around the spectral Doppler graph causing distortion. In the event of aliasing the user may initially change the baseline, followed by the velocity scale to attempt to optimise the graph.

The most common use of PW Doppler for POCUS users is to measure the left ventricular outflow tract (LVOT) flow velocity to calculate stroke volume and cardiac output. This will be discussed in more detail in the echocardiography chapter.

Continuous Wave Doppler

Continuous wave Doppler provides a similar signal to PW Doppler but is more suited to the higher velocity flow as it does not alias. CW functions by having crystals that continually transmit and receive signals at the same time. Unlike PW Doppler, it will therefore sample velocities from the entire length of the cursor and is unable to precisely localise where a velocity is originating from (Figure 1.27).

It is most commonly used for valvular assessment. Care must be taken if the cursor is crossing multiple structures that may generate different velocities as the high velocity will usually overlap and obscure the lower velocity.

Tissue Doppler Imaging

Tissue Doppler imaging is a less commonly used Doppler mode that applies a low-pass filter to returning Doppler signals so that only low velocity signals return. It is used for measuring the speed of tissue/muscle movement for assessment of diastolic function (Figure 1.28). It will not be discussed in detail in this textbook.

Ultrasound Artefacts

Artefact is the term used for structures or distortions that are not actually present. They are caused by the behaviour of sound waves passing through tissues with differing echogenicity. Artefact may be caused by technical imaging errors or due to the complex interaction of US with structures in the body. Some imaging modalities, such as thoracic US, principally rely on the interpretation of artefact patterns to identify pathology. Understanding, recognising and correcting reversible artefact is essential to generating good quality diagnostic imaging.

The most commonly encountered artefacts will be discussed and are listed in Table 1.4. When the user identifies artefact it is essential to assess the same structure using multiple views to ensure the finding is not pathological.

Acoustic Enhancement

This occurs when US waves pass through a structure with significantly lower attenuation such as blood- or fluid-filled structures. The area underlying the low attenuation zone will appear much brighter than the surrounding field. This is commonly seen deep to the bladder, gallbladder, cysts and vessels (Figure 1.29).

Table 1.4 Common imaging artefacts

Artefacts
Acoustic Enhancement
Acoustic Shadowing
Reverberation Artefact
Comet Tail Artefact
Ring Down Artefact
Mirror Image Artefact
Refraction Artefact
Edge Shadowing Artefact
Beam Width Artefact
Side Lobe Artefact

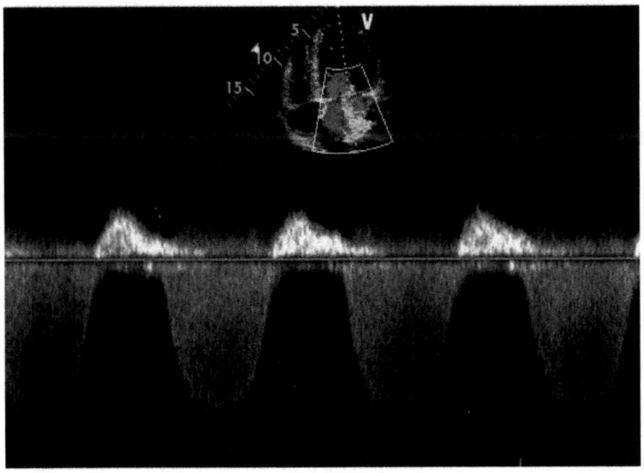

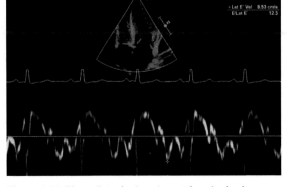

Figure 1.27 Continuous wave Doppler trace showing mitral regurgitation in a patient with dilated cardiomyopathy.

Figure 1.28 Tissue Doppler imaging at the mitral valve annulus.

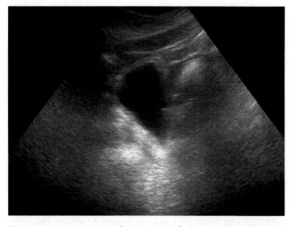

Figure 1.29 Acoustic enhancement of ultrasound waves through the bladder makes underlying tissue appear more hyperechoic.

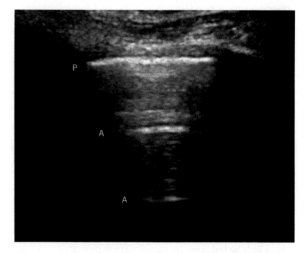

Figure 1.31 Reverberation artefact. The A lines (A) seen with lung ultrasound are examples of reverberation artefact from the pleural line (P).

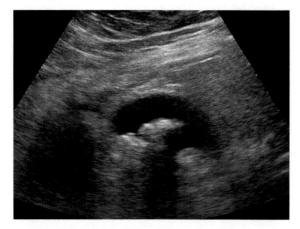

Figure 1.30 Acoustic shadowing due to the high acoustic impedance of a gallstone. Note the hypoechoic region directly underneath the stone.

Acoustic Shadowing

Highly reflective structures (hyperechoic) block US from penetrating any further. This causes shadowing in the far field distal to the structure. Whilst this may be problematic in some circumstances due to difficulty imaging beyond a reflective surface, in others it may aid with diagnosis due to shadowing behind an abnormal structure. An example of this is the image dropout seen beyond gallstones (Figure 1.30) and rib shadows.

Reverberation Artefact

Ultrasound can rebound between two strong reflectors before returning to the transducer. This increases the time taken to be detected and is therefore displayed as being further away from the probe. This causes 'ghost' images in the far field which will move in tandem with the original structure.

An example of this is the A lines seen with lung imaging, where US is reflected back and forth from the pleural line. These lines are equidistant and gradually decrease in intensity in the far field due to diminishing signal strength (Figure 1.31).

Comet Tail Artefact

This is a form of reverberation artefact. US will become trapped between two reflective surfaces that are close together and not parallel. A small amount of this energy will be reflected back to the probe. The signal is rapidly attenuated and reduces in intensity causing the artefact to fade with depth. This makes it different from a ring down artefact which does not fade with depth. These are commonly seen as small, triangular shaped downward deflections from the pleural line (Figure 1.32) and metal such as guidewires and valve replacements (Figure 1.32).

Ring Down Artefact

Ring down artefact is similar to comet tail artefact. Rather than occurring at the interface of two reflective surfaces, ring down artefact occurs at the interface between gas and liquid. As US reaches the gas bubbles it causes excitation of trapped liquid which begins to resonate. This creates lines or a series of bands extending parallel to the bottom of the screen. This

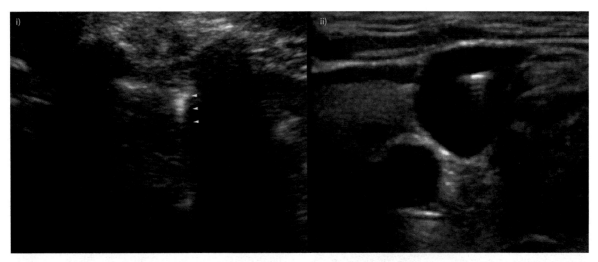

Figure 1.32 Comet tail artefact seen from (i) the hyper-reflective pleural line (arrows) and (ii) a metallic guidewire within the right internal jugular vein during central venous cannulation.

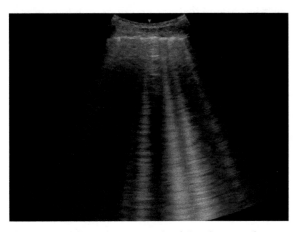

Figure 1.33 B lines are an example of ring down artefact.

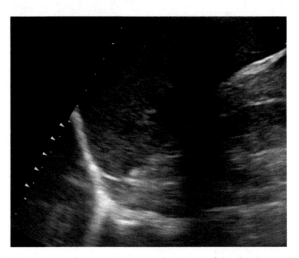

Figure 1.34 This right upper quadrant view of the diaphragm, liver and kidney demonstrates mirror artefact. An image of the liver is reflected across the diaphragm (arrows) giving the impression of two structures with similar echotexture either side of the diaphragm.

can be differentiated from comet tail artefact as it does not fade with depth.

This is most commonly seen as B lines in lung US signifying pulmonary oedema, inflammation or fibrosis (Figure 1.33).

Mirror Image Artefact

This forms when US hits a highly reflective structure but does not return directly to the receiver and instead takes an indirect path via another reflective surface. The machine cannot distinguish between the real image and artefact and generates a mirror image deep to the reflective surface. An example of this is in imaging the liver where structures may appear reflected on the thoracic side of the diaphragm due to mirror image artefact (Figure 1.34). The mirror image will appear more blurred and distorted than the original structure as the US will return via a longer pathway.

Refraction Artefact

Refraction occurs when the US strikes a surface at a non-perpendicular angle causing the direction of the wave to change. The transducer will assume all beams have travelled in a straight line and may cause deep structures to be mapped in an incorrect location (Figure 1.35).

Edge Shadowing

Edge shadowing occurs at the edges of curved, smooth walled structures. It is caused by reflection of the beam away from the surface edge and refraction of the beam as it passes through the structure. The resulting image is a shadow-like line of reduced intensity beyond the edges of these structures. This is often seen with vessel walls, gallbladder, bladder and cystic structures (Figure 1.36).

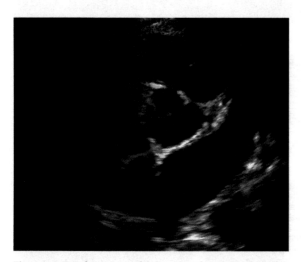

Figure 1.35 Refraction artefact creating the appearance of two aortic valves.

Beam Width Artefact

An US beam has a finite width and the machine has difficulty discerning whether a returning signal has arisen from the centre or edge of the probe. This is particularly problematic in the far field. Strong reflectors from the edge of the beam are displayed by the machine as originating from the centre, 'smearing' the displayed image creating false detectable echoes that overlap the structure of interest. This can be minimised by focusing. This is often seen with anechoic structures – see Figure 1.37 which shows the bladder which is being smeared with peripheral echoes from the bowel.

Side Lobe Artefact

The primary, central US beam is produced by expansion and contraction of piezoelectric crystals. These crystals also contract radially causing secondary, low-intensity beams that are known as side lobe beams. Side lobe artefact occurs when side lobes encounter a strongly reflective structure that is outside of the central beam. The returned signals are assumed to have originated from the central beam causing duplication, malpositioning or obscuration of structures.

This is commonly seen in echocardiography in the parasternal long axis (PLAX) view where there appears to be a moving structure in the left atrium, but it is actually a side lobe artefact from the mitral valve annulus (Figure 1.38). This is a very important artefact as these side lobes may be mistaken for masses, clots or foreign bodies.

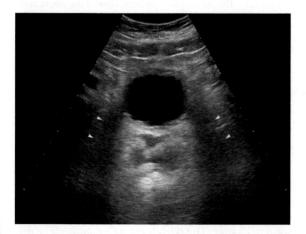

Figure 1.36 Edge shadowing can be seen on either side of the bladder (arrows).

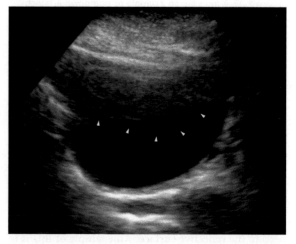

Figure 1.37 Beam width artefact commonly affects anechoic structures. Here, the anechoic bladder is being 'smeared' by peripheral artefact from the bowel (arrows).

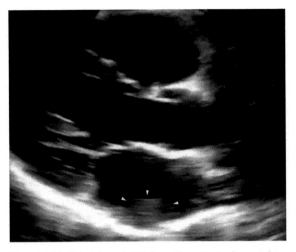

Figure 1.38 Side lobe artefact from the mitral valve causing the appearance of a structure (arrows) within the left atrium. *A video is available to view in the online video library.*

Step 5 – Image Optimisation

Familiarity with the basic controls and understanding knobology will allow users to rapidly transform the quality of the generated image. These settings will be available on all US machines regardless of the size, cost or complexity.

Depth

The first setting to adjust is the depth (Figure 1.39). The screen will display a scale that demonstrates how deep the US window is set to. Having excessive depth beyond the structure of interest is a common mistake for novice sonographers. This leads to wasted screen *'real-estate'*

and reduced frame rate due to the US having to travel further through the body prior to being displayed.

It is good practice to begin imaging with a larger depth to identify key anatomy prior to optimising the window to only display the structures of interest. This will ensure an optimal frame rate and magnification for US assessment.

Zoom

Zoom provides an opportunity to magnify small objects to assess in more detail (Figure 1.40). A key point is that zooming into an object does not improve frame rate or resolution as the full US sector is still being imaged by the machine. If the structure you wish to zoom into is shallow it is good practice to reduce the image *depth* prior to zoom as this will improve the overall quality of the image.

Sector Width

With phased array probes the sector width may be adjusted. This is demonstrated in Figure 1.41. Reducing the sector width, much like reducing the depth, will lead to a better quality image due to improved resolution and frame rate. Conversely, increasing the sector width degrades the image. The user must, however, ensure that adequate sector width is chosen to provide an acceptable window for interpretation of key structures.

Gain (Brightness)

Adjusting the gain will alter the display brightness of the received signals. It is important to remember that increasing the gain *does not* increase the strength of

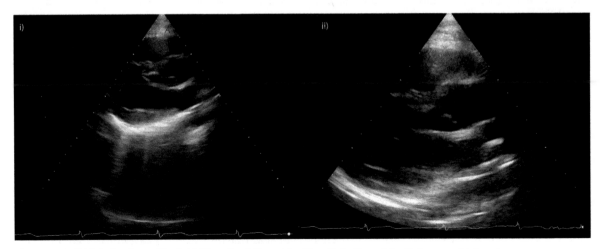

Figure 1.39 (i) High depth used for initial imaging followed by (ii) optimisation of depth for area of interest.

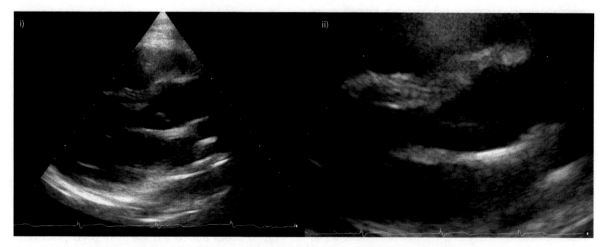

Figure 1.40 **(i) Normal PLAX view followed by (ii) a zoomed-in view of the aortic valve and ascending aorta.**

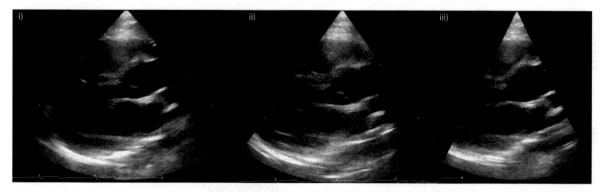

Figure 1.41 **Comparison between (i) wide; (ii) optimised; and (iii) narrow sector widths.** The wide sector width offers a large field of view but at the expense of frame rate. The narrow sector width will have an excellent frame rate but does not include all the key structures that need to be identified within the PLAX view.

the returning signal but simply amplifies whatever signal has already returned. Excessive gain is another very common mistake for novices and will lead to a bright, grainy image with more noise and artefact. Increasing the gain reduces the overall contrast of the image and may cause structures, such as valves, to appear significantly *thicker* than reality leading to incorrect interpretation.

Figure 1.42 shows an example of increased gain and decreased gain. Note how challenging both images are to interpret.

Time Gain Compensation

Time gain compensation (TGC) allows manual adjustment of the amount of gain at certain depths whilst leaving the remainder of the image unaffected. This is particularly useful when a highly echogenic

structure is causing artefact and obscuring the surrounding image. The pericardium beneath the left ventricular posterior wall on the parasternal long axis view in echocardiography is an example of a hyperechoic structure that may benefit from localised gain reduction. Many users will increase the gain of the far field due to concerns that attenuation will lead to weaker returning signals from deeper structures. Most US machines will compensate for this by automatically increasing the gain of returning signals. This means that users are applying a further gain amplification onto signals which potentially leads to image distortion. Figure 1.43 demonstrates TGC set with gain in far and near field high.

We would advise you to keep the TGC central as demonstrated in Figure 1.44 until you are proficient in scanning.

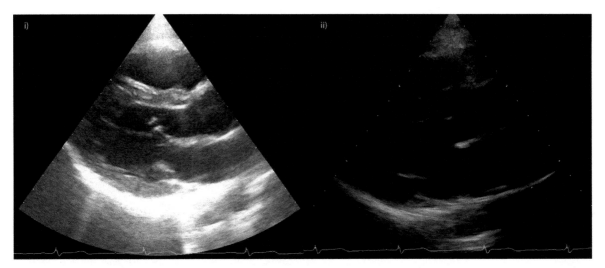

Figure 1.42 In these images the gain is set either (i) too high or (ii) too low. Note how challenging interpretation is for both images.

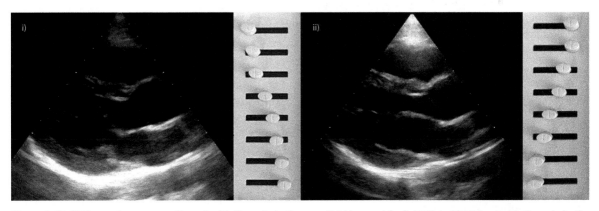

Figure 1.43 (i) Time gain compensation set with the gain in the near field low and far field high. (ii) TGC set with the gain in the near field high and far field low. Image (i) causes an imbalanced image with poor resolution in the near field and excessive brightness and distortion in the far field. Image (ii) causes a very bright region at the top of the screen with very poor definition of the right ventricular free wall.

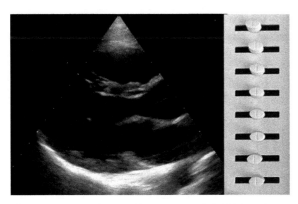

Figure 1.44 Neural TGC is the recommended initial setting.

Focus

Most probes have the ability to focus on a particular area of an image. Setting the focus level will lead to convergence of the US beam at that level leading to increased resolution. For normal imaging this should be kept at the centre of the US field (Figure 1.45). If you wish to interrogate a specific structure the focus may be adjusted to this level, e.g. for assessment of a valve.

Tissue Harmonic Imaging

The non-linear propagation of US waves within tissues causes distortion and generation of 'resonant frequencies'. This describes signals that are multiples

23

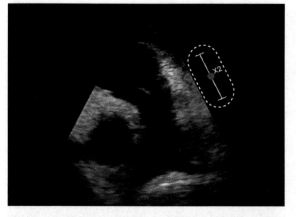

Figure 1.45 Focus set at the area of interest (circled). In this case – the pulmonary valve in the parasternal short axis view.

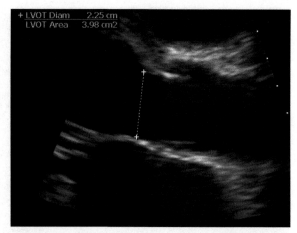

Figure 1.46 Frozen zoomed image of the PLAX view. Callipers have been used to measure the LVOT diameter and the machine has automatically calculated the LVOT area.

of the fundamental or transmitted frequency. Modern machines have the capability of using tissue harmonic imaging (THI) to detect these signals as 'harmonics' rather than true signals and generate a more accurate image with better resolution and fewer artefacts. This is typically switched on as default on most machines.

Compound Imaging

Compound Imaging is a broad bandwidth technology that combines multiple coplanar images combined from different beam angles from different US frequency spectra to create a single image in real time. Compound imaging reduces speckle artefacts and improves contrast resolution.

Step 6 – Saving Your Images

Image acquisition is essential to training and for quality assurance, governance and audit. This is described more in Chapter 13 – 'Governance and Quality Assurance'.

Freeze Image, Capture and Record

All machines will enable the user to freeze the frame, scroll through an automatically recorded loop and save images to the internal storage. Although many machines will differ in the description of these buttons, almost all machines will function in a similar way:

– Freeze – this will pause the image and allow the user to scroll backwards through an automatically recorded loop.

– Freeze and capture/record – pressing capture or record whilst the screen is frozen will save a still image with annotations if applied.

– Capture/record – pressing capture or record whilst scanning will save the video loop. The loop that is saved may be retrospective or prospective and tailored to a particular clip length/number of QRS complexes depending upon the preference of the user.

Measurements/callipers

After freezing an image, the user is able to select the callipers to perform basic numerical measures.

Most machines will also have inbuilt data analysis packages depending on the selected preset that will provide a list of measurement options. For example, selecting the LVOT diameter measure in the cardiac package will cause the machine to automatically calculate LVOT area that may be used in the stroke volume and cardiac output calculations (Figure 1.46).

Caring for Your Machine

The US machine should be respected and cared for and kept in a safe place. The probes must be placed carefully in the holders with particular attention to the cables. These commonly become trapped underneath the wheels when moving the machine and are exceptionally expensive to replace.

All probes and the machine should be cleaned regularly for infection control purposes. The probes must be cleaned with non-alcoholic wipes as alcohol may lead to degradation of the piezoelectric elements.

Summary

- A fundamental understanding of basic physics is critical for all clinicians practicing POCUS to appreciate how US images are created and how they can be optimised for accurate interpretation and reporting.
- Understanding, recognising and correcting reversible artefact is essential to generating good quality diagnostic imaging.
- Clinicians must be confident using the basic controls of the US machine to manipulate the resulting image. Scans must be saved, labelled and reported for governance and quality assurance purposes.

A full list of references and further reading is available at www.GeneralistUltrasound.com

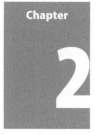

Echocardiography

Introduction

Echocardiography (echo) is an intimidating discipline that many clinicians avoid assuming it is too complex to acquire and interpret images. It is true that a comprehensive, 'formal' study is time consuming and requires a significant degree of expertise and training to be performed accurately. However, focused echo differs to departmental studies as only a few images need to be acquired to answer key clinical questions (Table 2.1). This reduces the inter-user variability, subjective bias and transforms echo into a diagnostic tool that is simple, accessible and easier to achieve the required competence and confidence.

Historically, echo has firmly been within the remit of cardiologists and echocardiographers. The utility of echo is increasingly being recognised by other specialties including Acute and General Medicine, Critical Care, Anaesthesia, Emergency Medicine and prehospital services. This growing trend has been recognised by a consensus document, endorsed by the American Society of Echocardiography (ASE) and the British Society of Echocardiography (BSE), advocating for focused echo in shock to be performed by frontline clinicians.

The utility of echo within the shocked, acutely unwell patient is clear: to identify key diagnoses that will rapidly transform the patient's management at the bedside. We believe that focused echo is equally mandated in patients with chronic disease. A five-minute study can identify individuals with ventricular dysfunction, valvular disease, pericardial collections or structural heart disease and facilitate appropriate referrals to specialist teams and for definitive investigations.

The key to point-of-care ultrasound (POCUS) is to formulate a question in the clinician's mind based upon conventional history and examination. This is particularly important for echo as findings may be compatible with multiple different pathologies depending on the pre-test probability for each. For example, right ventricular dilatation is likely to be present in the setting of an acute massive pulmonary embolism (PE), cor pulmonale due to chronic obstructive pulmonary disease (COPD) or in patients on mechanical ventilation with high inspiratory pressures. Performing the basic cornerstones of history and examination will dramatically improve the utility of POCUS and make it an indispensable tool for general clinicians.

Key indications for focused echo are listed in Table 2.2, and Table 2.3 lists some key indications that mandate an urgent echo. Although some of these diagnoses will be beyond the skill set of some POCUS users, performing a focused scan whilst awaiting definitive studies may identify key findings the clinician was not expecting or seeing that *something is not quite right*.

Additional indications that may aid with clinical decision-making are listed in Table 2.4.

Table 2.1 Key clinical questions for focused echocardiography

Questions to ask	Yes/No
Is the LV function impaired?	
Is there pericardial fluid?	
Is the RV dilated and/or impaired?	
Is there evidence of hypovolaemia?	
Is there any gross valvular pathology?	

Table 2.2

Indications for focused echo
Undifferentiated shortness of breath
New murmur
Chest pain
Features of heart failure
Haemodynamic instability

Table 2.3

Indications for urgent formal echo

Cardiac arrest at all pulse checks (PE, tamponade and hypovolaemia)

Hypotension of unknown cause (shock)

Suspected pericardial tamponade

Suspected massive/sub massive PE

Suspected aortic dissection

New murmur post MI (VSD or papillary muscle rupture leading to new acute MR)

Unstable patient in known endocarditis

Suspected pericardial effusion

PE: pulmonary embolism; MI: myocardial infarction; VSD: ventricular septal defect; MR: mitral regurgitation.

Table 2.4

Other indications and examples for bedside echocardiography

Looking at LV function to decide:

1. Escalation of treatment and care – are they candidates for Intensive Care?

2. Should we be withdrawing treatment?

3. Undifferentiated SOB:

– Look at LV function/PE/Pericardial or pleural effusion

SOB: shortness of breath; PE: pericardial effusion; LV: left ventricle.

This chapter is designed to provide the reader with a basic overview of how to perform focused echocardiography and the key indications. There will be cases discussed that are beyond the scope of basic accreditation pathways to give insight into where clinicians may develop their skills further.

Method

The phased array ('echo') probe (1–5 MHz, Figure 2.1) should be used due to its low frequency (enabling visualisation of deeper structures) and small footprint (to scan between the ribs). The probe will have a notch, light or dot to aid orientation when viewing the heart in different views. This light refers to the icon on the right-hand side of the ultrasound (US) machine screen to help orientate yourself. Note

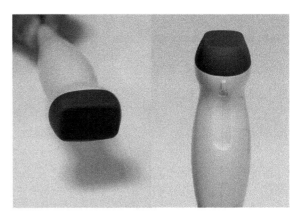

Figure 2.1 **The phased array probe.**

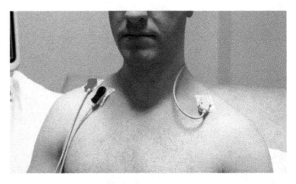

Figure 2.2 **Practical positioning of ECG dots during echo.**

that echo is the only US modality that has the icon on the *right-hand side* of the screen – for all other modalities this will be on the *left*. By selecting a cardiac preset the US machine should automatically change the marker location. This is purely due to convention and differs in other countries.

It is imperative an electrocardiogram (ECG) trace is attached to the patient to differentiate between systole and diastole. During arrest and peri arrest situations this clearly may not be viable but should be attempted in all but the most emergent settings. End-diastole corresponds to the Q wave when the mitral valve is maximally open and end-systole corresponds to the T wave. Although this may seem like a frustrating initial step, the ECG is particularly useful in identifying chamber collapse in cardiac tamponade or systolic anterior motion of the mitral valve. Furthermore, saved image loops are normally programmed to record based on a number of cardiac cycles which are identified based upon the ECG.

Placing the ECG dots onto the clavicles will ensure they do not impede the scanning locations (Figure 2.2).

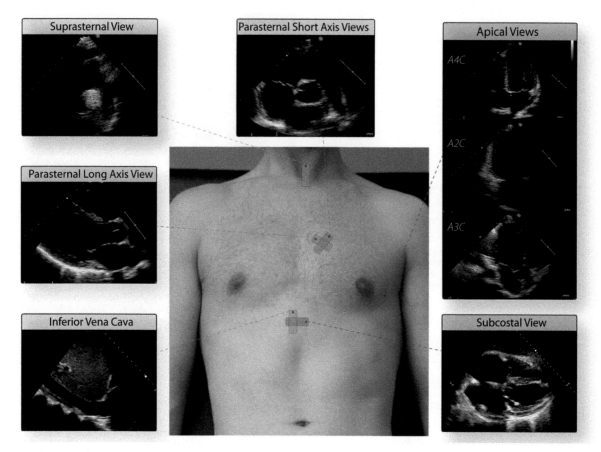

Figure 2.3 Probe placement and notch direction to achieve all basic echocardiography views. Each view will be discussed in more detail in the relevant section below.

A number of echo windows are available that allow good penetration of US without too much impedance by the lung or ribs. For focused echo we recommend that you view images for the following views as shown in Figure 2.3:

– Parasternal long-axis views (PLAX)

– Parasternal short-axis views (PSAX)

– Apical four-chamber view (A4C)

– Subcostal view (SC)

Axis simply refers to the plane that the US beam travels through the heart and therefore the cross-section image obtained.

We will describe other views that may help as you become more confident and advanced in your practice:

– Right ventricular inflow view

– Right ventricular outflow view

– Five-chamber view (A5C)

– Two-chamber view (A2C)

– Three-chamber view (A3C)

– Suprasternal view (SS)

You must be mindful that technically challenging scans are seen in the following groups of patients:

– Obese.

– Chest wall deformities.

– Chronic lung disease such as COPD or pulmonary fibrosis. The hyperinflation leads to a US barrier. This also explains the challenge of echo in patients on positive pressure ventilation (invasive or non-invasive).

– Acutely unwell patients who are unable to have their position optimised.

It is very rare that no imaging windows are available and a conclusion, albeit potentially limited, can be made even from a single imaging window.

Normal Echo Windows

When carrying out focused echo we suggest the following sequence of image acquisition.

1. Parasternal long-axis view (PLAX)
2. Parasternal short-axis view (PSAX)
3. Four-chamber view/apical view (A4C)
4. Subcostal view (SC)

Parasternal Long-Axis View

The first image to acquire in a stable patient is the PLAX. In a cardiac arrest or peri arrest situation the subcostal view would normally be acquired initially due to cardiopulmonary resuscitation (CPR) or the inability to reposition the patient.

The left parasternal window will be found in the second–fourth intercostal space, left sternal edge (Figure 2.4). If your patient is able to lie in the left lateral position this will be useful to bring the heart closer to the chest wall, limiting lung artefact. PLAX view is achievable in the supine position but may be more challenging.

We recommend you start higher than the second intercostal space and gradually move down rib spaces until you acquire the PLAX view. The marker/dot on the transducer points to the right shoulder. This image acquires an image of the heart in cross-section from the base to the apex of the heart – the so called 'long-axis'.

In this view you can see the left ventricular cavity, interventricular septum (IVS; LV anteroseptal segments), LV posterior wall (PW; LV inferolateral segments), LV outflow tract (LVOT), left atrium (LA), mitral valve (MV), aortic valve (AV), right

ventricular outflow tract (RVOT), pericardium and the ascending and descending aorta (Figure 2.5).

We suggest the following process for image interpretation:

Left Ventricular Cavity Size and Function

– This is a good view at assessing the left ventricular size and function. The walls should thicken and come towards each other into the centre of the cavity. This would indicate normal systolic function provided there are no regional wall motion abnormalities. This view only assesses the anteroseptal and inferolateral LV segments so regional impairment of other areas will not be visualised. Note the correspondence with the ECG trace.

Right Ventricular Size and Function

– The RVOT, ascending aorta and left atrium should all be equivocal in size. If the RV is dilated it will be seen to be notably larger than these other structures.

– Right ventricular function is challenging to assess and quantify in this view but the RV free wall should be seen to contract towards the interventricular septum.

Pleural and Pericardial Fluid

– Pericardial fluid will be seen as a hypoechoic space between the pericardium and the myocardial wall.

– The descending aorta is a key anatomical landmark for differentiating between pleural and pericardial fluid. Normally this will be directly

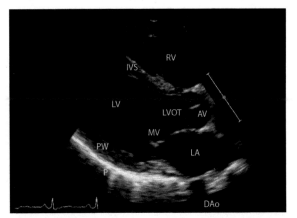

Figure 2.5 Normal PLAX view with structural annotations.
LV, left ventricle; LVOT, left ventricular outflow tract; AV, aortic valve; MV, mitral valve; PW, left ventricular posterior wall; LA, left atrium; P, pericardium; RV, right ventricle; DAo, descending aorta. *A video is available to view in the online video library.*

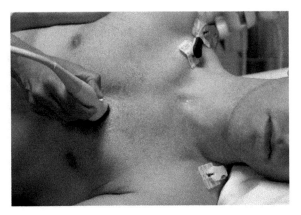

Figure 2.4 Typical probe position for the PLAX view. Note the probe marker is pointing towards the patient's right shoulder.

adjacent to the LA wall. If pericardial fluid is present the descending aorta will be pushed away from the LA wall because it is a structure located outside of the pericardial sac. If the fluid is pleural the descending aorta will remain adjacent to the LA.

Valvular Issues

- Parasternal long-axis view provides a good image of the aortic and mitral valves. They should each be assessed for any calcification, restriction in movement, masses or regurgitation using colour Doppler.

With increasing confidence, you can begin to take basic measurements assessing the LV internal diameter in diastole and systole (LVIDd and LVIDs) and the septal and posterior wall thickness in diastole (IVSd and LVPWd) (Figure 2.6). This can aid in diagnosis of LV dilatation and hypertrophy.

Please note that most normal values should now be indexed to either body surface area or height and gender. BSE guidance for normal internal LV dimensions in diastole are ≤ 5.6 cm for males and ≤ 5.1 cm for females.

Using M-mode can be useful to assess the motion of structures through time. M-mode is described in more detail in Chapter 1. As this will only assess a thin slice of the image, the frame rate will be excellent making it particularly suited to moving structures such as valves.

If the image is correctly aligned, M-mode may be used through the LV. Here you can appreciate the difference throughout the cardiac cycle with the LV thickening and diminishing the LV cavity size

indicating normal LV function. Normal motion of the MV is also seen within the LV cavity (Figure 2.7).

Modified Parasternal Windows

Tilting the tail of the probe either upwards (cephalad) or downwards (caudad) will reveal the modified parasternal windows. Tilting the tail of the probe upwards will reveal the right ventricle (RV) inflow view which provides excellent visualisation of the tricuspid valve (TV) and right atrium (RA) (Figure 2.8i).

Tilting the tail of the probe downwards will show the RV outflow view. This allows users to view the pulmonary valve (PV) and main pulmonary artery (PA) (Figure 2.8ii).

The modified parasternal windows are a more advanced technique but will allow the clinician to appreciate the surrounding anatomy. With practice they become an essential tool to assess tricuspid and pulmonary valve pathology.

Parasternal Short-Axis View

From the PLAX view rotate the transducer through 90 degrees so the marker is pointing towards the left shoulder (Figure 2.9).

- Now the heart is cut in the transverse, short-axis view. It is useful to consider various cross-sections through the PLAX view that are being assessed in turn. With the probe aimed cranially the 'basal structures' will be assessed. As the probe is gradually swept caudally it will pass through the mitral valve level, papillary muscle level and the apex. Each of these levels will be discussed in turn:

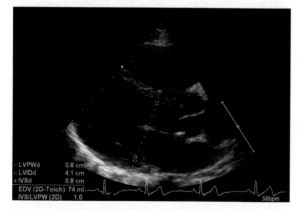

Figure 2.6 Calliper placement for PLAX measurement of IVSd, LVIDd and LVPWd.

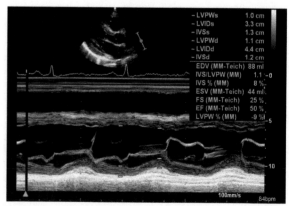

Figure 2.7 M-mode through the PLAX view at the mitral valve level.

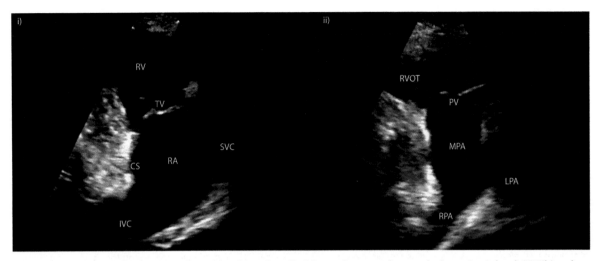

Figure 2.8 **(i) The RV inflow view is achieved by tilting the tail of the probe upwards towards the patient's head. (ii) Tilting the probe tail downwards will reveal the RV outflow view.** RV, right ventricle; TV, tricuspid valve; RA, right atrium; CS, coronary sinus; IVC, inferior vena cava; SVC, superior vena cava; RVOT, right ventricular outflow tract; PV, pulmonary valve; MPA, main pulmonary artery; RPA, right pulmonary artery; LPA, left pulmonary artery. *Videos are available to view in the online video library.*

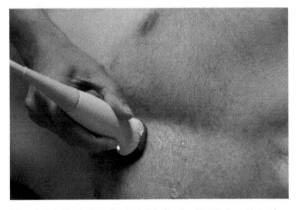

Figure 2.9 Typical probe location for the PSAX view. Note the probe marker is now pointing towards the patient's left shoulder.

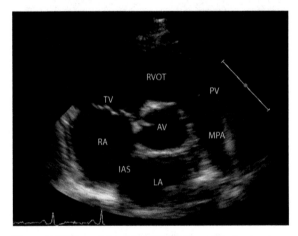

Figure 2.10 Normal basal level PSAX view with structural annotations. LA, left atrium; IAS, inter-atrial septum; RA, right atrium; TV, tricuspid valve; RVOT, right ventricular outflow tract; PV, pulmonary valve; MPA, main pulmonary artery. *A video is available to view in the online video library.*

Basal Level or 'Aortic Valve' Level (Figure 2.10)

In this view the left atrium (LA), right atrium (RA), RVOT, AV, pulmonary valve, tricuspid valve and the inter atrial septum are visualised. A normal AV is thin with three mobile leaflets (Mercedes sign). You may identify bicuspid (~1/100) or even a quadricuspid valve (1/1000–10,000). When the aortic valve is thickened and calcified you will see increased echogenicity with possible restriction in movement.

Mitral Valve Level (Figure 2.11)

This level provides excellent visualisation of the anterior and posterior mitral valve leaflets. The opening and closing of the valve is described to appear like a 'fish mouth' or 'skipping rope'. Contraction of the LV walls can be seen at this level and represents the LV 'basal' segments.

Mid-Papillary Level (Figure 2.12)

The mid-papillary level is excellent for assessing LV systolic function. This is the LV 'mid' level. The walls should be seen to thicken and move inwards towards the centre of the LV cavity. Placing your

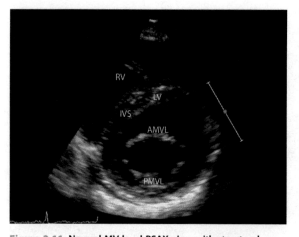

Figure 2.11 **Normal MV level PSAX view with structural annotations.** LV, left ventricle; IVS, inter-ventricular septum; AMVL, anterior mitral valve leaflet; PMVL, posterior mitral valve leaflet; RV, right ventricle. *A video is available to view in the online video library.*

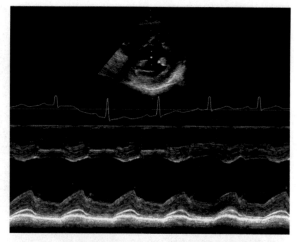

Figure 2.13 **M-mode placed through the LV showing thickening of the myocardium and a reduction in LV cavity size.**

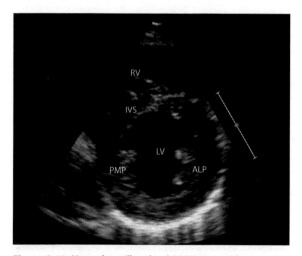

Figure 2.12 **Normal papillary level PSAX view with structural annotations.** LV, left ventricle; IVS, inter-ventricular septum; ALP, anterolateral papillary muscle; PMP, posteromedial papillary muscle; RV, right ventricle. *A video is available to view in the online video library.*

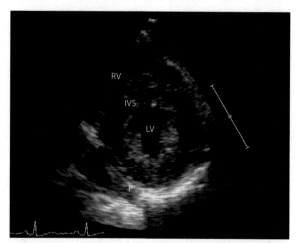

Figure 2.14 **Normal apical level PSAX view with structural annotations.** LV, left ventricle; IVS, inter-ventricular septum; P, pericardium; RV, right ventricle. *A video is available to view in the online video library.*

finger in the centre of the LV cavity on the US screen can be a useful tool to assess for regional wall motion abnormalities (RWMAs).

M-mode may also be placed through the LV to assess systolic function (Figure 2.13).

Apical Level (Figure 2.14)

The LV 'apical' level is the remaining region of the ventricle to assess for overall function. Although not routinely included in point of care studies, it is an important view to assess for apical regional wall

motion abnormalities and thrombus in the setting of apical akinesia.

The LV segments and regional coronary artery territories are essential to be familiar with if aiming to describe distribution of regional wall motion abnormalities. This will be discussed in more detail later in the chapter.

Apical Four-Chamber View

The probe is placed at the cardiac apex with the marker pointing towards the left shoulder (Figure 2.15). The

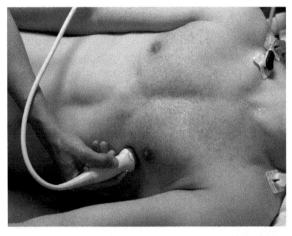

Figure 2.15 Typical probe location for the A4C view. Note the probe marker is pointing towards the patient's left shoulder with a fairly shallow US beam angle.

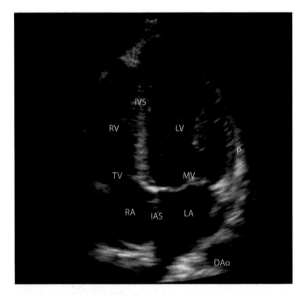

Figure 2.16 Normal A4C view with structural annotations.
LV, left ventricle; IVS, inter-ventricular septum; MV, mitral valve; RV, right ventricle; TV, tricuspid valve; LA, left atrium; IAS, inter-atrial septum; RA, right atrium; DAo, descending aorta; P, pericardium. *A video is available to view in the online video library.*

cardiac apex may be palpated to locate the initial location to place the probe. This is usually the most challenging view for novice sonographers to obtain.

This will give you the typical 'heart shaped' four-chamber view (Figure 2.16).

Here you can assess the following:

Left Ventricular Size and Function

– Are the walls contracting and thickening?

Size of the Right Ventricle

– The RV should be approximately two-thirds of the size of the LV. If it appears the same size as the LV it is *dilated*. If larger than the LV it is *severely dilated*.

Valvular Abnormalities

– The mitral and tricuspid valves should be assessed in turn for any obvious thickening, calcification, reduced mobility or masses.

– Colour Doppler may be used to assess for valvular insufficiency.

– Note that vegetations in endocarditis can adhere anywhere upon the valve and subvalvular apparatus including the papillary muscles and the LV walls.

Atrial Size

– Grossly dilated atria may signify valvular pathology or diastolic dysfunction and should prompt further investigation.

Five-Chamber View (Advanced Image)

The name 'five-chamber' is a misnomer as the 'fifth chamber' is actually the LVOT, AV and ascending aorta (Figure 2.17). The image is acquired by tilting the probe to scan more anteriorly (*shallower* probe angle) until the LVOT comes into view.

This is an important view to assess aortic valve function, haemodynamics and impact of hypertrophy

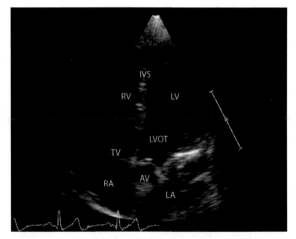

Figure 2.17 Normal A5C view with structural annotations.
LV, left ventricle; IVS, inter-ventricular septum; LVOT, left ventricular outflow tract; AV, aortic valve; RV, right ventricle; TV, tricuspid valve; LA, left atrium; RA, right atrium. *A video is available to view in the online video library.*

on LVOT obstruction – for example in hypertrophic cardiomyopathy (HCM).

Pulsed wave (PW) Doppler may be placed in the LVOT (~0.5–1 cm proximal to the AV) and Doppler envelope traced to calculate the *stroke distance*. When this is multiplied by the LVOT area (calculated from the LVOT diameter measurement) the *stroke volume* is calculated. This is an essential part of haemodynamic assessment in acutely unwell patients and will be discussed later in the chapter. PW Doppler may also be placed at various levels within the LVOT to assess for the high gradients seen with LVOT obstruction (LVOTO) in HCM.

Colour Doppler and continuous wave (CW) Doppler can be placed through the aortic valve to assess for any stenosis or regurgitation. The CW envelope is then traced and peak and mean valve gradients calculated. This is the cornerstone of severity grading for aortic stenosis.

Two-Chamber View (Advanced Image)

From the apical view you can rotate the probe by 45 degrees anticlockwise with the probe marker pointing towards the ceiling. Here you will see the LV and LA allowing for detailed assessment of the LV anterior and inferior walls (Figure 2.18).

Three-Chamber View (Advanced Image)

Continue to rotate the probe anticlockwise until the probe marker is pointing towards the left shoulder. The 'three-chamber' (another misnomer) or apical long-axis view (as the structures seen are the same as those seen in the parasternal long-axis view) allows assessment of the LV anteroseptal and inferolateral walls, mitral valve, LVOT, AV and ascending aorta (Figure 2.19). Occasionally the alignment of spectral Doppler with the LVOT in this view is better than the A4C and allows for more accurate assessment of AV pathology, haemodynamic assessment and LVOTO.

Subcostal View

The SC view is important in the acutely unwell patient as it is readily achievable with the patient supine. Similarly, in the event of cardiac arrest, the probe may be placed whilst chest compressions are being performed and an image taken immediately during a pulse check to minimise time delay.

The images obtained are similar to the A4C view but rotated 45 degrees clockwise. The probe should be placed flat to the skin surface (see image) with the US beam aiming towards the heart and probe marker directed towards the patient's left shoulder (Figure 2.20). The liver may be used as an acoustic window to improve visualisation if required.

If the patient has very tense abdominal muscles they can be asked to lift their knees to relax the

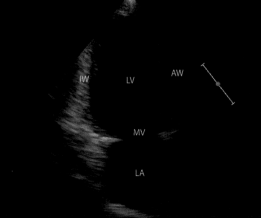

Figure 2.18 Normal A2C view with structural annotations.
LV, left ventricle; AW, left ventricular anterior wall; IW, left ventricular interior wall; MV, mitral valve; LA, left atrium. *A video is available to view in the online video library.*

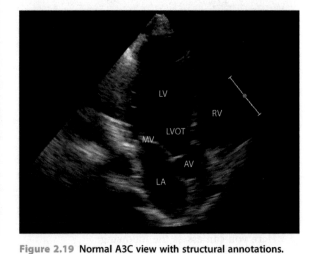

Figure 2.19 Normal A3C view with structural annotations.
LV, left ventricle; LVOT, left ventricular outflow tract; AV, aortic valve; MV, mitral valve; LA, left atrium; RV, right ventricle. *A video is available to view in the online video library.*

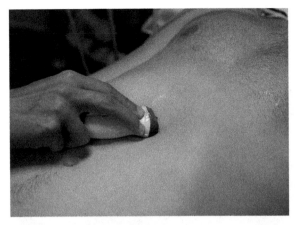

Figure 2.20 Typical probe location for the subcostal view. Note the probe marker is pointing towards the patient's left-hand side.

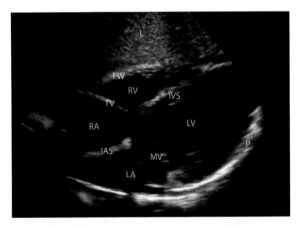

Figure 2.21 Normal subcostal view with structural annotations. LV, left ventricle; IVS, inter-ventricular septum; MV, mitral valve; LA, left atrium; RV, right ventricle; FW, right ventricular free wall; TV, tricuspid valve; RA, right atrium; IAS, inter-atrial septum; P, pericardium; L, liver. *A video is available to view in the online video library.*

musculature. The LV, RV, mitral valve, tricuspid valve and interatrial/interventricular septae may be assessed in this view (Figure 2.21).

The probe may be rotated 45 degrees anticlockwise from the SC view to obtain a subcostal short-axis image which demonstrates the same structures as the PSAX views. This is particularly useful in the setting of critical care where parasternal views may be unachievable and positive pressure ventilation causes downwards displacement of the thoracic structures.

Inferior Vena Cava

The inferior vena cava (IVC) is a useful structure to estimate RA pressure as part of a haemodynamic

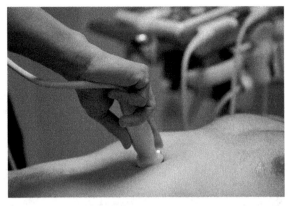

Figure 2.22 Typical location for the IVC view. Note the probe marker is pointing upwards towards the patient's head.

assessment. The probe is rotated anticlockwise 45 degrees so the probe marker is directed cranially with a steeper approach (Figure 2.22). The key structure to differentiate the IVC from is the abdominal aorta. This is discussed in detail in Chapter 4.

Although fraught with error, the IVC may be used to estimate volume status and right-sided pressure. It is dilated when it measures >2 cm and should normally compress >50% with inspiration. To make this assessment you can ask the patient to 'sniff' or take a deep breath to see this response. If the IVC does not compress with respiration it suggests raised right atrial pressure (Figure 2.23).

As with anything in medicine, the IVC should never be used in isolation to assess 'filling status'. It may be dilated for a multitude of reasons and will be dynamically affected by abdominal and thoracic pressures and structures. This will be discussed in more detail in the haemodynamic section of this chapter.

Suprasternal View (Advanced Image)

The probe is placed in the suprasternal notch with the probe marker pointing cranially (Figure 2.24). The patient should be asked to extend their neck and warned as it may be slightly uncomfortable.

By tilting the probe to the left and right the following structures may be seen as shown in Figure 2.25:

- Ascending aorta
- Aortic arch
- Descending aorta
- Right pulmonary artery
- Left main bronchus

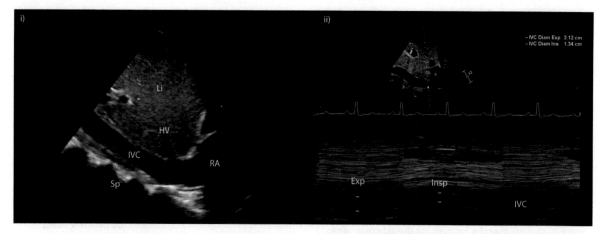

Figure 2.23 (i) Normal IVC view with structural annotations. (ii) M-mode IVC view showing IVC diameter change during respiratory cycle with inspiratory and expiratory measurements. IVC, inferior vena cava; RA, right atrium; HV, hepatic vein; Li, liver; Sp, spinous processes; exp, expiration; Insp, inspiration.

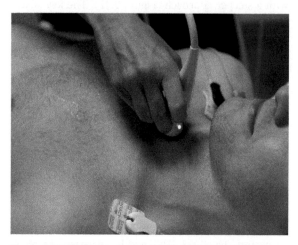

Figure 2.24 Typical probe position for the suprasternal view. The probe marker should point between the patient's head and left shoulder. Optimal direction for the marker is variable.

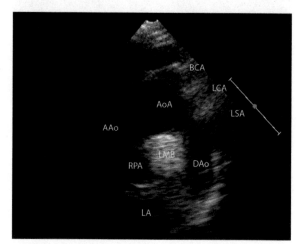

Figure 2.25 Normal suprasternal view with structural annotations. AAo, ascending aorta; AoA, aortic arch; DAo, descending aorta; BCA, brachiocephalic artery; LCA, left common carotid artery; LSA, left subclavian artery; LMB, left main bronchus; RPA, right pulmonary artery; LA, left atrium. *A video is available to view in the online video library.*

– Arterial branches from the aorta: the brachiocephalic artery, left common carotid, left subclavian artery.

This is a useful imaging view for the assessment of aortic dissection, coarctation and for severe aortic regurgitation.

Focused Echo in Cardiac Arrest

Echocardiography should be mandated as part of the cardiac arrest algorithm. This guides us on the potentially reversible causes of cardiac arrest: the four Hs and the four Ts (Table 2.5). The conditions highlighted in **bold** can be diagnosed with echo and treated at the bedside. Remember that tension pneumothorax may also be assessed using lung ultrasound which is described in Chapter 3.

The features of each of these will be described in the pathology section of this chapter.

Many resuscitation guidelines across the world now promote the use of echo during cardiac arrest to answer the following questions:

– Is the RV dilated? Could this be a massive pulmonary embolism?

Table 2.5

Reversible causes of cardiac arrest	
Hypovolaemia	**Cardiac Tamponade**
Hyper/Hypokalaemia	**Thromboembolism**
Hypoxia	Tension Pneumothorax
Hypo/Hyperthermia	Toxins

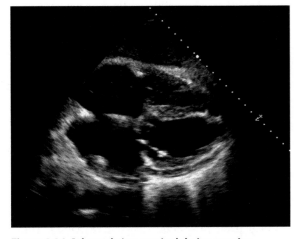

Figure 2.26 Subcostal view acquired during ongoing cardiopulmonary resuscitation. The probe has been correctly placed whilst CPR is being performed so the user can guide compressions and ensure an adequate window has been acquired for the pulse check. *A video is available to view in the online video library.*

– Is there pericardial fluid? If so this must be treated as tamponade and requires urgent pericardiocentesis.

– Are there signs of frank hypovolaemia? Fluid should be administered.

To perform echo in cardiac arrest the user should place the probe within the subcostal position whilst chest compressions are being performed. This will ensure that the moment chest compressions pause for a pulse check the probe is in the correct location and an image is available on screen. Although many clinicians will attempt to interpret the echo images during a pulse check, this may lead to unnecessary delays in restarting compressions.

We advocate for the US user to prepare the machine to record a minimum of a five-second image loop (Figure 2.26). The moment chest compressions cease they should optimise the image and press record. Instead of attempting to interpret the image during this window they should aim to acquire and save the best possible video that can be analysed in detail during the subsequent two-minute cycle of CPR.

Although five seconds is an arbitrary number, the key principles are to:

1. Make sure the US machine is recording based on time and not ECG rhythm which is likely not to be attached to the patient.
2. Save a long enough recording to capture a cardiac contraction in the event of severe bradyarrhythmia.
3. Review the images in a less time critical and pressured moment to ensure correct interpretation.

Accurate image interpretation is essential as there is growing evidence to suggest that echo during cardiac arrest may aid in prediction of long-term survival based on the presence of cardiac motion. Clinicians are generally poor at palpation of pulses during cardiac arrest and many patients who are profoundly hypotensive are labelled as having pulseless electrical activity (PEA). Echo has been suggested to be able to distinguish between PEA and 'pseudo-PEA' – the presence of organised electrical activity without a pulse but with cardiac motion on echo.

Although this may seem academic, the presence of cardiac activity is associated with a significantly higher probability of return of spontaneous circulation (ROSC) and improved survival to hospital admission. These improved outcomes are mirrored in asystolic patients with cardiac motion seen with POCUS.

Absence of cardiac activity during a pulse check is associated with a significantly reduced chance of survival. If no other reversible causes are identified and the echo demonstrates cardiac standstill this may inform the decision to discontinue CPR based on likely prognosis.

Echo is complementary to conventional clinical assessment and should never be used in isolation. Despite this, skilled users may aid in prognostication during these high stress clinical scenarios and provide additional evidence for deciding whether to continue or discontinue resuscitation.

Post Return of Spontaneous Circulation Care

The post ROSC phase of a resuscitation provides an opportunity for a more thorough assessment for potentially reversible causes. Identification of regional wall motion abnormalities is not possible if there is no cardiac contraction and RV dilatation is present in a high proportion of cardiac arrests. Following ROSC, the user is able to perform a more detailed study aiming to identify these features that may warrant further investigation or treatment e.g. CT pulmonary angiography or percutaneous coronary intervention (PCI).

The Left Ventricle

Left Ventricular Function

Left ventricular function is a vital element of any echocardiogram. The majority of requests for departmental studies are based upon LV contractility and POCUS users should expect the majority of questions to reflect this. LV function provides the clinician with essential information about how well the heart is able to pump blood around the body. This may be influenced by many variables and is a key marker for prognostication. Cardiovascular disease is the leading cause of death globally and it is essential that practitioners have considered cardiac disease regardless of the clinical setting. Identification within the General Practice setting will enable optimisation of medical therapy with significant improvement to life expectancy. In Emergency and Acute Medical Departments finding LV impairment provides key information for diagnosis and decision-making regarding ceilings of care. Patients on Critical Care are associated with a significantly higher incidence of cardiac dysfunction and LV impairment may lead to introduction of inotropy to optimise circulatory support.

The LV is a complex structure with fibres extending in many directions. During contraction, the LV myocardial fibres will shorten in a radial, longitudinal and circumferential manner leading to challenges when measuring LV systolic function.

Detailed studies will employ many techniques to estimate LV systolic function including Simpson's biplane ejection fraction, fractional shortening, fractional area change, mitral annular plane of systolic excursion, tissue Doppler, strain measurement and 3D echocardiography. These measurements are time consuming and require a level of expertise unachievable for most generalist clinicians. POCUS relies on the visual assessment of the LV in combination with the overall clinical picture to formulate a conclusion.

As a POCUS practitioner a subjective visual assessment must be evaluated in at least two views. All visualised walls of the ventricle should be seen to thicken symmetrically and move vigorously towards the centre of the chamber during systole. Basic level training pathways, such as Focused Ultrasound in Intensive Care (FUSIC), only expect the user to differentiate between normal and severely impaired systolic function. With experience, a more detailed interrogation of the myocardial function should be attempted including vigilance for large territory regional wall motion abnormalities. This will be discussed in more detail later in the chapter.

Ejection fraction (EF) is defined as the percentage of blood leaving the heart during systole and it is the most popular method of describing and quoting LV systolic function. Whilst important, this is a value that is highly subjective depending on the sonographer and can vary dramatically depending on the haemodynamic status of a patient. POCUS practitioners should not be attempting to estimate EF as it requires a high level of experience and familiarity to 'eyeball'. Novice POCUS users should aim to review as many images as possible, both normal and abnormal, to gain familiarity with the appearance of LV function.

One measure that is useful to attain is the mitral annular plane of systolic excursion (MAPSE). This is akin to the tricuspid annular plane of systolic excursion (TAPSE) measure taken to assess RV systolic function. The LV relies less heavily on the longitudinal fibres for contraction when compared with the RV (20% versus 80%) but is an easy measure to obtain and may help to justify reporting normal or impaired systolic function. Interestingly, longitudinal function may become impaired before radial function and can be a feature of early LV systolic dysfunction. This is performed by placing the M-mode cursor over the lateral mitral valve annulus in the A4C view and measuring the longitudinal excursion with a dedicated 'MAPSE' measurement selected (Figure 2.27). Normal value is >1.0 cm. A video describing this technique is available in the online video library.

The British Society of Echocardiography (BSE) has recently advocated to change the classification of EF from the previously used measures of normal (>55%), mildly impaired (45–55%), moderately impaired (35–45%) and severely impaired (<35%). This is due to the relative inaccuracy with differentiation between mildly impaired and moderately impaired. The new classification is:

- Hyperdynamic or normal – EF $\geq$ 55%
- Borderline low – EF 50–54%

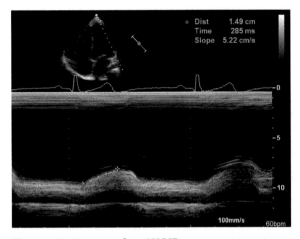

Figure 2.27 How to perform MAPSE measurement. *A video explaining this technique is available to view in the online video library.*

– Impaired – EF 36–49%
– Severely impaired – $\leq$ 35%

Whilst this has replaced the conventional categorisation in the UK, this change is not widespread and clinicians should be familiar with the recommended classification within their country of practice.

Diastolic dysfunction is recognised as being responsible for as many as one-third of all diagnoses of heart failure. Another term for this is heart failure with preserved ejection fraction (HFpEF). Diastolic dysfunction is due to the inability of the heart to adequately relax which impedes ventricular filling. The assessment of this is complex and will not be discussed in this chapter.

Left ventricular systolic dysfunction may be broadly categorised as *ischaemic* or *global*. These will be discussed below.

Ischaemic Left Ventricular Dysfunction

Ischaemic heart disease is a common clinical finding which is important to identify in the acute or chronic setting. It may progress to cause significantly reduced EF and ischaemic cardiomyopathy.

Knowledge of the terminology used to describe LV segments and the coronary artery distribution is essential when performing echocardiography in these patients. The most commonly used segmental pattern divides the LV into 17 distinct segments. These are demonstrated in Figure 2.28 with the associated coronary artery distributions. This is a simplified diagram and many territories will have overlap in their true coronary artery supply. The figure may appear complex,

but it essentially divides the LV into three distinct levels: the basal, mid and apical levels. Furthermore, remember that from all the apical views the segments on the *left* of the screen will be an *inferior* segment:

– A4C – the inferoseptal wall.
– A2C – the inferior wall.
– A3C – the inferolateral wall.

This will aid recall of the opposite LV wall.

The PSAX view is often the most useful view to identify for regional wall motion abnormalities and will allow assessment of every segment.

Any findings suggestive of regional wall motion abnormalities should prompt correlation with clinical features and ECG changes.

Each segment may be assessed and labelled as normal, hypokinetic, akinetic, dyskinetic or aneurysmal. This can be plotted using a 'bullseye' as demonstrated in Figure 2.28. Segment location when visualised from the apical views is also described.

Coronary artery supply is denoted by the colours of each segment. It is important to note the absolute coronary artery perfusion is highly variable between individuals with regions of 'cross-over'. This version of the perfusion distribution is described for simplicity and may be built upon with clinical experience.

The anatomy of the anterior and posterior leaflets of the mitral valve (A1– A3 and P1– P3), the anterolateral papillary muscle (ALP) and the posteromedial papillary muscle (PMP) are labelled in the relevant images.

Regional wall movement in each segment is reported as follows:

– Normal
– Hypokinesia – reduced thickening
– Akinesia – no thickening. Key to look for LV thrombus, particularly in an akinetic apex.
– Dyskinesia – abnormal motion of the myocardium, classically bulging outwards during systole.
– Aneurysmal – ballooning of weakened myocardium. This particularly predisposes the patient to thrombus formation, arrhythmia and sudden cardiac death.
– Hyperkinesia or hyperdynamic – increased contraction.

39

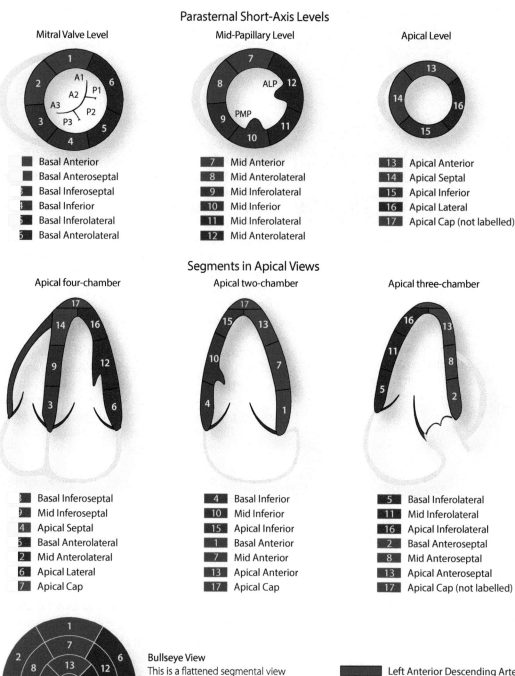

Parasternal Short-Axis Levels

Mitral Valve Level

■ Basal Anterior
■ Basal Anteroseptal
3 Basal Inferoseptal
4 Basal Inferior
5 Basal Inferolateral
6 Basal Anterolateral

Mid-Papillary Level

7 Mid Anterior
8 Mid Anterolateral
9 Mid Inferolateral
10 Mid Inferior
11 Mid Inferolateral
12 Mid Anterolateral

Apical Level

13 Apical Anterior
14 Apical Septal
15 Apical Inferior
16 Apical Lateral
17 Apical Cap (not labelled)

Segments in Apical Views

Apical four-chamber

3 Basal Inferoseptal
9 Mid Inferoseptal
4 Apical Septal
5 Basal Anterolateral
2 Mid Anterolateral
6 Apical Lateral
7 Apical Cap

Apical two-chamber

4 Basal Inferior
10 Mid Inferior
15 Apical Inferior
1 Basal Anterior
7 Mid Anterior
13 Apical Anterior
17 Apical Cap

Apical three-chamber

5 Basal Inferolateral
11 Mid Inferolateral
16 Apical Inferolateral
2 Basal Anteroseptal
8 Mid Anteroseptal
13 Apical Anteroseptal
17 Apical Cap (not labelled)

Bullseye View
This is a flattened segmental view combining all short-axis levels. It is available on most reporting software to map RWMAs.

■ Left Anterior Descending Artery
■ Circumflex Artery
■ Right Coronary Artery

Figure 2.28 The 17-segment model of the left ventricle. The LV is divided into 17 distinct segments which are named due to their level: whether basal, mid or apical; and for their location around the 'clock face'.

Examples of regional wall motion abnormalities (RWMA) will now be discussed. Figure 2.29 demonstrates anterior wall akinesia in a patient presenting with an anterior STEMI. Note the difference between the thickening of the walls when viewing using the online material.

Figure 2.30 shows an echo of a patient who presented with an inferior wall NSTEMI. Note the decreased thickening of the inferior walls which is described as hypokinesia. Compare the degree of thickening with the previous figure showing akinetic segments. It is useful to focus on each individual segment in turn to assess for contractility and thickening separately.

Figure 2.31 shows an example of dyskinesia in a patient following a large anterior MI. Dyskinesia is characterised by outward movement of a wall during systole. Look at the septal wall which creates a

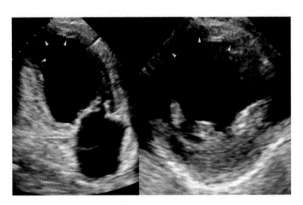

Figure 2.29 Anterior wall akinesis (arrows). Patients with this pattern of akinesia are at high risk of developing an apical thrombus. *Videos are available to view in the online video library.*

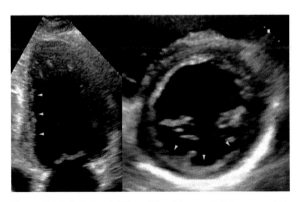

Figure 2.30 Inferior wall hypokinesis(arrows). *Videos are available to view in the online video library.*

'bounce' motion. The patient had left bundle branch block (LBBB) on the ECG.

Post Myocardial Infarction Complications

In addition to RWMAs and LV dysfunction there are several acute complications following a myocardial infarction (MI) which are important to diagnose in the acute setting and where echo plays a vital role.

Acute Mitral Regurgitation

Acute mitral regurgitation (MR) is a common complication post MI. Whilst some acute MR is due to tethering of valve leaflets or cardiac impairment and raised left ventricular end diastolic pressure (LVEDP) there are some causes that may be disastrous and lead to cardiogenic shock and death. Acute rupture of chordae tendineae or a papillary muscle causes catastrophic MR. The aetiology is due to ischaemia of the valve apparatus or papillary muscle. It is more common in posterior MI due to the singular blood supply of the posteromedial papillary muscle by the posterior descending coronary artery compared with the dual supply of the anterolateral papillary muscle.

Urgent surgical intervention is required in patients with acute papillary muscle or chordae rupture and 'medical optimisation' is unlikely to be successful due to the severity of MR. Figure 2.32 demonstrates acute rupture of the posterior mitral valve leaflet (PMVL) apparatus leading to a flail PMVL, prolapse and severe MR.

Ventricular Septal Rupture

Acute ventricular septal defect (VSD) post MI is fortunately rare. Despite this, mortality remains very high and percutaneous or surgical intervention is challenging due to the surrounding myocardium being very friable. Muscle necrosis leads to septal rupture and patients present with variable symptoms which range from angina and dyspnoea to severe cardiovascular collapse. Echo is key for diagnosis and colour Doppler may reveal a high velocity jet extending from the left to the right ventricle. Placing colour Doppler over the septum should be routine practice when scanning patients with shock post-MI. Figure 2.33 demonstrates an acute VSD in a patient who sustained a large anterior MI.

Ventricular free wall rupture is also a possible complication post MI. Unfortunately these patients

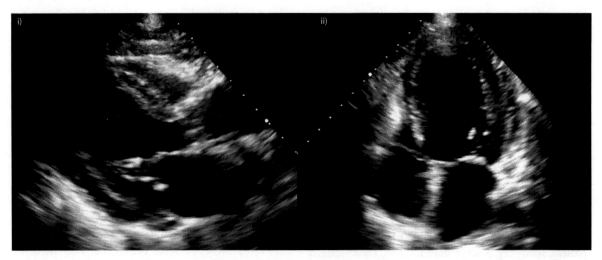

Figure 2.31 (i) PLAX and (ii) A4C views demonstrating anterior and septal dyskinesia following a large anterior myocardial infarction. *Videos are available to view in the online video library.*

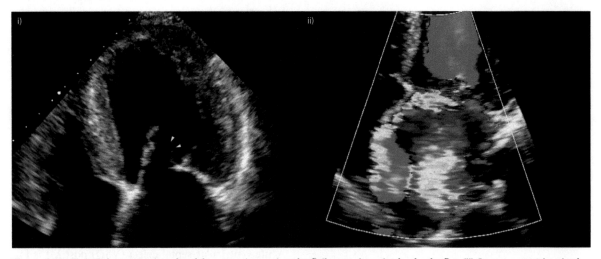

Figure 2.32 (i) A4C demonstrating chordal rupture (arrows) and a flail posterior mitral valve leaflet. (ii) Severe eccentric mitral regurgitation jet. The chroma colour was used as per the preference of the sonographer. *Videos are available to view in the online video library.*

rapidly develop cardiac tamponade and the mortality rate is extremely high.

Thrombus

Left ventricular thrombus formation is a recognised complication of MI and can occur as early as 24 hours post infarct. They tend to occur where there is blood stasis within large regions of akinesia or aneurysm. Studies suggest that up to 25% of anterior MIs develop thrombus with the majority occurring within the LV apex (Figure 2.34). This highlights the importance of incorporating the PSAX apical view into routine imaging of patients post MI. Particular care should

be taken in any region of akinesia or aneurysm as thrombus may occur in any region of the heart. Figure 2.34 demonstrates an apical thrombus in a patient who sustained a large anterior MI.

Global Left Ventricular Dysfunction

Global LV dysfunction describes poor LV contractility without any clear regional coronary artery distribution. The LV cavity is often dilated with thinned walls. Common clinical scenarios are in patients with either myocarditis or dilated cardiomyopathy (DCM). This is usually a very clear, easy diagnosis to make at the bedside and may alert the clinician to previously

Table 2.6

Causes of global left ventricular dysfunction

Viral infections (Coxsackie, EBV, Adenovirus, COVID-19, HIV)

Alcohol

Pregnancy – peri- and post-partum

Drugs – cocaine, amphetamines, doxorubicin.

Thyroid disease

Idiopathic

EBV: Ebstein Barr virus; HIV: human immunodeficiency virus; COVID-19: Coronavirus disease 2019.

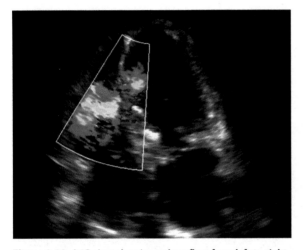

Figure 2.33 A4C view showing colour flow from left to right through a ventricular septal defect post MI. *A video is available to view in the online video library.*

unrecognised cardiac disease. Common causes are listed in Table 2.6.

Figure 2.35i demonstrates a PLAX view showing a dilated, thin-walled LV with poor contractility and pleural effusion in the setting of alcohol-related DCM. Figure 2.35ii uses M-mode imaging to show the minimal change in cavity size and wall thickening during the cardiac cycle.

The globally thinned walls and lack of regional distribution can clearly be seen in the PSAX view (Figure 2.36i) and the A4C further demonstrates global dysfunction (Figure 2.36ii). It is important to closely assess the RV to distinguish isolated LV failure from biventricular failure as this may have significant implications for long-term management.

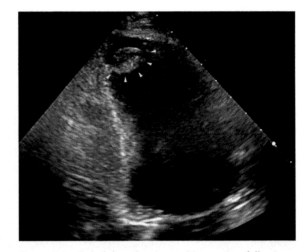

Figure 2.34 Apical thrombus (arrows) in a patient following a large anterior MI. *A video is available to view in the online video library.*

Case – Point-of-Care Ultrasound Is the Icing on the Cake

A 39-year-old female presented with acute shortness of breath for three days. The initial treatment within the Emergency Department (ED) was with intravenous antibiotics and fluids for bilateral pneumonia. Chest X-ray (CXR) revealed cardiomegaly with features of pulmonary oedema (Figure 2.37).

She was reviewed by the Acute Medicine Consultant where a pansystolic murmur and clinical features of fluid overload were identified. She was eight weeks post-partum. An urgent bedside echo was undertaken which demonstrated a dilated LV with severe global impairment as well as MR and TR. The PLAX and PSAX views are shown in Figure 2.38. A4C views with colour Doppler show significant MR and TR (Figure 2.39).

She was promptly commenced on diuretics, ACE inhibitor and a beta blocker and moved swiftly to the care of the cardiology team. She continued to make gradual improvement and serial echos have revealed an increase in her systolic function.

The diagnosis of post-partum DCM must be urgently identified during and after pregnancy. Aggressive fluid administration is disastrous in these patients leading to acute pulmonary oedema and respiratory failure. Bedside echo was key in this case for diagnosis and led to prompt referral to specialist teams.

Case – Not All Dyspnoea Is a Pulmonary Embolism

A 30-year-old male with a background of severe learning disability was admitted overnight with a two-week history of increasing shortness of breath

43

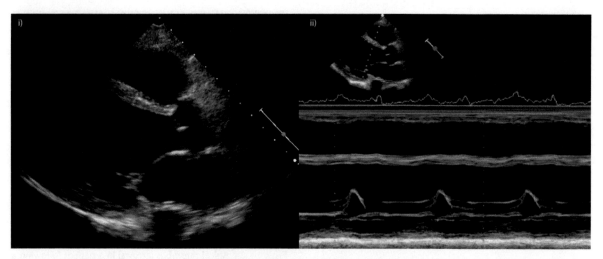

Figure 2.35 (i) PLAX showing a dilated, thin-walled LV with poor contractility. (ii) M-mode PLAX view demonstrating minimal cavity change during the cardiac cycle indicating poor LV function. *A video is available to view in the online video library.*

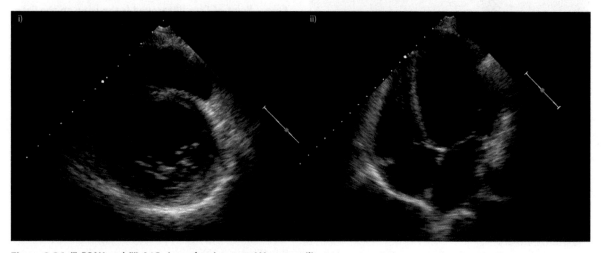

Figure 2.36 (i) PSAX and (ii) A4C views showing poor LV contractility. *Videos are available to view in the online video library.*

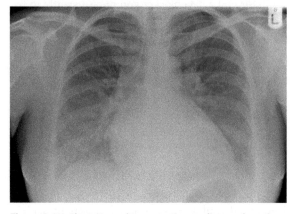

Figure 2.37 Chest X-ray demonstrating cardiomegaly and pulmonary oedema.

and was initially treated as a pulmonary embolism within the ED. Assessment by the medical team revealed profound shortness of breath on exertion, orthopnoea, paroxysmal nocturnal dyspnoea, and a recent history of viral illness.

Chest X-ray was performed that demonstrated severe cardiomegaly and pulmonary oedema. The key question at this point was whether there was a large pericardial effusion or significant cardiac failure contributing to this.

Bedside POCUS was performed overnight by the acute medical team revealing severe, globally impaired biventricular systolic function with a non-dilated cavity. There was no pericardial effusion

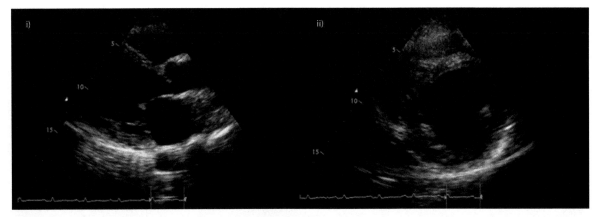

Figure 2.38 (i) PLAX and (ii) PSAX views showing severely impaired LV function. *Videos are available to view in the online video library.*

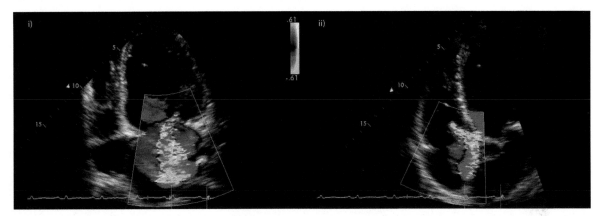

Figure 2.39 A4C view with colour Doppler showing (i) severe mitral regurgitation and (ii) eccentric tricuspid regurgitation. *Videos are available to view in the online video library.*

present. The images were saved and reviewed by the cardiology team during the morning post-take ward round and the diagnosis of viral-induced myocarditis was suspected. The PLAX and A4C views are shown in Figure 2.40.

This patient received no further definitive imaging and was started on diuretics, an ACE inhibitor and a beta blocker with a plan for outpatient follow-up with departmental echocardiography. He subsequently made a full recovery.

Taking a detailed history was cardinal in the diagnosis alongside the frontline medical team having the appropriate skills to make the diagnosis promptly at the bedside out of hours. If the team had followed the diagnosis of a pulmonary embolism this would have led to delay in diagnosis and possible harm to the patient.

Hypertension and Left Ventricular Hypertrophy

Hypertension (HTN) is a very common diagnosis and left ventricular hypertrophy (LVH) is one of the most common echocardiographic findings (Figure 2.41). Echo provides an insight into the degree of *end organ dysfunction* due to HTN and associated ECG changes may be seen. Measurements of the septum (IVSd) and posterior wall in diastole (LVPWd) on the PLAX view are the most common methods for identifying LVH. These are quick and easy measurements to perform and should not be 'eye-balled'. Other methods such as LV mass calculations are complex and not advised for POCUS users. Care should be taken not to include the RV trabeculations in the septal thickness as this will lead to a falsely high IVSd measurement.

45

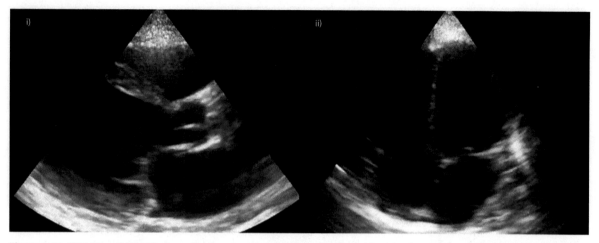

Figure 2.40 (i) PLAX and (ii) A4C views showing severely impaired biventricular function in a patient with suspected myocarditis. *Videos are available to view in the online video library.*

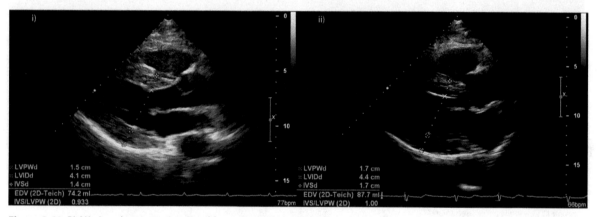

Figure 2.41 PLAX view demonstrating (i) mild concentric LV hypertrophy and (ii) moderate concentric LV hypertrophy. These images appear very similar 'by eye' and therefore actual measurements should be performed. The orange colour for the myocardium is a *chroma* setting that is available on most machines. It may aid with delineating the border between the interventricular septum and RV trabeculations. It is not required and was simply the personal preference of this sonographer.

Normal IVSd and LVPWd dimensions are < 1.2 cm.

The presence of significant LV hypertrophy warrants referral for formal echocardiography due to the association with diastolic dysfunction. Furthermore, in severe cases there may be associated LV outflow tract obstruction (LVOTO) and systolic anterior motion of the mitral valve.

Proximal Septal Hypertrophy – 'Septal Bulge'

Isolated proximal septal hypertrophy with a septal *bulge* or *knuckle* is a common finding – particularly in elderly females with hypertension (Figure 2.42). Although this is usually inconsequential, in severe cases it may lead to a systolic murmur due to turbulence around the LVOT and possible LVOTO. Colour Doppler should be used to visualise turbulent flow and PW Doppler to identify raised outflow gradients in the LVOT.

Hypertrophic Cardiomyopathy

Hypertrophic cardiomyopathy (HCM) is a genetic condition that must be considered in patients presenting with presyncope, syncope, murmurs and a family history of sudden death. It is characterised by gross LVH that is classically asymmetrical. Although most cases cause asymmetrical septal hypertrophy, hypertrophy may also be symmetrical, mid cavity or apical in distribution.

Due to severity of hypertrophy the LV cavity will often be completely obliterated during systole. Although this may preserve the *ejection fraction (EF)*,

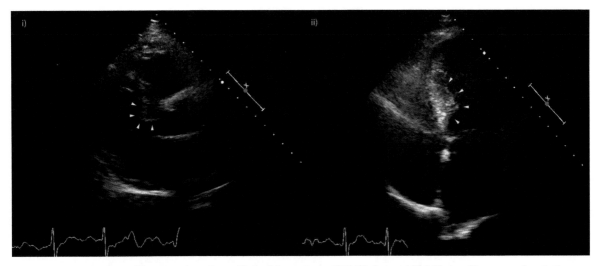

Figure 2.42 Proximal septal hypertrophy or 'septal bulge' shown in the (i) PLAX view and (ii) A4C view. The arrows denote the area of proximal hypertrophy. *Videos are available to view in the online video library.*

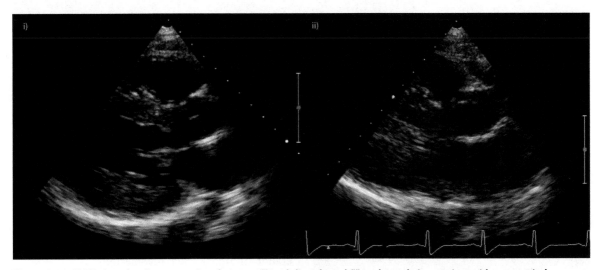

Figure 2.43 PLAX view showing comparison between (i) end diastole and (ii) end systole in a patient with symmetrical hypertrophic cardiomyopathy. Note the complete obliteration of the LV cavity during systole. *A video is available to view in the online video library.*

the systolic function is clearly abnormal with significantly reduced stroke volume. An example of symmetrical HCM is shown in Figure 2.43i *and* Figure 2.43ii shows complete obliteration of the LV cavity during systole. An example of asymmetrical HCM is shown in Figure 2.44.

Syncope in these patients is either arrhythmogenic or due to systolic anterior motion (SAM) of the mitral valve obstructing the outflow tract. This may be seen by using M-mode through the mitral valve leaflets on the PLAX view. Figure 2.45i demonstrates the finding of SAM and includes a normal case for comparison (Figure 2.45ii).

The arrows denote the systolic anterior motion of the mitral valve seen during the systolic phase of the cardiac cycle. The normal mitral valve motion is highlighted in (ii). Systole can be identified using the ECG QRS complexes.

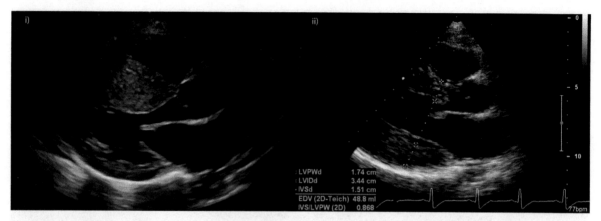

Figure 2.44 Comparison of the PLAX view in (i) asymmetrical versus (ii) symmetrical hypertrophic cardiomyopathy. *Videos are available to view in the online video library.*

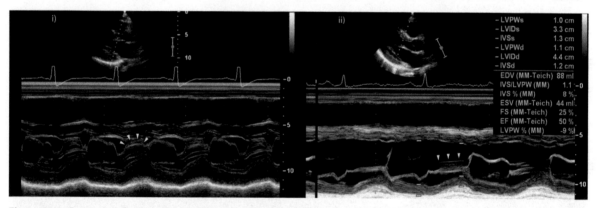

Figure 2.45 Comparison between systolic anterior motion seen in (i) hypertrophic cardiomyopathy PLAX M-mode and (ii) normal PLAX M-mode.

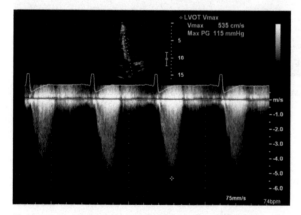

Figure 2.46 CW Doppler performed in the A5C view demonstrating raised LVOT gradient due to LVOT obstruction.

resulting 'dagger sign' and raised outflow velocities. Figure 2.46 demonstrates a severely raised LVOT gradient in an 18-year-old patient with HCM who presented with dizziness. She was referred for consideration of urgent septal myomectomy.

Severe obstruction is defined as a gradient of >50 mmHg. In this image the gradient is 115 mmHg.

Left Ventricular Non-Compaction Cardiomyopathy

Left ventricular non-compaction cardiomyopathy (LVNCC) or 'spongy myocardium' is a rare congenital cardiomyopathy that can be diagnosed at any age. It is characterised by large LV trabeculations and may be mistaken for LVH or DCM (Figure 2.47).

These patients should be urgently referred for definitive investigations including cardiac MRI.

Systolic anterior motion leads to turbulent LVOT flow and subsequent LVOTO. This is measured by placing spectral Doppler in the LVOTO with a

Arrhythmogenic Right Ventricular Cardiomyopathy

Arrhythmogenic right ventricular cardiomyopathy (ARVC) is one of the most common undiagnosed causes of cardiac sudden death in a young person. If the echo reveals RV dilatation with akinesia, dyskinesia or aneurysm then urgent specialist input is required.

It is a difficult diagnosis to make based purely on echocardiographic features but is included here due to the increasingly recognised frequency and clinical significance.

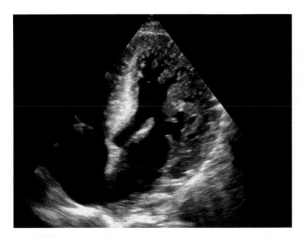

Figure 2.47 Hypertrabeculation of the LV seen in LVNCC. *A video is available to view in the online video library.*

Valvular Heart Disease

Assessment and quantification of valve dysfunction is complex and requires the use of spectral Doppler, colour Doppler and numerous calculations. This is beyond the scope of most POCUS practitioners and the aim of focused studies is not to grade severity. Understanding the appearance of severe valvular lesions and using basic colour and spectral Doppler can aid diagnosis. If there is a suspicion of significant valvular dysfunction the patient should be referred urgently for a departmental study.

Basic accreditation pathways, such as FUSIC, do not advocate for the use of colour Doppler. Whilst this is useful to focus the trainee on achieving good quality views early in the learning process, it is difficult to gauge function of the ventricles without visualising the direction of blood flow. For example, torrential mitral regurgitation (MR) may cause LV function to appear 'normal' despite the majority of the LV stroke volume flowing backwards into the LA rather than the systemic circulation. Regurgitation is easily seen by placing colour Doppler over the valve in question. Figure 2.48 demonstrates a MR jet seen on the PLAX and A4C views.

Aortic stenosis (AS) is one of the most commonly diagnosed valvular disorders. This is commonly calcific in aetiology causing thickening and bright echogenic appearance of the valve. Reduced excursion may be seen. To assess for raised outflow gradients CW Doppler is placed across the AV in the A5C view as seen in Figure 2.49. Quantification of AS using

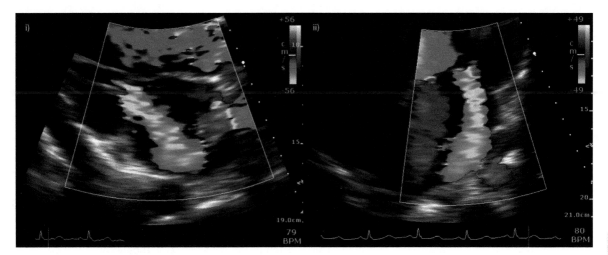

Figure 2.48 Mitral regurgitation jet shown in the (i) PLAX and (ii) A4C views. *Videos are available to view in the online video library.*

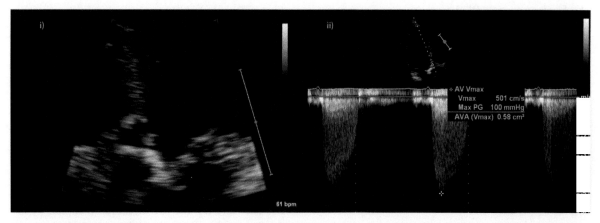

Figure 2.49 **(i) A5C view showing calcified, stenotic aortic valve. (ii) CW Doppler trace through the AV in the A3C view measuring a high transvalvular gradient.** Severe aortic stenosis is diagnosed with a peak pressure gradient of >65 mmHg. In this case it is measured at 102 mmHg. *A video is available to view in the online video library.*

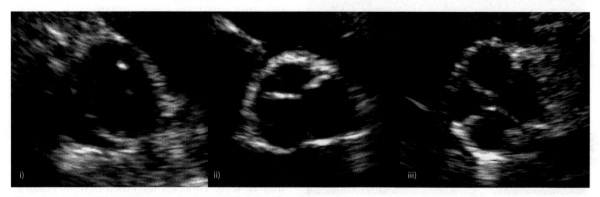

Figure 2.50 **Congenital variation in the number of aortic valve leaflets: (i) bicuspid aortic valve (open); (ii) normal, tricuspid valve (closed); (iii) rare quadricuspid valve (closed).** Note the eccentric, oval shaped orifice of the bicuspid aortic valve and the additional leaflet in the quadricuspid valve. *Videos are available to view in the online video library.*

outflow velocity, gradients, valve area and other measures is beyond the scope of this book.

Typically, the AV has three leaflets. Occasionally, using the PSAX view at the AV level you may identify either two leaflets (bicuspid) or four leaflets (quadricuspid). Bicuspid AV is the most common congenital valve malformation with an incidence of 1–2% of the population. It leads to AS, aortic regurgitation (AR) and is the most common reason for patients under 60 years old to require an aortic valve replacement. Quadricuspid valves are significantly less common affecting 1 in 1000–10,000 of the population. Figure 2.50 shows a bicuspid, tricuspid and quadricuspid valve.

Mitral stenosis (MS) is much less common. The normal excursion of the valve is restricted and may appear to *bow* during atrial systole – commonly described as a '*hockey stick*' appearance. There is invariably LA dilatation and associated MR. Figure 2.51 demonstrates a PLAX view and appearance of MS with LA dilatation. Figure 2.52 is an A4C view; note the coexisting MR picked up on colour Doppler.

Pericardial Effusion and Cardiac Tamponade

A pericardial effusion is an abnormal collection of fluid within the pericardial cavity. A small amount of pericardial fluid (~15–50 ml) is normal and reduces friction between the fibrous and serous pericardial layers during contraction. Larger volumes should be considered pathological. Limited space within the pericardial sac means that as fluid develops there is an increase in intrapericardial pressure. As

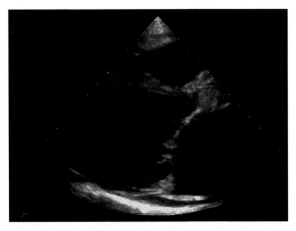

Figure 2.51 **PLAX view of a patient with mitral stenosis.** Note the poor excursion of the mitral valve, thickened leaflets and severely dilated left atrium. *A video is available to view in the online video library.*

Table 2.7

Causes of pericardial effusion
Inflammation (pericarditis, rheumatoid arthritis, SLE)
Infection (TB)
Malignancy (lymphoma)
Drugs
Uraemia
Radiation

SLE: systemic lupus erythematous; TB: tuberculosis

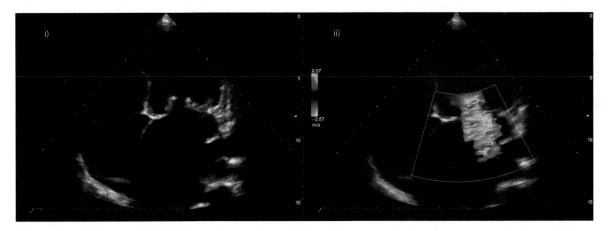

Figure 2.52 **(i) A4C view of mitral stenosis with grossly dilated LA. (ii) Colour Doppler showing coexisting mitral regurgitation.** *Videos are available to view in the online video library.*

this progresses, the intrapericardial pressure may begin to exceed the end diastolic pressure of the heart chambers, particularly the lower pressured right-sided chambers, causing diastolic collapse, reduced cardiac filling and subsequent cardiovascular collapse and cardiac arrest. This is pericardial tamponade. Rapid diagnosis with echo in this instance is critical and potentially life saving. Common causes of pericardial effusions are listed in Table 2.7.

Pericardial effusions frequently present with shortness of breath on a background history suggestive of infection or inflammation. The commonest misdiagnosis is pulmonary embolism and empirical anticoagulation in these patients can be disastrous.

Beck's triad is a collection of three clinical key signs indicative of cardiac tamponade: raised jugular venous pressure (JVP), soft heart sounds and reduced blood pressure. Other signs of pericardial effusion include a pericardial friction rub (often associated with pericarditis) and pulsus paradoxus. Pulsus paradoxus describes a drop in blood pressure of >10 mmHg during inspiration and has been shown to be more than 80% sensitive for the presence of tamponade.

The CXR will reveal a *globular heart* as the surrounding pericardial fluid increases the overall size of the cardiac shadow (Figure 2.53). The ECG may demonstrate small QRS complexes (Figure 2.54) or *electrical alternans*. This describes QRS complexes that alternate in amplitude, direction and duration (Figure 2.55). This is due to the heart swinging back and forth on its axis within the large volume of pericardial fluid.

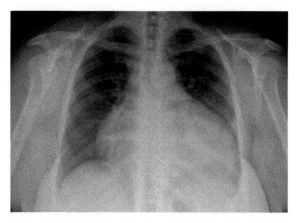

Figure 2.53 Chest X-ray showing globular heart suggestive of pericardial effusion.

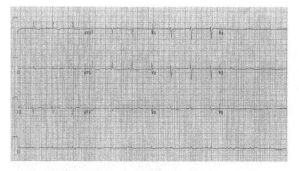

Figure 2.54 ECG showing small QRS complexes seen in pericardial effusion.

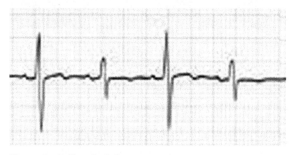

Figure 2.55 Electrical alternans.

Echo Findings

A pericardial effusion will appear as an anechoic strip between the myocardial wall and the pericardium. This should be visualised in as many echo windows as possible to describe the size and distribution of the effusion. As previously mentioned, the PLAX view is key to differentiating between pericardial and pleural effusion due to the location of the descending aorta. Figure 2.56 demonstrates the difference in appearance

between a pleural effusion (Figure 2.56i) and a pericardial effusion (Figure 2.56ii). Note that in the pericardial effusion the anechoic strip is seen to extend between the descending aorta and left atrium and causes separation of these structures.

Measurements of the size of pericardial effusion should be taken in end-diastole guided by the ECG. Taking a measurement in systole will artificially overestimate the size of a pericardial effusion. Figure 2.57 demonstrates the method for measuring a pericardial effusion at the LV posterior wall. It measures 24.9 mm at end diastole equating to a *large* pericardial effusion.

The pericardial effusion may be seen in all windows. Figure 2.58 shows the entire heart surrounded by fluid in the PSAX view.

The A4C again reveals a global pericardial effusion (Figure 2.59). In this view the heart may be seen to swing back and forth within the pericardial cavity – demonstrating how electrical alternans occurs.

The subcostal image is important for multiple reasons. Firstly, it may be the only attainable view in critically unwell or cardiac arrest patients. Secondly, it is the most common site for pericardiocentesis and therefore important to be able to demonstrate a significant sized effusion anterior to the RV free wall. Figure 2.60 shows a 26.6 mm effusion measured anterior to the RV free wall.

Cardiac Tamponade

Cardiac tamponade is a life-threatening condition. The rate of accumulation of fluid is more important than the absolute volume which limits the utility of *small*, *moderate* and *large* size categories. As little as 100 ml of fluid is needed to cause cardiac tamponade if it accumulates rapidly enough. Conversely, several litres of fluid may be present in a chronic effusion that develops slowly due to the ability of the elastic fibrils of the pericardium to stretch over time. This causes the volume-pressure curve to be shifted to the right allowing a larger volume prior to haemodynamic compromise.

Although cardiac tamponade is a clinical diagnosis there are certain features on echo that are frequently relied upon prior to the diagnosis being made.

Is There Right Atrial or Right Ventricular Diastolic Collapse?

As discussed earlier in this chapter, chamber collapse is the hallmark feature of cardiac tamponade and represents the intrapericardial pressure exceeding

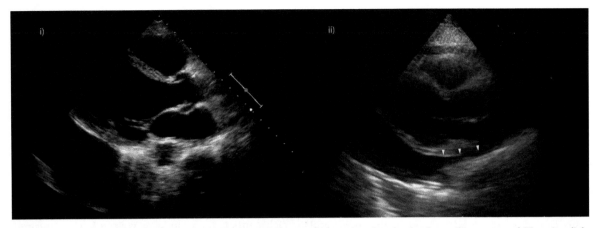

Figure 2.56 Comparison between (i) pleural effusion with the anechoic region deep to the descending aorta and (ii) pericardial effusion seen to extend between the descending aorta and left atrium. The extension of the anechoic pericardial effusion between the LA and Desc Ao is highlighted with arrows. The pericardial fluid is also visible anterior to the RV in the near field. *Videos are available to view in the online video library.*

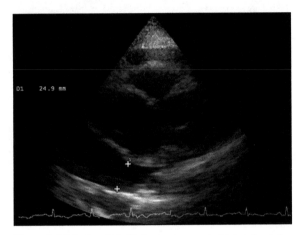

Figure 2.57 Pericardial effusion measurement taken in end diastole. In this case the effusion measures 2.5 cm and is classified as a large pericardial effusion.

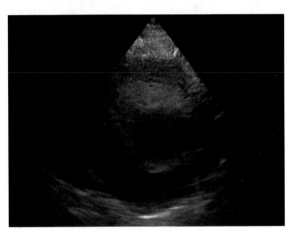

Figure 2.58 PSAX view of a pericardial effusion. *A video is available to view in the online video library.*

the end diastolic pressure of the heart chambers. The earliest chamber to collapse will be the RA due to the lowest end diastolic pressure. Note that the lowest RA pressure is seen during ventricular, not atrial diastole and therefore the collapse will be seen in the *atrial systole* which occurs in late *ventricular diastole*.

The RV is the next chamber that will demonstrate collapse. This will occur during diastole and is almost always associated with haemodynamic compromise. The PLAX view is usually the best view to assess for collapse and the M-mode may be utilised to visualise collapse over time. The ECG is essential to this assessment. Figure 2.61 demonstrates RV diastolic collapse (Figure 2.61i) in comparison to no RV diastolic collapse (Figure 2.61ii).

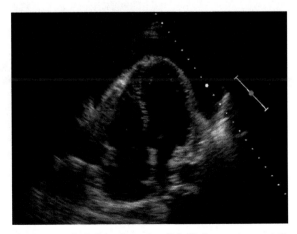

Figure 2.59 A4C view of a pericardial effusion. *A video is available to view in the online video library.*

Left atrial and LV collapse occur much later in the tamponade process and will likely be associated with significant cardiovascular compromise.

Is the Inferior Vena Cava Dilated and Fixed?

A fixed and dilated IVC is a very sensitive sign (>92%) for tamponade. Clearly there are many causes for a patient to have a dilated IVC but it may be used as an additional feature. Figure 2.62 shows the IVC is dilated at 26.5 mm with minimal inspiratory variability.

Elevated Mitral Valve and Tricuspid Valve Inflow Variability

This is a more advanced assessment that is beyond the scope of POCUS clinicians. PW Doppler is placed at either the MV or TV leaflet tips and the variability of inflow velocities measured during the respiratory cycle.

Exaggerated inflow variability is a sonographic representation of *pulsus paradoxus* (Figure 2.63). Normal MV inflow variability is <20% and is abnormal when >30%. Normal TV inflow variability is <30% and abnormal when >40%. Note that these features are abolished during mechanical ventilation and the user must rely on haemodynamic stability and chamber collapse.

The key role of focused echo is to identify the effusion and escalate to the cardiology team for specialist input. As a clinician your role is to integrate this finding with the history and haemodynamic

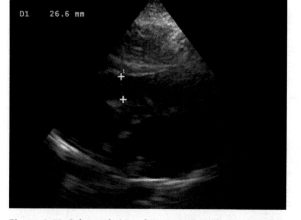

Figure 2.60 Subcostal view of a pericardial effusion with the measurement taken in end diastole anterior to the RV free wall. *A video is available to view in the online video library.*

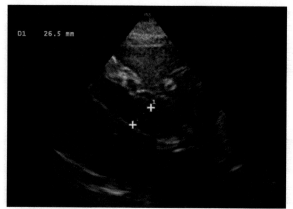

Figure 2.62 Dilated IVC seen in a patient with cardiac tamponade. This is not a specific finding but may be used as a supporting feature in the event of suspected tamponade.

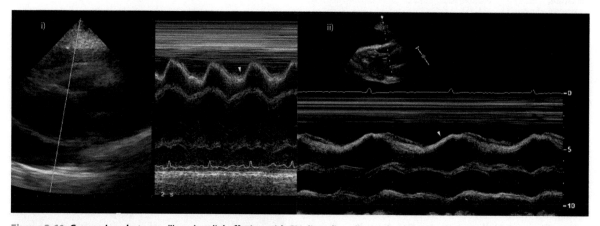

Figure 2.61 Comparison between (i) pericardial effusion with RV diastolic collapse demonstrated on PLAX M-mode suggesting tamponade and (ii) PLAX M-mode taken in patient with pericardial effusion with no RV diastolic collapse. The key points to highlight are labelled with arrows. In (i) there is downward notching of the RV free wall trace at end diastole as indicated by the ECG p wave. Image (ii) shows a gradual rise in the RV free wall during diastole suggesting unimpeded ventricular filling.

status of the patient. Is there pulsus paradoxus? The following echo findings should be communicated:

- Position – Is it localised or circumferential?
- Size in end diastole? *See Table 2.8 for reporting of size.*
- Haemodynamics on echo
- Is there RA or RV diastolic collapse?
- Is the IVC fixed and dilated?
- Is there any significant variation at MV/TV flow? (advanced assessment).

The Right Ventricle

The right ventricle (RV) is a complex, crescent-shaped structure that wraps around the LV. It is notoriously difficult to assess with 2D echocardiography and the optimal method for quantification of size and function is debated. Despite this, basic visual assessment of size and function can be assessed in all echocardiographic views. The PSAX view is

particularly suited to comparing right-sided pressure with left-sided pressure.

On echo, the RV should usually be around two-thirds the size of the LV depending on the views achieved. If the RV is the same size as the LV cavity, particularly in the A4C or subcostal views, this equates to it being dilated. If the size of the RV exceeds the LV this is severely dilated. Although measurements may be taken, this is a conclusion that can be made by eye.

Typical measurements taken include the RV internal diameters at the base (RVID1), mid (RVID2) and RV length (RVID3), the RV end systolic area (RVESA) and the RV outflow tract measures. The RVID1 basal measure can be compared with the LVIDd to calculate a RV:LV size ratio.

Assessment of RV systolic function is challenging due to its unique geometry. Measures such as EF cannot be estimated due to insufficient visualisation with 2D echo. The most common methods for measuring RV function include tricuspid annular plane of systole excursion (TAPSE) and fractional area change (FAC). Both of these measures have been demonstrated to correlate well with cardiac MRI calculations of RV ejection fraction.

Fractional area change requires the user to trace around the RV cavity in diastole and systole in the A4C view. The difference in these measures is the area change with a normal value being >30%. This measure is akin to the *Simpson's Biplane* measure but only relates to *area* due to inconsistency of the RV shape. FAC is a more time-consuming measure and requires good quality images for adequate endocardial

Table 2.8 Classification of pericardial effusions by size

Size	Depth (mm) end diastole	Volume (ml)
Small	<10	<200
Moderate	10–20	200–500
Large	>20	500–2000

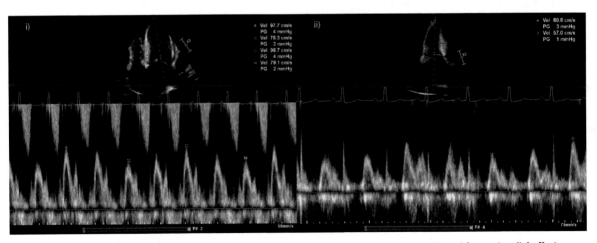

Figure 2.63 Exaggerated (i) mitral valve and (ii) tricuspid valve inflow variability trace in a patient with a pericardial effusion. The highest and lowest E wave velocities have been measured throughout several respiratory cycles. The inflow velocity variation may then be calculated.

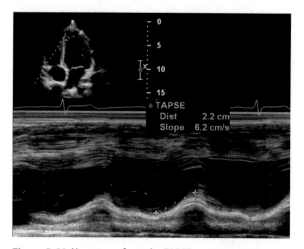

Figure 2.64 How to perform the TAPSE measurement. *A video explaining this technique is available to view in the online video library.*

definition. Care should be taken not to trace the RV trabeculations as this may result in an artificially small RV cavity size. Most point of care accreditation pathways do not recommend the user performs FAC.

Tricuspid annular plane of systole excursion, by comparison, is much easier to measure and reflects the RV longitudinal function. The RV relies more heavily on longitudinal contraction than the LV (around 80% of its overall function) meaning TAPSE is a reasonably reliable measure of RV systolic function. Users should place the M-mode cursor on the tricuspid valve lateral annulus and measure the height of excursion during systole. By using a 'TAPSE' measurement on the machine the hyperechoic line (representing the lateral annulus) may be traced and a distance calculated (Figure 2.64). Normal TAPSE is ≥1.7 cm.

Pulmonary Embolism

Acute pulmonary embolism (PE) is common and is a frequent consideration in the shocked patient. Rapid identification of features consistent with massive PE may prompt treatment with thrombolysis which is potentially lifesaving.

Massive PE may be defined as:

- Pulmonary embolism that leads to haemodynamic compromise. Sustained hypotension <90 mmHg for at least 15 minutes and requiring inotropic support not due to any other cause.

- Cardiac arrest.

- Profound bradycardia (HR < 40 bpm with signs or symptoms of shock).

Sub-massive PE is defined as a PE causing right heart strain but without systemic hypotension. Common features of RV strain will be described below. This is a challenging subtype of PE to manage and patients should be clearly counselled about the risks of thrombolysis versus conservative management. Thrombolysis is associated with a 9% risk of significant bleeding and 1.5% risk of intracranial haemorrhage but may reduce the long-term risk of pulmonary hypertension and morbidity. Current recommendations suggest that due to this risk, thrombolysis may be reserved for patients with massive rather than sub-massive PE. Thrombolysis may be administered up to 48 hours after initial presentation and if a patient with sub-massive PE develops haemodynamic instability this should be considered.

The vast majority of pulmonary emboli are neither massive or sub-massive and cause no cardiovascular complications. These are unlikely to reveal any echocardiographic features.

Echo Features of Acute Pulmonary Embolism

The echo features of PE reflect the raised pulmonary vascular resistance, right ventricular and right atrial pressures. None of these are sensitive or specific enough to either diagnose or exclude PE. They must be interpreted within the clinical context to gauge the likelihood of a significant pulmonary embolism being present. Identification of these findings should prompt further investigation, notably computerised tomography pulmonary angiogram (CTPA), or guide emergency management such as thrombolysis in the setting of a convincing clinical history.

The key findings that may be seen are listed in Table 2.9.

Prior to performing an echo, clinical signs should be sought suggestive of massive PE. These include features of right-sided heart failure and ECG changes including tachycardia, right bundle branch block (RBBB) and S1, Q3, T3 (Figure 2.65).

Right Ventricular Dilatation

Right ventricular dilatation is a common finding in acute PE. It may be seen initially within the PLAX view with a dilated RVOT. Remember the rule of thirds – the RVOT, LVOT/ascending aorta and LA should all be similar sizes. This should be confirmed on the PSAX, A4C and subcostal views. As previously mentioned, there are many different causes of RV

Table 2.9

Sign of acute pulmonary emobolism on echo
RV dilatation
Septal flattening (D-Shape)
McConnell's sign (regional RV dysfunction with apical sparing)
Tricuspid regurgitation
'60/60 sign'
Shortened pulmonary acceleration time with 'notching'.
IVC dilatation with minimal respiratory variation.
Visualising clot in the MPA, RVOT, RA or IVC

RV: right ventricle; IVC: inferior vena cava; MPA: main pulmonary artery; RVOT: right ventricular outflow tract; RA: right atrium.

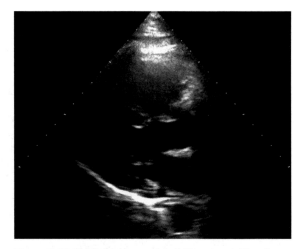

Figure 2.66 PLAX showing a dilated RV and septal bowing due to RV overload. *A video is available to view in the online video library.*

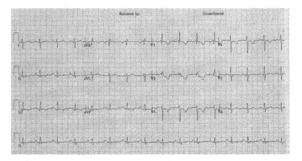

Figure 2.65 ECG showing signs of right heart strain in a patient with acute massive pulmonary embolism.

dilatation and findings should be interpreted within the clinical context. See Figure 2.66.

Septal Flattening

Normally the LV shape and structure are preserved throughout the cardiac cycle as the pressure exceeds that of the RV. When there is an increase in RV pressure or volume to a degree where there is equalisation between chambers, the septum may become flattened or even deviate inwards into the LV cavity – this is known as *septal flattening*.

This is best assessed within the PSAX view where the normally round LV cavity is distorted by the flattened septum. This may occur within systole or diastole. Systolic flattening is classically associated with *RV pressure overload* and diastolic flattening with *RV volume overload*. Of course, both pressure and volume overload may coexist causing septal flattening throughout the cardiac cycle. Figure 2.67

demonstrates the difference between the normal LV shape and flattening due to RV overload.

There are many causes of raised right-sided pressures and the key question in PE is whether this has occurred acutely due to significant clot burden. This may be challenging to differentiate particularly when patients may have acute on chronic insults. The presence of RV hypertrophy, assessed by measuring the thickness of the RV free wall in the subcostal view (Figure 2.68), is indicative of a more chronic process. RV free wall thickness of >5 mm is abnormal.

McConnell's Sign

McConnell's sign is the presence of regional RV dysfunction with sparing of the RV apex. It occurs due to sudden dilatation of the ventricle compromising the reduced blood supply to the RV basal wall. This is a more specific sign for an acute PE but is also seen in conditions such as RV myocardial infarction so should be interpreted with caution.

Tricuspid Regurgitation

Acute dilatation of the RV will lead to failure of coaptation of the tricuspid valve leaflets. This incompetence will cause a significant degree of TR which can be assessed using colour Doppler (Figure 2.69). Clearly the presence of TR is not a specific sign for PE but may add supporting evidence to the overall clinical picture.

Placing CW Doppler through the TR jet will allow measurement of the maximal jet velocity and maximal pressure gradient. This may be used in combination with the estimated right atrial pressure to

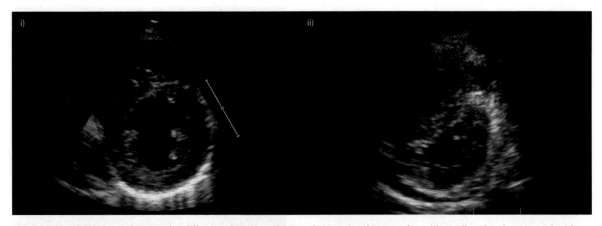

Figure 2.67 PSAX views showing the difference between (i) normal LV cavity shape at the mid papillary level compared with (ii) septal flattening, or 'D-shaped septum', seen in a patient with acute massive pulmonary embolism. *Videos are available to view in the online video library.*

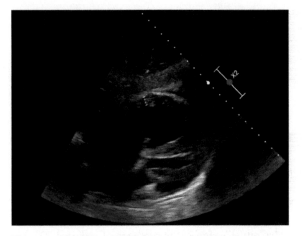

Figure 2.68 Subcostal view demonstrating RV hypertrophy. **This is suggestive of chronically elevated right heart pressure.** Callipers highlight the normal place for measuring RV free wall thickness. Normal diameter is <0.5 cm. Here, it measures 1.3 cm. *A video is available to view in the online video library.*

Figure 2.69 Tricuspid regurgitation jet in a patient with acute pulmonary embolism.

infer pulmonary artery systolic pressure. The '60-60 sign' is an echocardiographic finding which has been reported to be sensitive for acute PE and includes the following assessments:

- The TR max pressure gradient should be *less than* 60 mmHg in acute PE. In chronic pulmonary hypertension the RV will remodel and lead to higher RV pressure. In an acute insult this remodeling has not occurred and therefore pressure gradients of >60 mmHg are extremely unlikely to be present.

- The second '60' describes a shortened *pulmonary acceleration time* of <60 ms. This measurement is taken using PW Doppler of flow through the RV outflow tract and using the callipers to measure the time taken for the flow to reach a maximal velocity. Normal measurement is ≥ 110 ms with shorter durations or 'notching' seen in cases of raised PA pressure.

The 60-60 sign is a more advanced echo assessment but has been included here for interest and to explain the possible additional findings in this common clinical condition.

Dilated Inferior Vena Cava

A dilated IVC, as discussed in the section on tamponade, will be present in any cause of raised right-sided

Table 2.10

Other causes of right ventricular dilatation on echo

Any cause of cor pulmonale

– Chronic thromboembolic disease

– COPD

– Primary pulmonary hypertension

– OSA

Left heart failure

Positive pressure ventilation (invasive or non-invasive)

COPD: chronic obstructive pulmonary disease; OSA: obstructive sleep apnoea.

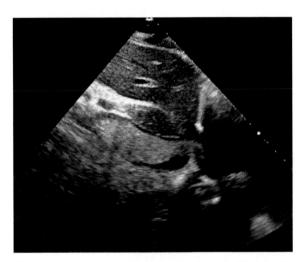

Figure 2.70 Large thrombus extending from the IVC into the RA. *A video is available to view in the online video library.*

pressure. This is an additional feature that should be communicated with the medical team to raise the suspicion of acute cor pulmonale.

Thrombus

Visualising thrombus within the right heart (MPA, RVOT, RV or RA) and IVC is diagnostic of acute pulmonary embolism. Figure 2.70 shows an extensive clot within the IVC. This is rarely seen and is associated with a very poor prognosis. Urgent anticoagulation, thrombolysis or thrombectomy is needed.

There are many other causes of RV dilatation (see Table 2.10) and these must be interpreted with history and examination.

Shock, Hypovolaemia, Fluid Responsiveness and Fluid Overload

The use of bedside echo is a mandatory part of the assessment of any shocked patient. We have already discussed multiple scenarios that may lead to shock and therefore these will not be discussed in further detail.

Point-of-care ultrasound will be able to distinguish between the different forms of shock:

– Hypovolaemic shock – will reveal a small LV cavity with hyperdynamic function. This will be discussed in more detail below.

– Cardiogenic shock – poor LV systolic function with reduced stroke volume.

– Obstructive shock – causes such as cardiac tamponade or massive pulmonary embolism will usually be evident on bedside echo.

– Distributive shock – the LV function will be 'hyperdynamic' – the LV end diastolic volume will often be normal, but the ejection fraction is significantly higher than 65% causing a small end systolic volume.

Assessment of fluid status in a patient is one of the most common requests for bedside echo. It is a challenge that is often underestimated by inexperienced users. 'Fluid status' should be differentiated into multiple questions and *always preceded by a detailed clinical examination*. These key questions include:

– Is there evidence of *frank hypovolaemia*?

– Is there evidence of significantly impaired systolic function?

– Are there features suggesting the patient is not *fluid tolerant*?

– Could this patient be fluid *responsive*?

– Is there evidence of significant *fluid overload*?

Frank Hypovolaemia

A combination of features can assure the clinician that the patient is profoundly hypovolaemic requiring fluid resuscitation. These features include:

– Small LV end diastolic diameter (LVIDd). Figure 2.71 shows a PLAX view in a shocked patient with a small LV end diastolic and end systolic diameter with hyperdynamic contractility. A measured diameter of <4.2 cm in males and <3.9 cm in females would suggest this. Where

59

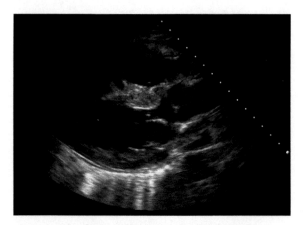

Figure 2.71 A small IVC with near-complete respiratory collapse measured using an auto-IVC tool (GE Venue).

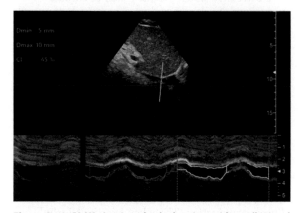

Figure 2.72 PLAX view in a shocked patient with small LV end diastolic and end systolic diameter with hyperdynamic contractility. *A video is available to view in the online video library.*

possible measurements should be indexed against body surface area. A value of <2.2 cm/m^2 equates to frank hypovalaemia (FH).

- The LV end diastolic area is measured by tracing the endocardial wall in the PSAX view at the mid-papillary level in diastole. An area of <9 cm^2 or indexed measure of <5.5 cm/m^2 is consistent with frank hypovolaemia.

- Small LV end systolic area and papillary apposition – this is where the walls of the LV 'kiss' one another during systole.

- Inferior vena cava diameter of <1.5 cm with $>50\%$ inspiratory collapse (Figure 2.72).

Users must be cautious when interpreting LV cavity size in the setting of severe LV hypertrophy.

These patients will commonly have a small cavity and tolerate fluid loading very poorly.

Impaired Systolic Function

If there is significantly impaired LV function, the predominant cause of shock is unlikely to be due to hypovolaemia. Although this sounds like an obvious statement, many patients are exposed to unnecessary harm by fluid administration without consideration of their cardiac function.

Concepts of Fluid Responsiveness and Fluid Tolerance

Differentiating between fluid tolerance and responsiveness is a key principle in POCUS fluid assessment. Fluid responsiveness is defined as the *increase in cardiac output or stroke volume by 10–15% following administration of a 500 ml fluid bolus over 10–15 minutes.* The best method to identify patients who are likely to respond to fluid is unclear and subject to much debate.

The initial step in assessing haemodynamics is to calculate the stroke volume (SV) and cardiac output (CO). Stroke volume is calculated using echo by performing two key measures:

- Measurement of the LVOT diameter in systole on the PLAX view. This should be taken 0.5–1 cm proximal to the aortic valve annulus when the valve is open (Figure 2.73i). The machine will automatically calculate the LVOT area based upon this measurement. Care should be taken to ensure this is accurately measured as any error is *squared* during the area calculation.

- Measurement of stroke distance. This is performed by placing the PW Doppler within the LVOT (0.5cm proximal to the valve) in the A5C view. This will produce a Doppler envelope that should be traced using the LVOT VTI measurement (Figure 2.73ii). VTI stands for velocity time integral and essentially describes the 'area under the curve'. Normal stroke distance is 18–22 cm.

Left ventricular outflow tract area and stroke distance are multiplied together to calculate stroke volume (SV). This can be multiplied by the heart rate (HR) to calculate cardiac output (CO).

To assess fluid responsiveness the CO measurement should be performed before and after a fluid challenge to identify an increase in SV. The least harmful method of assessing this is through a passive

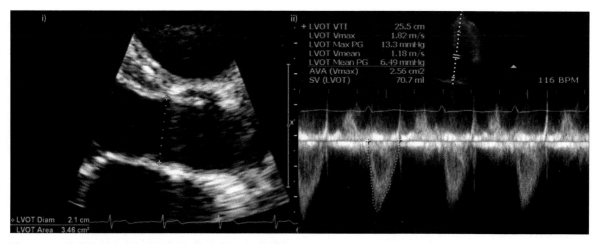

Figure 2.73 Images demonstrating how to perform the stroke volume calculation. (i) LVOT diameter measured proximal to the AV annulus when the valve is open. This measure is squared during the LVOT area calculation. (ii) PW Doppler envelope with the cursor placed in the LVOT. This may be traced to calculate the stroke distance. Note that the machine has automatically calculated the stroke volume using the LVOT area measurement performed earlier in the study. *The alternative method of measuring stroke volume is to measure LV end diastolic and end systolic volumes using Simpson's biplane in the A4C and A2C views. This method is more prone to error and less reliable in the point-of-care setting. A video demonstrating this technique is available to view in the online video library.*

leg raise. This is performed by raising the legs, holding the position for 90–120 seconds and repeating stroke volume assessment after a further 30–60 seconds. An increase in SV of **>12%** is suggestive of fluid responsiveness.

Variation in LVOT velocity, VTI or SV over time is a commonly performed measure in critical care (Figure 2.74) but is only accurate in the setting of invasive mandatory ventilation due to the impact of heart–lung interaction in normal respiration.

Fluid tolerance is a very different principle. This describes whether it is safe to administer fluids to your patient without significant complications. Features suggesting fluid tolerance include:

– Normal or hyperdynamic LV systolic function.

– Non-dilated LV cavity.

– Normal LV wall thickness – patients with LV hypertrophy will tolerate fluid very poorly.

– Absence of a B line profile or pleural effusions on lung ultrasound (please see thoracic chapter for more information).

– Lack of features suggesting hypervolaemia e.g. dilated IVC (discussed below).

Point-of-care ultrasound users should integrate multi-system assessment to identify features suggesting a patient is becoming fluid intolerant. Development of B line pattern on lung ultrasound

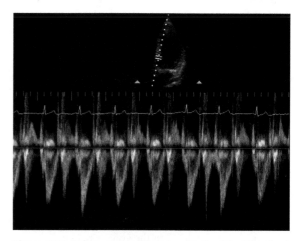

Figure 2.74 Pulse wave Doppler placed in the LV outflow tract showing variation in blood flow velocity and stroke distance.

(LUS) should alert the clinician that the patient is developing pulmonary oedema and fluid should be urgently discontinued.

Hypervolaemia

Identifying features of hypervolaemia is equally as important as identifying the presence of hypovolaemia. These patients will not tolerate further fluid administration and may develop pulmonary oedema, right-sided heart failure and congestive liver or renal failure.

Although the systemic circulations are intrinsically linked, the left and right heart may be assessed in turn to identify features of hypervolaemia.

Numerous methods may be used to assess for raised LV end diastolic pressure (LVEDP). Many of these are beyond the scope of this book. Understanding those patients who are at risk of raised LVEDP is important and a simple visual assessment should aid in identification of these. Findings include:

– Left ventricular hypertrophy – these patients usually have significantly raised LVEDP and tolerate excessive fluid administration extremely poorly.

– Left ventricular impairment.

– Atrial dilatation – this may indicate either valvular insufficiency or diastolic dysfunction.

A visual inspection of the interatrial septum will rapidly inform the clinicians as to whether the RA or LA is exposed to a higher pressure. The interatrial septum is a thin, mobile structure that should typically swing to and fro during the cardiac cycle. In the setting of raised atrial pressure, the septum will bow outwards into the atrium with the lower pressure (Figure 2.75).

Venous congestion is a common finding on POCUS. The IVC is a commonly assessed structure to infer right atrial pressure based on its diameter and degree of inspiratory collapse. Although the absolute values used may vary, the British Society of Echocardiography (BSE) suggest the values listed in Table 2.11.

Whilst these are a useful guide, the reality is that these measurements are likely to be vastly inaccurate in the majority of patients. Furthermore, many confounding factors may influence the diameter of the IVC and it cannot be solely used as a marker of fluid status. This is discussed in more detail in the abdominal chapter.

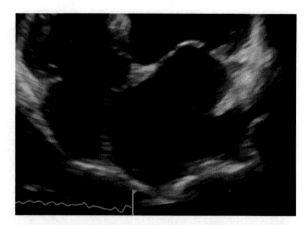

Figure 2.75 Image showing bowing of the inter-atrial septum into the RA suggesting elevated left atrial pressure.

The use of PW Doppler analysis of the hepatic veins, portal veins and intraparenchymal renal vessels has grown in popularity over recent years. This has been termed 'Venous Excess Ultrasound' or 'VEXUS' assessment. The aim is to provide a more detailed assessment of flow characteristics within the right-sided circulation and may be a guide to the *degree* of venous congestion that can be used to monitor response to treatment.

The hepatic veins are seen to drain into the IVC just proximal to the RA. Their appearance can be differentiated from the portal veins due to the absence of the thick, hyperechoic wall seen in the portal venous system. Normal PW Doppler flow consists of a dominant systolic peak (S wave), smaller diastolic peak (D wave) and brief flow reversal during atrial systole (A wave). The S and D wave are separated by a transitional inflection point known as the V wave which may rise above the baseline (Figure 2.76i). With increasing venous congestion, the S wave becomes blunted and smaller than the D wave (Figure 2.76ii). As this progresses the systolic flow may in fact *reverse* with the PW Doppler trace seen to rise above the baseline (Figure 2.76iii). The ECG is essential in this assessment for the timings of systole and diastole.

The portal venous system can be most reliably assessed from the right upper quadrant abdominal view. Normal portal venous flow should be continuous and antegrade with minimal variation between systole and diastole (Figure 2.77i). With increasing congestion there is progressive pulsatility within the portal vein. When mildly abnormal, this is limited to ~30–50% pulsatility (Figure 2.77ii). In severe cases this may exceed 50% and even reverse causing biphasic flow (Figure 2.77iii).

Table 2.11 Estimated right atrial pressure based upon inferfior vena cava calibre and collapsibility

Inferior vena cava size (cm)	Inferior vena cava change with inspiration (%)	Estimated right atrial pressure (mmHg)
<1.5	Collapse	0–5
1.5–2.5	>50%	5–10
1.5–2.5	<50%	10–15
>2.5	<50%	15–20
>2.5	No change	>20

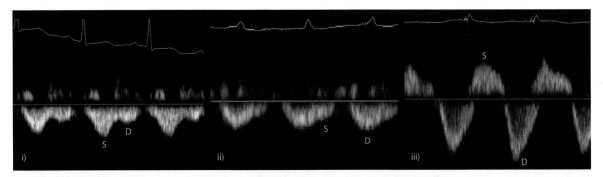

Figure 2.76 Comparison of different hepatic venous Doppler flow profiles: **(i) normal systolic dominant flow with a brief A wave reversal that is barely visible in this clip; (ii) blunting of the systolic flow with the largest peak representing the diastolic flow; (iii) complete reversal of the systolic flow as seen by the wave rising above the baseline.** Although experienced users may be able to infer the S and D waves by eye alone, we recommend using the ECG trace to better delineate between systole and diastole.

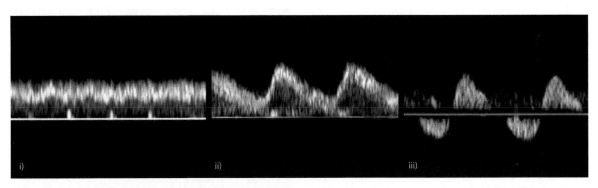

Figure 2.77 Comparison of different portal venous Doppler flow profiles: **(i) normal continuous antegrade flow; (ii) reduced systolic flow leading to portal venous pulsatility; (iii) systolic flow reversal.**

Assessment of the renal intraparenchymal vessels is more challenging for the novice user and will not be considered here.

Whilst these measures provide an opportunity to gain more insight into the flow characteristics of the venous system, they remain prone to misinterpretation due to other physiological factors. Furthermore, 'VEXUS' is currently only validated in post cardiac surgery patients with RV impairment which potentially limits its utility in other acutely unwell patient cohorts. The key finding that must be noted in the presence of abnormal Doppler studies is TR. Hepatic venous Doppler assessment is used in the severity assessment of TR and the utility of this measure is likely to be limited in severe TR.

If significant fluid overload is present the patient will require diuresis to reduce the risk of congestive organ injury. As with any POCUS finding, this should be balanced with overall clinical assessment of the patient.

Cardiac Masses

Cardiac masses, including thrombi, neoplasm and vegetations may be identified on focused echo. It is important that these are appropriately and accurately described within reports and referred for specialist opinion and imaging.

Thrombus

Thrombus may be seen in left- or right-sided disease. Left-sided thrombus typically relates to pathology such as atrial fibrillation, prosthetic valves and ischaemic heart disease. Right-sided thrombus is usually related to venous thromboembolism or right ventricular impairment or infarction.

The left atrial appendage is a structure within which thrombus may form. It is poorly visualised using transthoracic imaging and transoesophageal echo is required to definitively exclude clot which is particularly relevant during preparation for DC

63

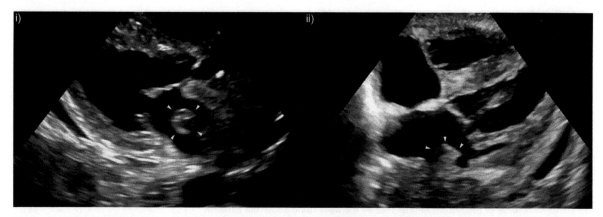

Figure 2.78 **A left atrial mass visualised on the (i) PLAX and (ii) subcostal views.** *Videos are available to view in the online video library.*

cardioversion. Figure 2.78 shows a left atrial mass in keeping with a thrombus. As previously discussed, ischaemic heart disease may cause thrombus to form in regions of akinesia and is most commonly visualised in the apex following anterior wall infarction.

Tumours

Primary cardiac tumours are rare with a prevalence of 0.05%–0.1% of the population. Of these, only 10% are malignant. Cardiac myxomas are the most common cause of primary cardiac tumour and, although most commonly seen within the left atrium, they may occur in the ventricles. They are gelatinous and friable which causes a significant risk of systemic embolism. Secondary cardiac tumours are estimated to occur in 2.3–18.3% of extracardiac malignancies. Figure 2.79 shows a large mobile LV mass adherent to the LV posterior wall.

Any patient with a previously unidentified cardiac mass requires urgent referral to specialist teams for further investigation and management discussions.

Endocarditis

Infective endocarditis is a common differential diagnosis and is primarily identified using echo. Transthoracic echo has a diagnostic sensitivity of approximately 50–60% but a negative study does not *exclude* endocarditis.

The most common locations for vegetations to form are on the upstream side of the valve. They may, however, develop on the papillary muscles, chordae, chamber walls or within the apex. If identified, they should be reported by describing the

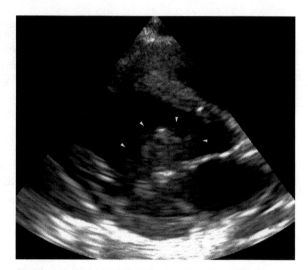

Figure 2.79 **Large mobile LV mass adherent to the LV posterior wall.** *A video is available to view in the online video library.*

location, size, shape, motion and any complications such as valve incompetence, rupture or abscesses.

Using focused echo provides the clinician with an opportunity to diagnose endocarditis in the acute setting. Many echo departments are too busy to provide urgent, same day studies and diagnostic delay in patients with severe endocarditis may be disastrous. There is often an understandable reluctance to perform focused studies for endocarditis due to the challenge of identifying discrete vegetations. However, many vegetations are large and difficult to miss even for inexperienced sonographers and the benefit from early recognition cannot be understated. These patients will often undergo formal departmental echocardiography even if the focused study is negative and so little is lost by simply *'having a look'*.

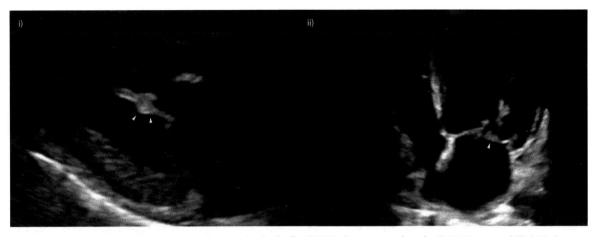

Figure 2.80 Vegetation noted on the posterior mitral valve leaflet (PMVL) demonstrated on the (i) PLAX view and (ii) A4C view. The location of the vegetation is highlighted by the arrows. *Videos are available to view in the online video library.*

Figure 2.80 demonstrates a vegetation identified on the posterior mitral valve leaflet. If something abnormal is seen, then the image should be zoomed and colour applied to assess for turbulence. This patient was diagnosed with MV infective endocarditis. As with any echo abnormality it is essential to confirm the finding on multiple views. Figure 2.80 shows the vegetation confirmed on PLAX and four-chamber view.

Case – An Unmissable Finding

A 35-year-old female with a background of intravenous drug use presented overnight to ED with sepsis of unknown source. She was treated with broad spectrum antibiotics and intravenous fluids by the ED team and referred for medical admission.

On assessment by the medical team she was found to be drowsy, febrile with a labile blood pressure. A pansystolic murmur was audible on auscultation.

Bedside echocardiogram was performed in the ED by the medical junior doctor due to the strong differential diagnosis of infective endocarditis. This revealed a large mitral valve vegetation with mitral regurgitation and a smaller aortic valve vegetation with severe aortic regurgitation (Figure 2.81). CT brain imaging was performed revealing several small septic emboli.

She required transfer to the regional cardiothoracic centre due to haemodynamic instability and severe valvular dysfunction. The acquired images were of high quality and the cardiology team did not require further imaging prior to the transfer. She

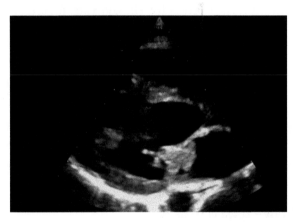

Figure 2.81 PLAX view demonstrating a large vegetation on the mitral valve. *A video is available to view in the online video library.*

underwent a mitral valve and aortic valve replacement and required septal repair due to the mitral valve vegetation eroding through the septal wall. She was discharged, cognitively intact, after completing a six-week course of antibiotics for methicillin susceptible staphylococcus aureus (MSSA).

Focused echo enabled diagnosis and accelerated the patient journey, facilitating early transfer to a specialist centre. Without this, the patient may have waited several days for a departmental study thus delaying life-saving interventions.

Aortic Dissection

Type A aortic dissection may be identified on bedside echo. This is not a sensitive enough assessment to exclude dissection but is useful to identify complications such as severe aortic regurgitation and cardiac tamponade.

Dissection appears as a flap within the ascending aorta, root or descending aorta seen on the PLAX and suprasternal views. It is important to note the descending aorta on PLAX as type B dissection flaps may be visualised.

Case – Gastritis Disguised as Dissection

A 62-year-old female presented to the ED with symptoms of indigestion. Examination was otherwise unremarkable but due to severity of symptoms she was investigated for an acute MI revealing a raised troponin. She had transient periods of hypotension that were unexplained and bedside echo was therefore performed.

This revealed a type A dissection flap with moderate AR and a pericardial effusion with features of early cardiac tamponade. Figure 2.82 is a PLAX view showing a dilated aortic root with visible dissection flap originating from the coronary ostia. Pericardial fluid and AR may be seen. Note the significant dilatation of the descending aorta with visible dissection flap suggesting extension beyond the aortic arch. Figure 2.82 is a modified zoomed view of the ascending aorta clearly showing the dissection flap.

The patient was urgently transferred to cardiothoracic critical care and stabilised prior to undergoing aortic surgery.

Case – Listen to My Heart

A 19-year-old female had been visiting her GP for over six months with symptoms of lethargy and being generally unwell. She had been diagnosed with anxiety but continued to visit the ED on several occasions with vague symptoms. On the third occasion she was referred into the medical team with raised inflammatory markers a C-reactive protein (CRP) of 55 mg/L and erythrocyte sedimentation rate (ESR) of 47 mm/hr. On assessment by the senior physician a diastolic murmur, weak left brachial and radial arteries and bilateral subclavian and carotid bruits were identified. A bedside echo was undertaken which demonstrated a dilated aortic root with moderate aortic regurgitation (AR) with no vegetations.

Parasternal long-axis view showing a dilated aorta and AR is seen in Figure 2.83. The A5C view in Figure 2.84i confirms the finding of AR and Figure 2.84ii demonstrates a dilated ascending aorta and aortic arch on the suprasternal view.

Transoesophageal echo (TOE) was performed confirming moderate AR and root dilatation without features of dissection. CT angiogram confirmed thickening of the left carotid artery with 80% stenosis. A diagnosis of Takayasu Arteritis was made and the patient was commenced on immunosuppressant therapy.

This case highlights the importance of history and examination of the cardiovascular system in a young patient presenting with non-specific symptoms. Patients should not be labelled with *medically unexplained symptoms* until pathology has been excluded. Bedside echo complimented the detailed clinical examination and expedited more detailed investigations, in this case TOE, allowing the complex diagnosis to be promptly made.

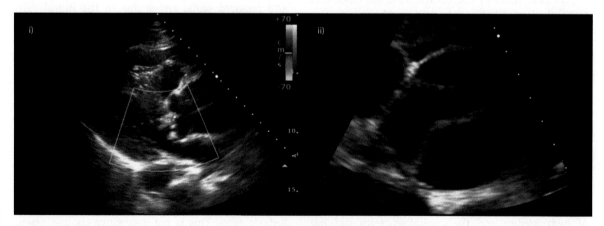

Figure 2.82 (i) PLAX view showing dilated ascending aorta with visible dissection flap, aortic regurgitation colour jet and a pericardial effusion. (ii) Modified aortic view clearly demonstrating dissection flap. *Videos are available to view in the online video library.*

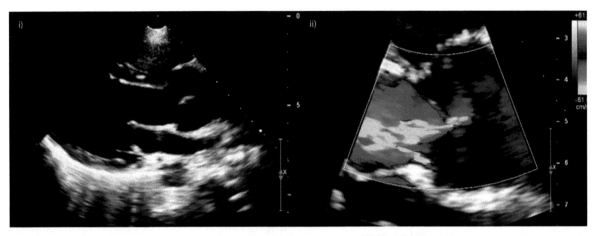

Figure 2.83 PLAX views showing (i) a dilated aortic root and (ii) aortic regurgitation colour jet. *Videos are available to view in the online video library.*

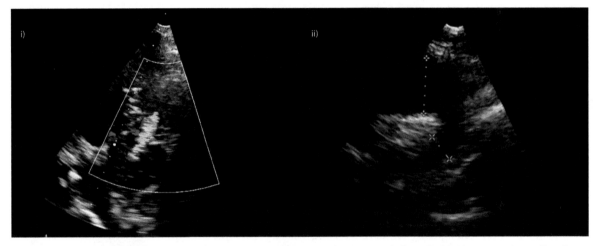

Figure 2.84 (i) A5C view confirming significant aortic regurgitation jet. (ii) Suprasternal notch view demonstrating a dilated ascending aorta and aortic arch. *Videos are available to view in the online video library.*

Normal Useful Reference Ranges

LVIDd (LV Internal Dimension in Diastole):

Male ≤ 5.6 cm

Female ≤ 5.1 cm

LV Septum: ≤ 1.2 cm

LV Posterior Wall: ≤ 1.2 cm

TAPSE: ≥ 1.7 cm

MAPSE: ≥ 1.0 cm

Summary

- Focused echocardiography aims to answer a few key clinical questions and can be critical in diagnosis and management of both the acutely unwell and the chronic patient.

- Echo is essential in the shocked and arrested patient as reversible causes such as hypovolaemia, embolism, and tamponade can be diagnosed.

- Left ventricular function is an important measure for clinicians as treatment can be titrated and prognosis or ceilings of care ascertained.

- Once basic views and competence is acquired we recommend clinicians move to the more advanced views.

- Echo is a challenging discipline with an unlimited degree of complexity. Many findings require close correlation with clinical features as interpretation may differ based upon indication.

A full list of references and further reading is available at: www.GeneralistUltrasound.com

Thoracic Ultrasound

Introduction

Lung ultrasound (LUS) is regarded as one of the simplest forms of ultrasound (US) to learn and requires the understanding of ten signs. We recommend this to be the first POCUS competency to acquire due to its relatively fast learning curve and frequency of use within clinical medicine. The speed of performing an assessment, typically less than five minutes, renders it a fundamental skill for all clinicians.

Once you have appreciated these ten signs you will have the knowledge and skills to make prompt diagnoses including pulmonary oedema, consolidation, pneumothorax and pleural effusions. Some of the findings in this chapter have more utility in daily practice than others, however, a thorough understanding of the less frequent findings will allow for more accurate and comprehensive diagnosis.

Lung ultrasound has been reported to detect pneumothorax with a sensitivity and specificity of 92–96% and 93–100% respectively. LUS is more accurate than chest radiography in differentiating between consolidation and pleural effusion without risking harm to your patients by exposing them to radiation. It has also been invaluable in the COVID-19 pandemic in triage, diagnosis and medical management which is described further in Chapter 12.

Lung ultrasound has become a requirement for performing procedures such as pleural aspiration and chest drain insertion in a safe and confident manner.

Probe Selection

The beauty of LUS is that **all probes** can be used.

Initially, we recommend the use of the **curvilinear probe** (3–5 MHz, Figure 3.1). The low frequency provides good tissue penetration for identifying effusions, consolidation and deep structures (e.g. the diaphragm), whilst maintaining adequate resolution for pleural assessment. This makes the curvilinear probe a good 'all-rounder', particularly in time-critical scenarios.

The **linear probe** (8–12 MHz, Figure 3.2) has very good resolution of superficial structures and gives excellent images of the pleural line and sliding sign. If specifically attempting to identify a pneumothorax this probe is ideal. Due to reduced tissue penetration deeper structures are poorly imaged.

Basic Views

Normal healthy lung will reflect 99.9% of transmitted US and the only visible structure is the pleural line.

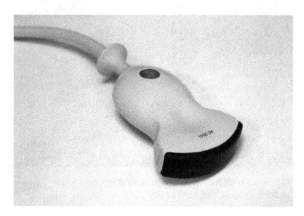

Figure 3.1 **The curvilinear probe.**

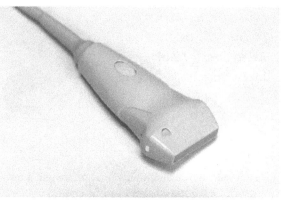

Figure 3.2 **The linear probe.**

No US will penetrate below the pleural line and therefore only artefact is seen. The key to success in LUS is the ability to **interpret this artefact**.

Lung-Specific Ultrasound Signs

There are **ten key LUS signs** listed in Table 3.1 that you must be able to interpret.

Each of these signs will be discussed in further detail later in the chapter. We will then address the specific lung pathology that can be identified by the presence and distribution of these signs.

Table 3.1 Ten key lung ultrasound signs

Lung ultrasound signs
1. **Rib shadows (bat wing sign)**
2. **Sliding sign**
3. **Sea-shore sign**
4. **Stratosphere/bar code sign**
5. **Lung point**
6. **A lines**
7. **B lines**
8. **Consolidation (tissue/hepatisation and shred sign)**
9. **Pleural fluid (quad and sinusoid sign)**
10. **Spine sign**

Chest Lung Anatomy

It is important for you to appreciate the anatomy of the lungs and pinpoint the location of pathology when scanning the lungs (Figure 3.3 and Figure 3.4).

Method

There are **two methods** we advocate for scanning the lungs: the comprehensive *'lawnmower' technique* and the *'BLUE protocol'*.

The **first method** is a comprehensive examination and can be carried out in the relatively well patient. It will take five to ten minutes to execute and will provide detailed information.

The **second method** is the BLUE protocol and is recommended in the acutely unwell patient in respiratory distress. It will take less than five minutes to perform with the patient placed in whichever position they are most comfortable.

Method selection depends upon the acuity of the scenario. Users should aim to perform a study that is as comprehensive as required for the clinical situation.

Method 1 – 'Lawnmower' Technique

In a relatively well and mobile patient we recommend they are seated in the upright position. The probe is initially placed longitudinally in the second intercostal space at the parasternal edge (Figure 3.5). The probe

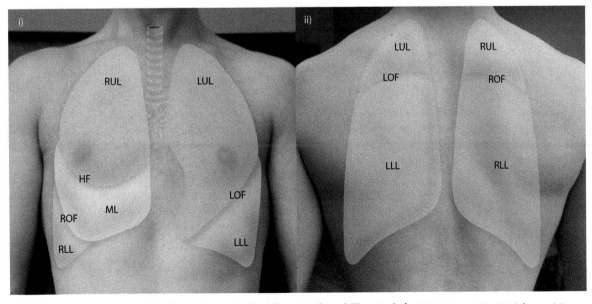

Figure 3.3 Surface anatomy of the lungs when visualised (i) anteriorly and (ii) posteriorly. RUL, right upper lobe; LUL, left upper lobe; HF, horizontal fissure; ML, middle lobe; ROF, right oblique fissure; LOF, left oblique fissure; RLL, right lower lobe; LLL, left lower lobe.

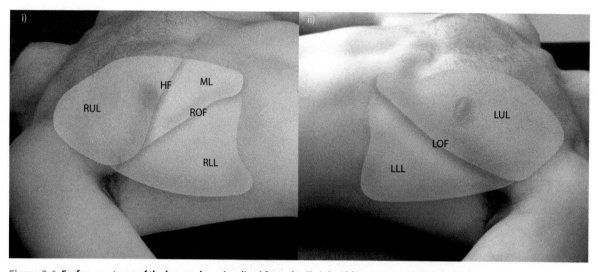

Figure 3.4 Surface anatomy of the lungs when visualised from the (i) right oblique view and (ii) left oblique view. RUL, right upper lobe; HF, horizontal fissure; ML, middle lobe; ROF, right oblique fissure; RLL, right lower lobe; LUL, left upper lobe; LOF, left oblique fissure; LLL, left lower lobe.

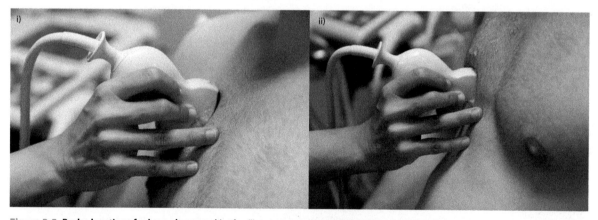

Figure 3.5 Probe locations for lung ultrasound in the (i) upper anterior and (ii) lower anterior regions. Note the positioning of the hand to stabilise the probe on the chest. *A video describing this technique is available to view in the online video library.*

is gradually moved inferiorly to assess each rib space in turn until the user reaches the diaphragm. The same process is then sequentially repeated with the probe placed more laterally until the mid-axillary line is reached (Figure 3.6).

Each rib space should be assessed with the probe in longitudinal and transverse approach.

The posterior chest is then scanned along the paravertebral line, linea scapularis and posterior axillary lines (Figure 3.7). The process for anterior and posterior assessment should be repeated for both lungs. The patient may be asked to lift their arms and place their left or right hand behind their head to aid access for the axillary region.

We advocate you scan cephalad to caudad (top to bottom) and identify the normal anatomy as landmarks. The liver, right kidney and diaphragm will be found at the base of the right lung and the spleen, left kidney and diaphragm at the base of the left lung. The spleen and liver have near identical acoustic impedance and therefore can function as similar landmarks bilaterally.

Tip

When scanning the lungs a lot of gel is required which can result in unintentional sliding of the probe and poor acquisition of images. We recommend you

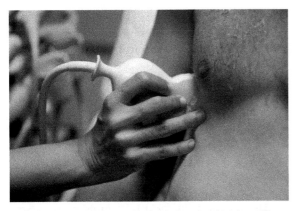

Figure 3.6 **Probe location for lung ultrasound in the axillary region.** *A video describing this technique is available to view in the online video library.*

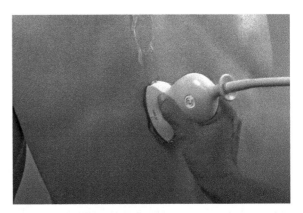

Figure 3.7 **Lawnmower technique on the posterior chest wall.** *A video describing this technique is available to view in the online video library.*

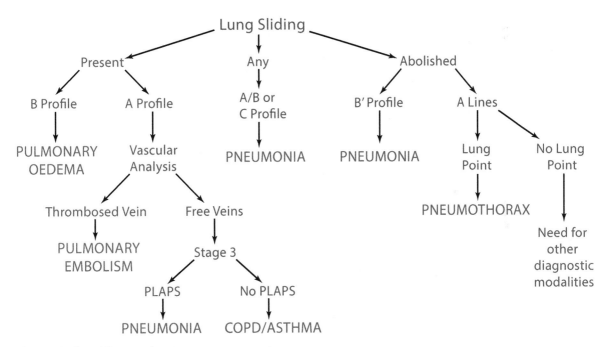

Figure 3.8 **The BLUE protocol**. Adapted from Lichtenstein and Mezière, 2008.

stabilise the probe by using your little finger (demonstrated in Figure 3.6) on the chest like holding a pen. Keeping the probe as still as possible is essential for all US imaging modalities.

Method 2 – The BLUE Protocol

The BLUE protocol (Figure 3.8) was created by Lichtenstein et al. in 2008 and is a systematic approach to US assessment in patients presenting with **acute shortness of breath**. It is incorporated into most POCUS accreditation pathways. It aims to provide a specific pathway to perform LUS in a logical manner which is reported to provide up to a 90.5% diagnostic accuracy.

Whilst initially described in acutely unwell patients this is a fairly intuitive and simple method upon which clinicians can build upon even in the well, ambulatory patient. This protocol can be utilised as a simple 'screen' for key pathology, however, it is important to emphasise that if your clinical suspicion suggests there is 'something to find' this must be extended to a more detailed assessment.

The first step for this method is to locate the **four** 'BLUE points', two on each lung, which mark the starting positions for performing the scan.

Place four fingers (excluding the thumb) of your left hand below the patient's right clavicle with fingers extending over the sternum. The upper 'BLUE point' is located at the base of the second/third fingers.

Next, place your right hand immediately below your left so the forefingers are adjacent to each other. The lower blue point is in the middle of your right palm (Figure 3.9).

Repeat the process on the other side to find all four anterior 'BLUE points'. For each point the probe should be placed at 90 degrees to the skin looking directly into the lung (Figure 3.10). All views are longitudinal, not transverse, with the probe marker pointing towards the patient's head.

The BLUE protocol requires you to initially identify **lung sliding** anteriorly which, if present, rules out a pneumothorax. Subsequently you must identify A lines or B lines in the two anterior points of each hemi-thorax.

If no causative pathology can be found in the four anterior points the protocol suggests scanning the lower legs to rule out a deep vein thrombosis (DVT) which would provide indirect evidence of pulmonary embolism (PE).

The final step in the BLUE protocol is to scan the base of the lungs which are, in reality, where the majority of pathology is likely to be identified. To find this point you must move from the lower anterior 'BLUE point' around the chest wall laterally to the posterior axillary line (Figure 3.11). In practice, given that the patient is supine, the aim is to move the probe as **posteriorly** as possible to see the thoracic/abdominal border. This will give you images of the lower lobe.

In this region the protocol aims to identify 'posterolateral alveolar and/or pleural syndromes', abbreviated to PLAPS. A positive PLAPS will suggest pneumonia and negative is most likely asthma or chronic obstructive pulmonary disease (COPD).

Lung Ultrasound Signs

This section is focused on the specific signs identified on lung ultrasound.

Rib Shadows ('Bat Wing' Sign)

Ribs and rib shadows are used as landmarks when scanning the lungs. Bone will reflect US waves back to the probe and therefore causes a post-acoustic shadow.

It is good practice to acquire an image with two ribs aligned centrally whether using a linear or curvilinear probe. The pleural line can be seen stretching between the two rib shadows approximately 0.5 cm below the rib line. The pleural line is a bright white line which moves with inspiration. Beneath this is an individual lung window where pathology may be identified. The combination of these signs in an image is referred to as the **'bat wing' sign** (Figure 3.12).

Sliding Sign

The parietal and visceral pleurae are closely opposed to each other with a tiny quantity of fluid between the

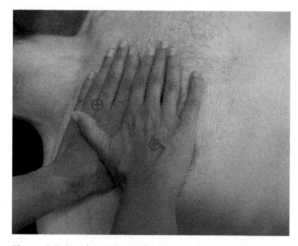

Figure 3.9 **Hand position to find the anterior 'BLUE Points'.**

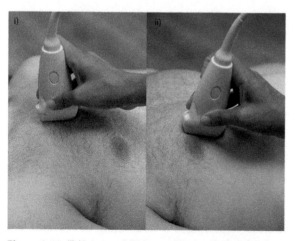

Figure 3.10 **(i) Upper and (ii) lower anterior 'BLUE Points'.**

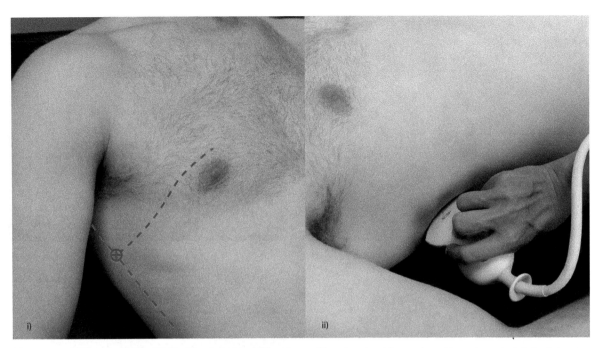

Figure 3.11 (i) Location of the 'PLAPs Blue Point' and (ii) probe position. Note the oblique probe position to image through the rib spaces.

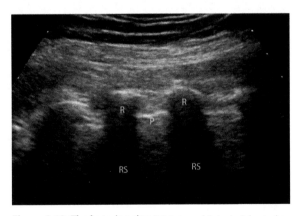

Figure 3.12 The bat wing sign This is termed 'bat wing' due to the shadows behind the ribs. R, rib; P, pleural line; RS, rib shadow.

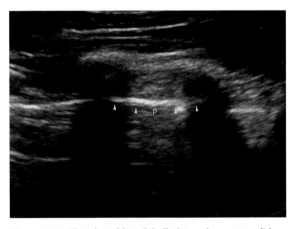

Figure 3.13 The pleural line (labelled) may be seen to slide backwards and forwards during respiration. Arrows demonstrate the length of the pleural line between rib shadows. *A video is available to view in the online video library.*

layers allowing them to slide across one another with respiration (Figure 3.13). This is a normal finding.

The pleurae can be seen as a bright white line adjacent to the rib shadows with the two pleurae 'shimmering' as they slide during inspiration and expiration. Small blebs may be seen moving from side to side and are sometimes referred to as 'ants crawling' across the pleural line (Figure 3.14). These are not thought to be clinically significant and must be differentiated from 'B lines' which will be discussed later.

The high frequency linear probe provides the best resolution for superficial structures and is therefore ideal to appreciate lung sliding when you first begin scanning.

Be aware that the bright white nature of the pleural line is due to the interface between the parietal and visceral pleurae and thus with pathology such as

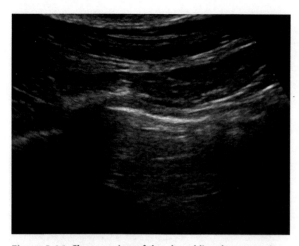

Figure 3.14 Close up view of the pleural line demonstrating pleural sliding. *A video is available to view in the online video library.*

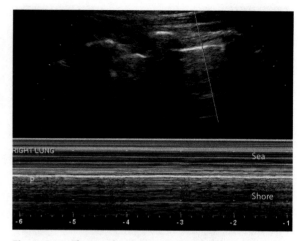

Figure 3.15 The sea-shore sign. The M-mode cursor has been placed through the middle of the pleural line. The pleural line is seen as the bright line in the middle of the M-mode trace (labelled). The sea is above the pleural line and grainy shore is below.

pleural effusions, where the layers are separated, it is unlikely to be visualised.

Various pathology may affect the ability of the pleurae to slide across one another. There are circumstances where the pleurae are **not opposed**, e.g. pneumothorax; **stuck together**, e.g. pneumonia, pleurodesis or acute respiratory distress syndrome (ARDS)/ acute lung injury (ALI), or there is **no lung ventilation**, e.g. breath holding or severe asthma.

The pleural line may be identified but the parietal and visceral pleurae will not slide across each other during respiration. This is an important sign which marks the first step of the BLUE protocol. These will be discussed with examples later.

Sea-Shore Sign (M-Mode)

We recommend using M-mode to reassure yourself the patient has normal lung sliding. This is acquired by placing the cursor through the pleural line. Where pleural sliding is present the resulting image is termed the 'sea-shore' sign (Figure 3.15).

Subcutaneous tissue above the pleura generates horizontal straight lines whereas the pleural sliding will result in a grainy, 'sandy' appearance below it. The resulting image is described as appearing like a **sandy beach** with the horizontal lines representing the sea and the grainy image of the sand. This is a reassuring sign suggesting normal pleural sliding.

A Lines

A lines are horizontal lines representing **reverberation artefact** from the pleural line (Figure 3.16).

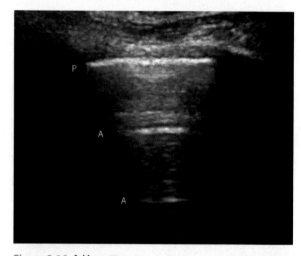

Figure 3.16 A Lines. The A lines can be seen equidistant from the pleural lines. P, pleural line; A, A lines. *A video is available to view in the online video library.*

As previously discussed the pleural line reflects US waves back to the probe and thus deeper structures cannot be identified in a normal lung. The probe itself may also act as a reflective surface causing US waves to bounce back and forth between the probe and the pleural line. This manifests as horizontal lines seen below the pleurae at regular intervals with diminishing amplitude. The interval between these lines will be the same as between the probe and the pleural line.

A lines indicate the presence of **air** beneath the pleurae and are therefore typically associated with normal lung. A caveat to this is with pneumothoraces as the air within the pleural space will also cause A lines.

Stratosphere Sign/Bar Code Sign (M-Mode)

In the absence of pleural sliding, e.g. in pneumothorax, the M-mode image will consist only of horizontal lines which is termed the 'stratosphere' or 'bar-code' sign (Figure 3.17).

It is good practice to confirm absence of pleural sliding using 2D imaging prior to utilising M-mode due to various pitfalls with this method. Prior identification of the pleural line is essential as in circumstances where US waves do not reach the pleural line, e.g. subcutaneous emphysema, a similar image to the stratosphere sign will be present.

The **lung pulse** is an additional sign that may be present in M-mode if the stratosphere sign is seen. It is created by the cardiac impulse being transmitted through the thorax causing small vertical lines to appear on the M-mode trace (Figure 3.18). The significance of the lung pulse is that it is only transmitted when the pleura are opposed and therefore is absent in pneumothorax. If a lung pulse is identified the user should consider an alternative to pneumothorax as the cause of absent pleural sliding.

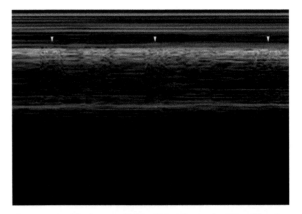

Figure 3.18 The lung pulse can be seen on the M-mode trace as regular vertical deflections (arrows). This represents transmitted cardiac impulses through the lung.

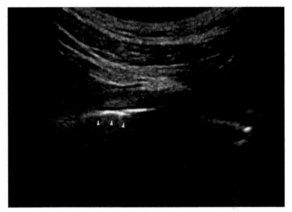

Figure 3.19 Lung point. The lung point may be seen as the location where pleura meet at the border of a pneumothorax. The arrows highlight the downward deflection that is called the lung point. *A video is available to view in the online video library.*

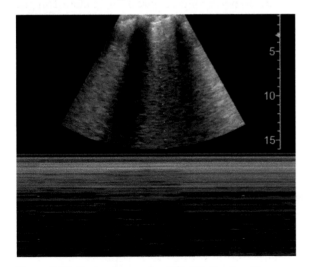

Figure 3.17 Stratosphere or barcode sign. The clear difference between the 'sea' and the 'shore' is lost in this case of pneumothorax. This creates a 'sea' picture throughout the M-mode image.

Lung Point

If a pneumothorax is suspected from the absence of sliding sign and presence of A lines then the clinician should attempt to identify a **lung point** (Figure 3.19). This can typically be identified by moving the probe laterally. With larger pneumothoraces the lung point will be located more **laterally**.

The lung point represents the location where the pleural layers re-join one another and marks the border of the pneumothorax.

It is seen as a downward deflection of the pleural layer with the sliding sign present on one side but not the other. The lung point will frequently move with respiration and it can move in and out of view during the respiratory cycle.

The lung point is the **most specific sign** for pneumothorax and is unlikely to be present in other causes of absent pleural sliding.

B Lines (Comet Tails)

B lines are vertical lines that extend from the pleura to the bottom of the screen. They erase A lines and will move with lung sliding (Figure 3.20). They are sometimes referred to as comet tails.

B lines are artefact resulting from the combination of air in the alveoli and thickening of the interlobular septa due to fluid or fibrosis. The US waves reverberate at the interface between the alveoli and the interlobular septa creating a line for each reverberation.

There is a consensus that the presence of **three or more** B lines is pathological due to disease of the interstitium. This disease may represent fluid, e.g. pulmonary oedema, ARDS, fibrosis or interstitial pneumonia/pneumonitis. Interstitial syndrome is a sonographic diagnosis which describes the presence of B lines and incorporates the above diagnoses. These may be distinguished by various additional features which will be discussed in more detail later in the chapter.

The most common cause of B lines is pulmonary oedema and they are the US equivalent of Kerly-B lines seen on chest radiographs. With increasing severity of pulmonary oedema the number of B lines increases and may become confluent filling the entire space between the rib shadows (Figure 3.21). This has been described as the waterfall sign.

Serial US examinations may be used to tailor management of pulmonary oedema without the need for repeat chest radiography in both inpatient and outpatient settings.

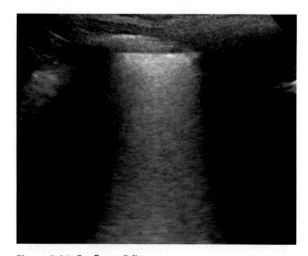

Figure 3.21 Confluent B lines. Individual B lines have now coalesced to form a bright lung window. Note the thin pleural line. This is a key differentiating feature between severe pulmonary oedema and ARDS. *A video is available to view in the online video library.*

Consolidation (Shred and Tissue Signs)

Consolidated lung is highly fluid rich and tends to extend to the pleura making it readily identifiable on US. Its appearance may be extremely difficult to differentiate from atelectasis.

Fluid bronchograms are black in appearance and specific to pneumonia (Figure 3.22i). Colour Doppler is useful to distinguish them from blood vessels.

Air bronchograms can be present, as with chest radiography, and appear white within consolidated tissue. Depending on the orientation of the probe the air bronchograms are linear or seen in cross section. Air bronchograms may be present in either pneumonia or atelectasis but if they are dynamic and move with respiration it is highly suggestive of pneumonia (Figure 3.22ii).

Three distinct patterns of consolidation may be seen:

Anterior/Subpleural Consolidation

Small pockets of echo-poor areas may be visible beneath the pleura and may abolish the pleural line (Figure 3.23).

Lines similar to B lines may be seen from the lower border of the consolidated tissue. These are not strictly speaking B lines as they do not originate from the pleurae.

Marginal borders of the consolidation are not well demarcated and can be described as appearing 'moth eaten'.

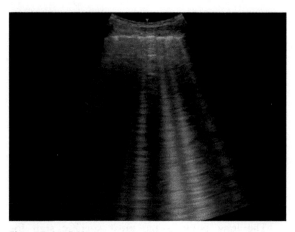

Figure 3.20 B Lines. Note that the bright lines extend from the pleural line to the base of the screen. *A video is available to view in the online video library.*

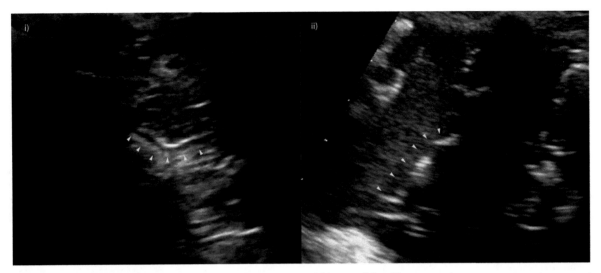

Figure 3.22 (i) Fluid bronchogram and (ii) air bronchogram seen within consolidated lung parenchyma. Note the hypoechoic centre of the fluid bronchogram and the hyperechoic, irregular air bronchogram. The pockets of air within the air bronchogram are seen to move with respiration. *Videos are available to view in the online video library.*

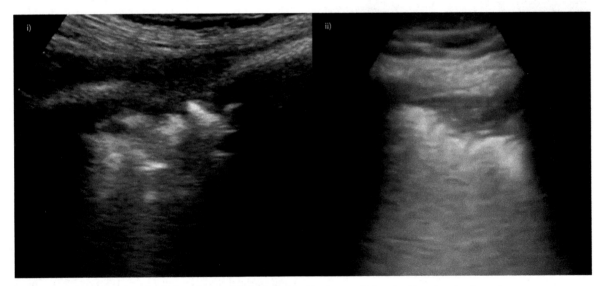

Figure 3.23 **Two examples of subpleural consolidation.** The pleural line become thickened and irregular or 'moth eaten'.

Shred Sign

In regions where consolidation is less extensive it can be bordered by normal lung. In these circumstances it may appear that chunks have been removed from the lung. This is known as the 'shred' sign and is highly diagnostic of pneumonia (Figure 3.24).

As with the anterior consolidation the border between the consolidation and normal lung may have B-type lines and be poorly demarcated.

Tissue Sign/Hepatisation

As previously considered, normal lung cannot be visualised on US due to high air content. Consolidated lung has significantly higher fluid content and thus may become visible on US. The echogenicity of consolidated lung is similar to the liver and thus is referred to being **'hepatisised'** (Figure 3.25).

The consolidated lung may act as an acoustic window making the opposite pleural line and mediastinal vessels visible. A pleural effusion often

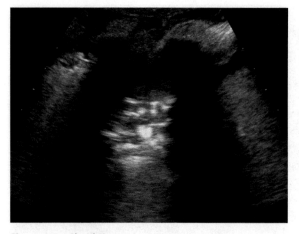

Figure 3.24 **Shred sign.** Small areas of focal consolidation may appear to have had 'chunks' removed from the lung. *A video is available to view in the online video library.*

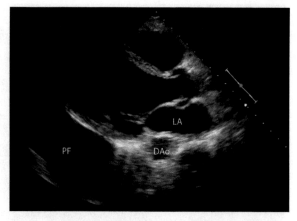

Figure 3.26 **Parasternal long-axis echocardiography view showing a large pleural effusion.** Pleural fluid (PF) sits beneath the descending aorta (DAo) without causing displacement of the aorta away from the left atrium (LA). Please see the echocardiography chapter for more detail. *A video is available to view in the online video library.*

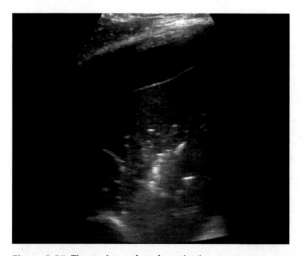

Figure 3.25 **Tissue sign or lung hepatisation.** High fluid content within the consolidated lung causes it to have a similar echogenicity to the liver. A parapneumonic effusion is also seen superiorly to the consolidation. *A video is available to view in the online video library.*

accompanies the consolidation which will further amplify these features.

Pleural Fluid

Lung ultrasound has a sensitivity approaching 100% for identification of pleural fluid. This makes it an extremely powerful tool when compared with chest radiography where up to 500ml may easily be missed.

Pleural fluid appears anechoic and therefore black on the display and one can often differentiate between exudate, transudate and haemothorax.

Fluid is dependent upon gravity and will accumulate inferiorly and posteriorly allowing easy identification above the diaphragm. Atelectatic lung is frequently seen floating within the effusion.

A pleural effusion may be incidentally identified when performing a focused echo (Figure 3.26). Fluid will appear deep to the descending aorta in the PLAX view. Differentiating pleural from pericardial effusion is discussed in more detail in Chapter 2. If a pleural effusion is identified on echo it should be interrogated in more detail using LUS.

Although identification of pleural fluid is usually clear, two different signs have been described that may also aid the user.

Quad Sign

The quad sign describes the rectangular shape caused by a pleural effusion that is bordered by rib shadows and parietal and visceral pleura (Figure 3.27). This is most useful in the setting of small pleural effusions.

Sinusoid Sign

In the presence of a pleural effusion the lung will move towards the pleural line during inspiration. M-mode may demonstrate this against time and appears as a sinusoidal wave (Figure 3.28).

Spine Sign

The thoracic spine sign on LUS is an indirect indicator of the presence of a pleural effusion or haemothorax (Figure 3.29).

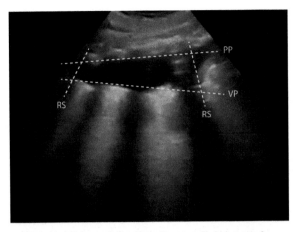

Figure 3.27 The quad sign describes a well demarcated pleural effusion. The borders of the 'quad' are the parietal pleura (PP), visceral pleura (VP) and two rib shadows (RS).

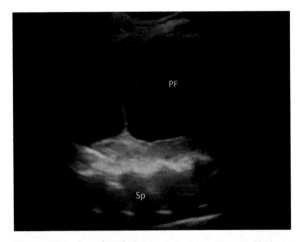

Figure 3.29 The spine sign. The spinal vertebrae (Sp) are visible due to the pleural fluid (PF) allowing transmission of ultrasound through to the posterior thoracic cavity. *A video is available to view in the online video library.*

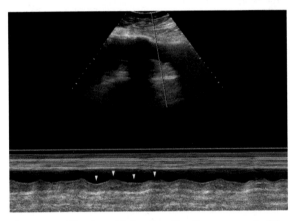

Figure 3.28 The sinusoid sign describes the movement of the lung towards the probe during inspiration seen on M-mode.

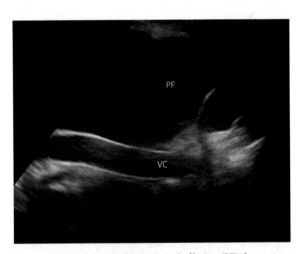

Figure 3.30 Due to the large pleural effusion (PF) the vena cava (VC) or aorta may be visible. *A video is available to view in the online video library.*

In a patient without a pleural effusion the aerated lung fills the costo-phrenic angle and therefore the spine above the diaphragm is not visualised – i.e. a negative spine sign.

In the presence of a pleural effusion the costo-phrenic angle is filled with fluid allowing US waves to reach the spine and therefore it is seen above the diaphragm.

The thoracic aorta or vena cava may also be seen due to the presence of pleural fluid (Figure 3.30).

Thickened and Irregular Pleural Line

Normally the visceral and parietal pleurae are opposed and approximately 0.2–0.3 mm in thickness. Pleural line thickening is defined as being >3 mm in width (Figure 3.31). The causes of pleural line thickening are varied and include acute viral infections (including COVID-19), pulmonary fibrosis, TB, haemothorax and acute respiratory distress syndrome (ARDS).

It is important on US to describe this as 'pleural *line* thickening' rather than 'pleural thickening'. Thickened pleura on other forms of imaging may signify extremely different, significant pathology such as mesothelioma and therefore being precise with reports is essential.

The Diaphragm

The diaphragm is very important in LUS for orientation and identification of pathology. It is a

79

dome-shaped structure that lies higher anteriorly and lower posteriorly. It is often visualised far higher than expected in the thorax causing many US users to be cautious when performing thoracocentesis.

On LUS the diaphragm is a bright white structure that moves up and down with respiration. It is commonly obscured by aerated lung causing it to be challenging to identify unless there is pathology such as pleural fluid or consolidation.

If no fluid is present the 'curtain sign' may be seen. This describes the abdominal organs, usually the liver or spleen, becoming obscured by lung during inspiration and reappearing with expiration (Figure 3.32). This is a normal finding. Paradoxical diaphragmatic movement may indicate the presence of phrenic nerve palsy.

If fluid is present this will allow visualisation of the diaphragm. The liver will be visible when imaging the patient's right side (Figure 3.33i) and the spleen when imaging the left side (Figure 3.33ii). The underlying lung will often be collapsed within the fluid.

Lung Pathology

This section will describe the signs seen in lung pathology and will act as a quick reference for the combination of signs in each condition. Case examples will highlight the LUS changes and how POCUS guides management and treatment.

Pneumothorax

Lung ultrasound is highly sensitive for identification of pneumothorax with the key finding being the absence of pleural sliding. In a supine patient the highest point of the anterior chest is usually where this will be seen.

As previously mentioned, the parietal and visceral pleurae are separated by a thin layer of fluid allowing them to slide across one another. With a pneumothorax the pleural layers are no longer opposed abolishing the sliding sign (Figure 3.34).

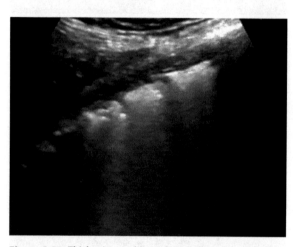

Figure 3.31 Thickening and irregularity of the pleural line.
A video is available to view in the online video library.

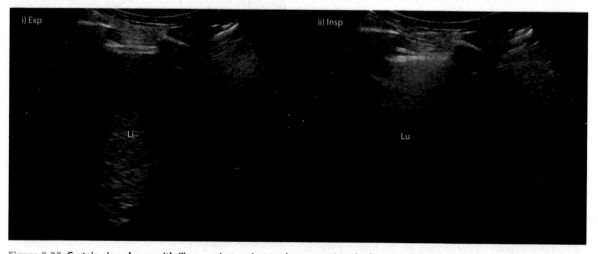

Figure 3.32 Curtain sign shown with (i) an expiratory image demonstrating the liver (Li), followed by (ii) an inspiratory image showing the lung parenchyma (Lu) expanding to obscure the liver. The diaphragm is not visible throughout the respiratory cycle.
A video is available to view in the online video library.

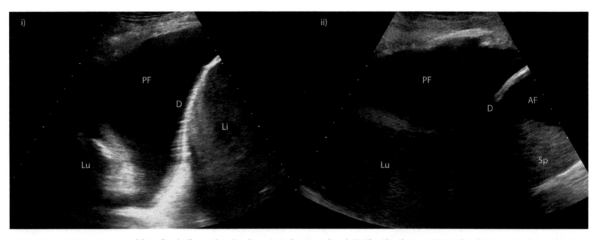

Figure 3.33 The presence of free fluid allows the diaphragm to be visualised. (i) The diaphragm (D) is clearly seen overlying the liver (Li) due to pleural fluid (PR). Collapsed lung (Lu) may be seen within the pleural effusion. (ii) The diaphragm is surrounded by pleural fluid (PF) and ascitic fluid (AF). The spleen (Sp) may be noted inferior to the diaphragm. *Videos are available to view in the online video library.*

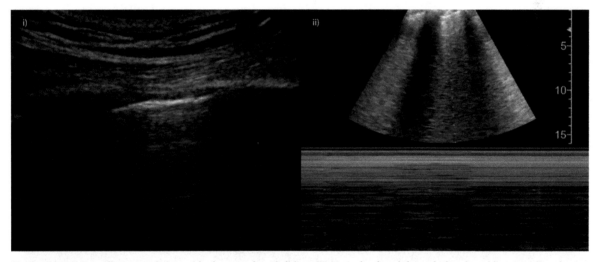

Figure 3.34 (i) Two-dimensional view with absence pleural sliding. (ii) M-mode placed through the pleural line revealing the stratosphere or barcode sign. *Videos are available to view in the online video library.*

It is important to identify the pleural line prior to looking for pleural sliding, particularly for the stratosphere/bar code sign, as subcutaneous emphysema may produce a similar appearance.

There are various additional causes of absent and reduced pleural sliding which are listed in Table 3.2. It is possible to artificially create this sign by asking the patient to hold their breath.

Figure 3.35 shows you pleural sliding versus absent pleural sliding. This can only be appreciated when viewing the online videos.

Once absence of pleural sliding has been confirmed the next step is to move the probe laterally to identify a lung point which is the most specific sign for pneumothorax. This is the point at which the two pleural layers re-join one another. It will be more lateral with increasing pneumothorax size and so should be searched for by moving the probe laterally. This point will move with lung inflation and deflation resulting in an area at which sliding will appear and disappear.

If a lung point cannot be localised then the user may attempt to identify a lung pulse. This has been described earlier and if present will prompt the user to consider diagnoses other than pneumothorax.

Case – Ultrasound Provides the Answer

A 32-year-old gentleman with a background of asthma presented to the ED with increased shortness of breath. His asthma was well controlled with no previous hospital admissions.

Observations identified a respiratory rate of 35 with heart rate, oxygen saturations and blood pressure within normal range. Examination revealed equal but poor air entry bilaterally.

He had no history of fevers or cough and therefore was managed as a non-infective exacerbation of asthma and received no chest imaging as per hospital protocol.

There was no improvement following nebulised B-agonists with the patient reporting increased shortness of breath.

Lung ultrasound was performed at the bedside revealing absence of pleural sliding in the left anterior

Table 3.2 Causes of absent or reduced lung sliding

Absent	Reduced
Pneumothorax	Hyperinflation (COPD, asthma)
ARDS/ALI	Low tidal volumes (during ventilation)
Pneumonectomy	ARDS
Severe consolidation	Pulmonary fibrosis
Atelectasis	
Endobronchial intubation	

'BLUE point' and a lung point was located laterally suggesting a spontaneous pneumothorax (Figure 3.36).

A chest drain was inserted after confirmation on chest radiograph with an improvement in symptoms.

Lung ultrasound enabled rapid identification of an alternative diagnosis in a patient assumed to be having an exacerbation of asthma. Chest radiography was requested due to widespread familiarity with this imaging modality and to aid in management decisions.

Interstitial Syndrome

Interstitial syndrome is a sonographic diagnosis encompassing all the conditions producing B lines.

B lines are likely to be present with cardiogenic or non-cardiogenic pulmonary oedema (acute respiratory distress syndrome (ARDS), acute lung injury (ALI)), lung fibrosis or interstitial pneumonia/pneumonitis. Additional features may assist in distinguishing between these causes.

Cardiogenic

Pulmonary oedema is by far the most common cause of interstitial syndrome and demonstrates correlation between the severity of oedema and number of B lines present. As oedema worsens the number of B lines increases (Figure 3.37i) and may begin to coalesce forming a homogeneous 'white out' at its most severe (Figure 3.37ii). This will correlate with deterioration in the clinical status of the patient.

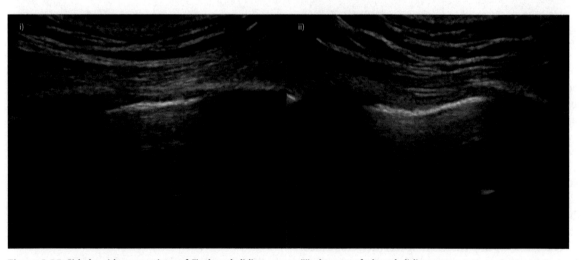

Figure 3.35 Side-by-side comparison of (i) pleural sliding versus (ii) absence of pleural sliding. This can only be visualised if viewing the online material. *Videos are available to view in the online video library.*

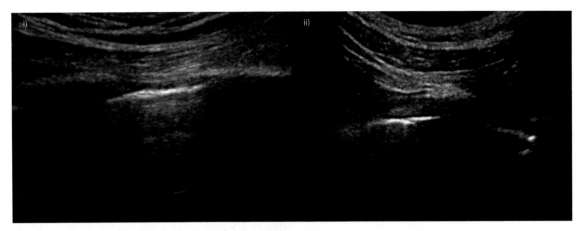

Figure 3.36 **(i) Absent pleural sliding. (ii) Lung point identified after sliding the probe laterally.** *Videos are available to view in the online video library.*

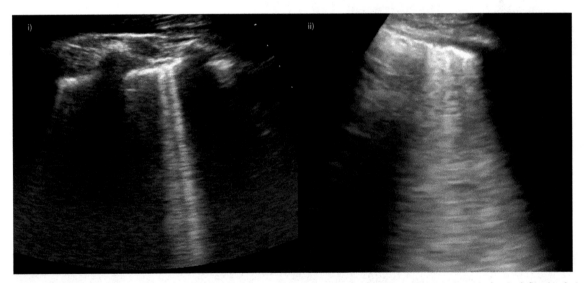

Figure 3.37 **Pulmonary oedema causes B lines to increase in number with severity. (i) ≥ 3 B lines in one window is defined as being pathological. (ii) With increasing severity the B lines will coalesce to form a 'waterfall'.** *Videos are available to view in the online video library.*

The pattern of B lines in pulmonary oedema is likely to follow a typical pattern becoming more numerous towards the bases of the lungs. This will be a gradual change with no regions spared. If upper regions of the lungs are affected this reflects a more severe degree of pulmonary oedema. Pleural effusions will often be present bilaterally with regions of collapsed parenchyma floating within the fluid (Figure 3.38). This may be termed the 'jellyfish sign' and will be discussed later. Where visible, the pleural line will remain normal in appearance when compared with the thickening present in other causes of B line profiles.

Case – Diagnosis in the Patient's Own Home

An 83-year-old female nursing-home resident received a home visit from the GP as she complained of increased shortness of breath. She had multiple comorbidities including hypertension, type 2 diabetes mellitus, COPD and congestive cardiac failure.

She had experienced no change in her productive cough but described an increasing severity of shortness of breath at night. Observations were all within normal range. She had significant peripheral oedema.

Lung ultrasound revealed a significant number of B lines bilaterally throughout the lower lung fields (Figure 3.39i) with bilateral pleural effusions (Figure 3.39ii).

The case was discussed with the community heart failure team and she was given a three-day course of intravenous diuretics within the nursing home. She made a gradual improvement in symptoms during the subsequent days without the need for hospital admission.

This case identified the key pathology in the patient's own home allowing appropriate management without referral to a hospital setting. Whilst this is a relatively simple case the presence of multiple comorbidities created diagnostic uncertainty.

Non-Cardiogenic

Conditions producing non-cardiogenic pulmonary oedema, such as ARDS/ALI, will have differing patterns to that seen in pulmonary oedema. There will be patchy regions where B lines are present interspersed with unaffected areas with normal pleura and no B lines. In affected regions, often dependent areas of the lung, the pleural line is thickened and irregular with associated subpleural consolidation. This can impact the ability to see the sliding sign which may become less pronounced (Figure 3.40).

Acute respiratory distress syndrome is characterised by diffuse alveolar damage with an increase in alveolar and capillary permeability leading to accumulation of fluid in the alveolar space and interstitium. LUS may be useful in diagnosis and differentiation from alternative causes of interstitial syndrome.

Although ARDS was seldom seen outside of the ICU prior to COVID-19, the radiological signs may have an unpredictable course in survivors with persistent long-term fibrotic changes. Given that these patients may be susceptible to future respiratory

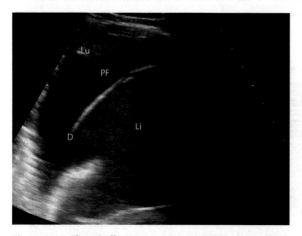

Figure 3.38 Pleural effusion secondary to pulmonary oedema. Atelectatic lung (Lu) may be seen floating in the pleural fluid (PF). This is known as the 'jellyfish sign'. The liver (Li) and diaphragm (D) are also labelled for reference. *A video is available to view in the online video library.*

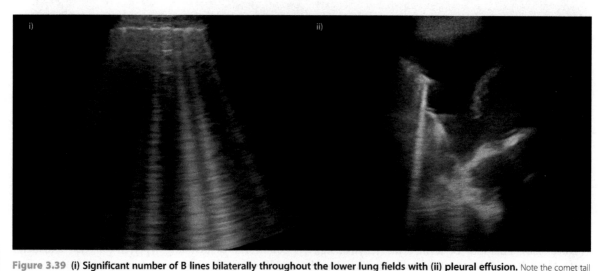

Figure 3.39 (i) Significant number of B lines bilaterally throughout the lower lung fields with (ii) pleural effusion. Note the comet tail artefact seen within the lung base adjacent to the pleural effusions. *Videos are available to view in the online video library.*

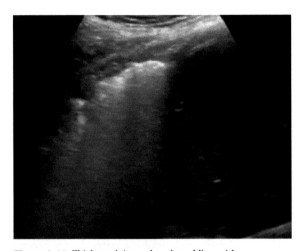

Figure 3.40 **Thickened, irregular pleural line with subpleural consolidation and B lines seen in ARDS.** P, pleural line; Lu, lung; Li, liver; D, diaphragm. *A video is available to view in the online video library.*

Table 3.3 Differences between acute respiratory distress syndrome and pulmonary oedema on lung ultrasound

	ARDS/COVID-19	Pulmonary oedema
Pleural line	Irregular and thickened	Thin
B lines	Multiples throughout lung B Lines do not improve with diuresis	Predominate at bases Number of B lines decreases with diuresis
Lung parenchyma	Sub pleural and lobar consolidation	No consolidation
Effusions	Rarely seen <10%	Common at bases

comorbidities and complications it is at least feasible to expect clinicians to understand that chronic findings may be present and not necessarily represent new changes. Furthermore, the COVID-19 pandemic has highlighted the impact on viral illnesses causing an 'ARDS-type' illness with very similar lung features. Differentiation between ARDS and pulmonary oedema can be identified with LUS (Table 3.3). This is discussed in more detail in Chapter 12.

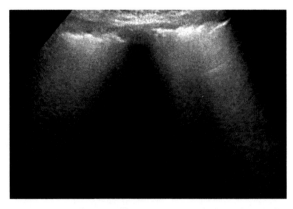

Figure 3.41 **Pulmonary fibrosis causing a thickened, irregular pleural line with nodules and coalescent B line pattern.** *A video is available to view in the online video library.*

It is worth noting that patients with chronic scarring of their septa from pulmonary fibrosis, old infections or interstitial lung disease have chronically widened/thickened septae that also create B lines. Not all B lines mean pulmonary oedema.

Lung fibrosis will cause widespread B lines which are frequently severe and will coalesce. The pleural line is fragmented and irregularly thickened with subpleural cysts and nodules differentiating from other causes of interstitial syndrome. Pleural sliding will be reduced or absent (Figure 3.41).

Different causes of interstitial syndrome can be challenging to distinguish from one another and are beyond the scope of current POCUS training programmes. It is, however, important to appreciate that B lines are not specific to pulmonary oedema and that combined clinical examination and sonographic assessment of other systems are required.

Alveolar Syndrome

Alveolar syndrome is a sonographic diagnosis encompassing the findings of consolidation and atelectasis. As previously discussed, fluid bronchograms are highly suggestive of pneumonia whilst air bronchograms may be present with consolidation or atelectasis. Moving air bronchograms suggest airway patency and therefore are more likely to represent consolidation rather than a cause of atelectasis such as airway obstruction from mucus plugging or tumour.

The LUS changes with consolidation can often be seen to progress with the severity of disease. The key stages that may be seen are listed and described below:

85

Stage 1 – Subpleural consolidation

Stage 2 – Shred sign

Stage 3 – Severe consolidation

Stage 4 – Hepatisation of the lung

Stage 1 – Subpleural Consolidation

The majority of community acquired pneumonia (CAP) causes peripherally located consolidation making it readily detectable on LUS. In early pneumonia, fluid can accumulate in pockets of peripheral alveoli causing

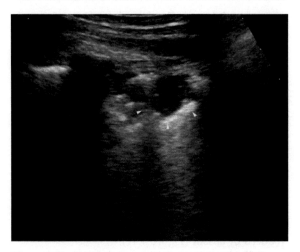

Figure 3.42 **Subpleural consolidation with localised B lines.**
A video is available to view in the online video library.

patches of subpleural consolidation (Figure 3.42). Reverberation artefact, similar to B lines, may be seen from the border of the consolidation.

Stage 2 – Shred Sign

As the regions of consolidated lung increase in size the shred sign becomes apparent on LUS. This is demonstrated in Figure 3.43 where the shred sign was seen in a patient with patchy consolidation on chest X-ray (CXR) (right upper zone, right lower zone, left lower zone).

Stage 3 – Severe Consolidation

Within severe consolidation the alveoli are progressively fluid-filled and the lung parenchyma become more visible on LUS. Small airways may retain small amounts of air that are visible as hyperechoic bubbles that are aligned within the small bronchioles. This is known as the sonographic air bronchogram. When the small bubbles in an air bronchogram can be seen moving with each breath the term 'dynamic air bronchogram' is used.

In time, the air within the bronchioles is replaced with fluid leading to a hypoechoic branched structure with echogenic walls. This is known as a fluid bronchogram. The use of colour Doppler can help to differentiate between fluid bronchograms and blood vessels.

Figure 3.44i shows CXR with dense right basal consolidation and small basal consolidation and

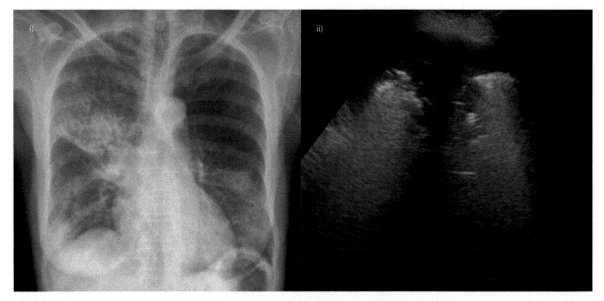

Figure 3.43 **(i) Chest X-ray features of pneumonia with (ii) lung ultrasound revealing the shred sign.**

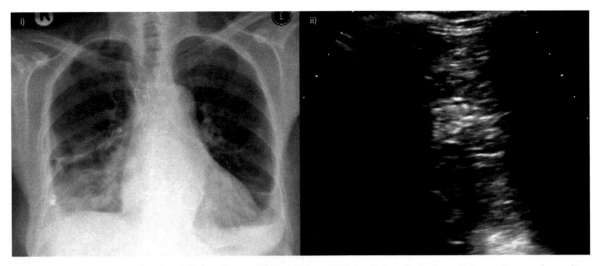

Figure 3.44 **(i) Chest X-ray showing right basal consolidation and small bilateral pleural effusions. (ii) Lung ultrasound revealing severe consolidation with air and fluid bronchograms.** *A video is available to view in the online video library.*

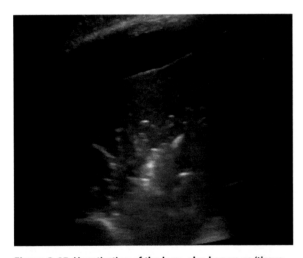

Figure 3.45 **Hepatisation of the lung, also known as 'tissue sign', in a patient with severe pneumonia.** Note the parapneumonic effusion and air bronchograms. *A video is available to view in the online video library.*

Figure 3.44ii shows air and fluid bronchograms on LUS.

Stage 4 – Hepatisation of the Lung

With dense consolidation or complete atelectasis the lung parenchyma can have a similar echogenicity to the liver. This is described as hepatisation. Bronchograms and a pleural effusion may also be present (Figure 3.45).

An additional method for differentiating between consolidation and atelectasis is by visually assessing

the lung volume. In consolidation, the lung parenchyma is filled with inflammatory liquid leading to the lung volume remaining unchanged or increasing. In atelectasis, the alveoli are collapsed causing lung volume to be reduced. Other features, such as a large pleural effusion, may also be present and explain the aetiology for the atelectasis.

Case – Essential Pre-Procedure Ultrasound

A 74-year-old woman presented with fever, dyspnoea and chest pain. Her family also reported poor appetite and confusion. She was reviewed in the ED where a new pleural effusion was diagnosed based on radiographic findings suggesting a meniscus (Figure 3.46i). Due to the worsening oxygen requirement and drowsiness the medical team prepared to perform an urgent intercostal drain. LUS was performed prior to the procedure being undertaken and this demonstrated severe consolidation with only a small parapneumonic effusion not amenable to drainage (Figure 3.46ii). Instead of an intercostal drain she was commenced upon IV antimicrobial therapy and continuous positive airway pressure (CPAP) to aid oxygenation.

This case highlights the superiority of LUS for the diagnosis of pneumonia compared with clinical examination and radiography. It is plausible that the team may have attempted to insert a drain into consolidated lung parenchyma causing unnecessary complications in an acutely unwell patient. In modern clinical practice the use of US guidance prior to drain

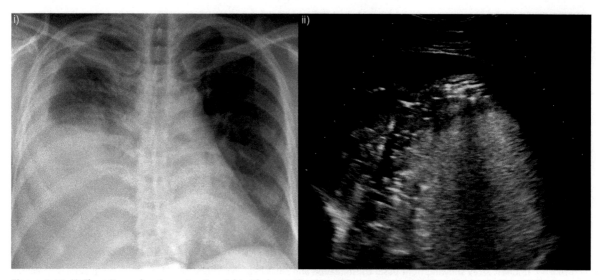

Figure 3.46 (i) Chest X-ray showing extensive right-sided opacification with meniscus suspicious of a large pleural effusion. (ii) Lung ultrasound revealed severe consolidation with only a small parapneumonic effusion. Air and fluid bronchograms can be seen within the consolidated lung. *A video is available to view in the online video library.*

insertion should be considered as mandatory to ensure correct diagnosis, optimal location and to reduce the risk of complications.

Pleural Effusions

Pleural effusions are common and typically accumulate at the base of the lungs. LUS is significantly more sensitive than CXR at the detection of pleural effusions and it has been reported to be able to detect 5–20 ml in comparison with 175 ml on a CXR.

A pleural effusion appears as an anechoic space between the parietal and visceral pleurae. They are categorised as simple or complex/complicated depending on their appearance. Simple effusions are anechoic, homogeneous and usually transudative. Complex effusions have an extremely varied appearance: hypoechoic, particulated, septated or hyperechoic. Complex effusions are much more likely to be exudates. The appearance of the effusion on LUS can guide the user to the aetiology (Table 3.4).

Size of Effusions

There are a number of published sizing techniques for effusions which vary significantly as an accurate volume is difficult to define with LUS. The most used is the formula by Balik et al. It involves measuring the maximal effusion diameter (in millimetres, mm)

Table 3.4 Appearance of different types of pleural effusions

Appearance	Nature
Anechoic	Transudate
Echoic (uniform or particles) or septated	Exudate
Echoic (uniform or particles) or anechoic of acute	Haemothorax

between the diaphragm and the base of the lung in a supine position and multiplying that number by 20.

$$\text{Pleural volume (ml)} = (\text{measured distance from diaphragm in mm}) \times 20$$

However, in clinical practice It is more practical and clinically relevant to classify an effusion volume as small, moderate or large. As a rule of thumb, an effusion depth of 4–5 cm at the widest point equates to an effusion of >1000 ml.

With large pleural effusions the underlying lung parenchyma can collapse and appear like a *jellyfish* moving with respiration. The mobility of the lung may guide to the nature of the effusion. If the fluid is thin and non-viscous, suggesting a simple or transudative effusion, the lung parenchyma will be highly

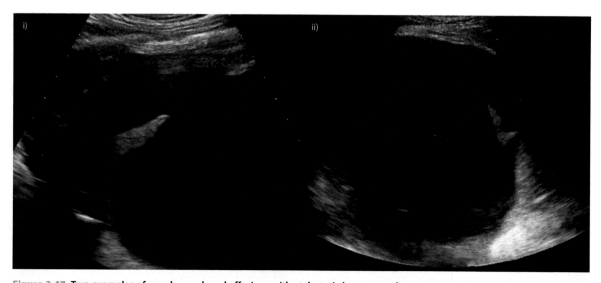

Figure 3.47 Two examples of very large pleural effusions with atelectatic lung parenchyma. The collapsed lung is highly mobile within the fluid which is suggestive of a low density transudative pleural effusion. *Videos are available to view in the online video library.*

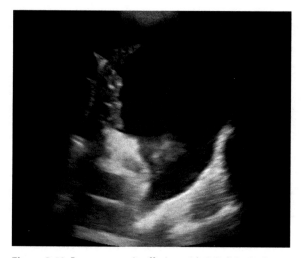

Figure 3.48 Parapneumonic effusion with 'jellyfish sign'. This collapsed lung parenchyma is far less mobile within the pleural fluid. This may reflect a higher density fluid which is suggestive of an exudative pleural effusion. *A video is available to view in the online video library.*

mobile within the fluid (Figure 3.47). In comparison, if the fluid is highly viscous, suggesting a complex or exudative effusion, there will not be significant movement of the lung (Figure 3.48).

After diagnosing a pleural effusion the maximum anterior-posterior (AP) depth should be measured to gauge amenability for drainage. The clip should be frozen and callipers used to measure depth. If you wish to aspirate the effusion, the patient should not move position as this will change the location and depth of effusion. Using a sterile probe cover will allow real time imaging of the effusion during the procedure and will therefore produce the most accurate information.

Small effusions of >1 cm have been described to be safe to aspirate by experienced clinicians. Figure 3.49 shows two pleural effusions; the first measures 2.2 cm in depth and the second measures 11 cm in depth. The distance between the skin and the pleural cavity can also be measured to guide the user to the expected depth of needle insertion to achieve an aspirate.

Case – Decreasing Length of Stay and Improving Patient Journey

A 76-year-old man presented with acute dyspnoea on a background of lifelong smoking. He had significant red flag features including a persistent cough with occasional haemoptysis and weight loss. His CXR revealed a complete white out of the right lung. LUS demonstrated a large right-sided effusion and an inverted diaphragm due to pressure from the pleural fluid (Figure 3.50).

Urgent thoracocentesis was performed which immediately relieved his shortness of breath (Figure 3.50). Pleural fluid was blood tinged and

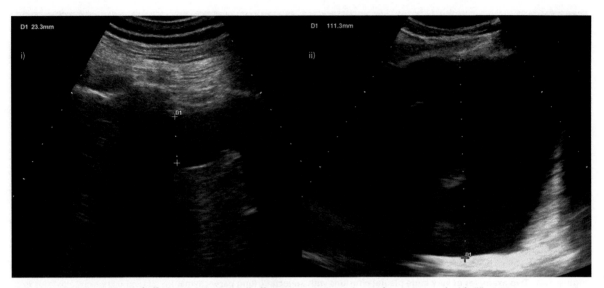

Figure 3.49 Measurement of effusion depth. (i) Small effusion measuring 2.3 cm when compared with (ii) at 11.1 cm. Measuring the depth of the subcutaneous tissue above the thoracic cavity will guide the user to the expected depth of needle insertion prior to obtaining an aspirate.

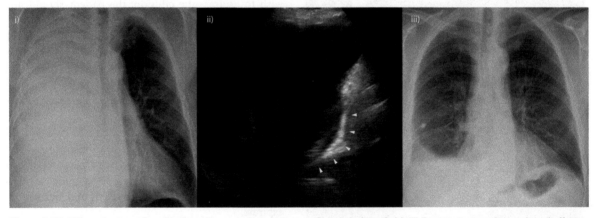

Figure 3.50 This patient was found to have (i) a complete whiteout of his right lung field. (ii) Demonstrates a large pleural effusion with deviation of the diaphragm (arrows). (iii) CXR showing resolution of the fluid after insertion of an intercostal drain.

exudative. The drain was in situ for <24 hours and he was discharged home with an urgent CT request and follow-up with the lung cancer team.

Pleural fluid analysis confirmed a small cell lung cancer and he was promptly referred to the oncology team for further treatment and management. This case highlights the importance of urgent thoraco-centesis for symptomatic and diagnostic purposes, expediting discharge and avoiding unnecessary hospital stay. US empowered the frontline clinicians to perform the procedure promptly and fast-track his pathway through the hospital and outpatient settings.

Parapneumonic Effusions, Complex Effusions and Empyema

Parapneumonic effusions occur in up to 40% of patients with pneumonia and are associated with a higher mortality rate due to development of empyema or lung abscess.

Small parapneumonic effusions tend to resolve with basic antibiotic therapy. Larger effusions often require drainage which, if complex, may need fibrinolytic therapy or surgical intervention. All significant parapneumonic effusions should be aspirated to exclude biochemical features of empyema (low pH < 7.2; low glucose <3.4 mmol/l; high lactate dehydrogenase (LDH) > 100 IU/l).

An empyema may appear as a simple pleural effusion that is only diagnosed following pleural aspirate and fluid analysis. In other cases, debris may be seen swirling within the effusion. This is known as the **plankton sign** (Figure 3.51) and is highly suggestive of an exudative pleural effusion, empyema or haemothorax.

If left untreated an empyema can become purulent, thick and loculated with fibrinous strands and adhesions (Figure 3.52). These effusions are challenging to manage as thoracocentesis is often unsuccessful and fibrinolytics/surgery may be required.

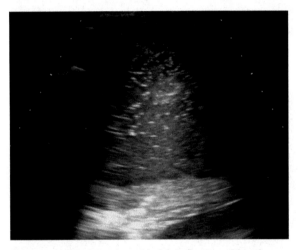

Figure 3.51 Plankton sign with debris floating within the effusion. *A video is available to view in the online video library.*

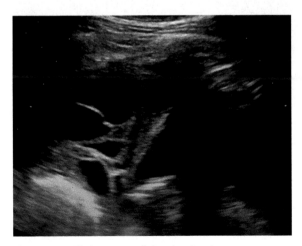

Figure 3.52 Fibrinous strands in a loculated empyema.

A loculated effusion is an example of a **complex effusion**. These are typically associated with causes of intense pleural inflammation such as empyema, tuberculosis and haemothorax. The gold standard for analysis of a complicated effusion is CT imaging and requires multidisciplinary input for management.

Case – Empyema

A 54-year-old man presented with fevers, cough and left-sided pleuritic chest pain. He was diagnosed with pneumonia with a CURB-65 score of 0. He mounted an appropriate inflammatory response and his observations were all within normal range. He was commenced on a regime of oral antibiotics by the GP as per regional antimicrobial guidelines.

Forty-eight hours later the patient presented to Ambulatory Care with worsening symptoms despite appropriate antibiotic therapy. He continued to spike temperatures and his inflammatory markers were significantly elevated.

Chest X-ray revealed left-sided basal and upper zone consolidation and a moderate left-sided pleural effusion (Figure 3.53i). LUS examination revealed an effusion measuring 5 cm in maximal depth and anterior consolidation (Figure 3.53ii). There was no evidence of fibrinous strands or loculations within the effusion.

A LUS-guided aspiration revealed a pH of 6.9 and pleural fluid glucose of 0.6 mmol/L consistent with an empyema. A chest drain was inserted in Ambulatory Care and the patient's condition improved over the course of 24–48 hours.

Lung ultrasound was instrumental in this case highlighting a cause for this gentleman's lack of response to conventional treatment. There is often difficulty in differentiation between consolidation and effusion on a CXR, whilst LUS is significantly more sensitive in detecting the presence of fluid.

Case – Ultrasound Is Critical in Challenging Thoracentesis

A 45-year-old man presented after 3 weeks of being unwell with cough, fevers and left-sided chest pain. He had a dislike of hospitals and was not keen to be admitted. His CXR revealed a left-sided moderate effusion (Figure 3.54i) and LUS demonstrated a very complex effusion with loculations and fibrinous strands (Figure 3.54ii).

Pleural aspiration was initially unsuccessful and the intercostal drain required multiple attempts prior

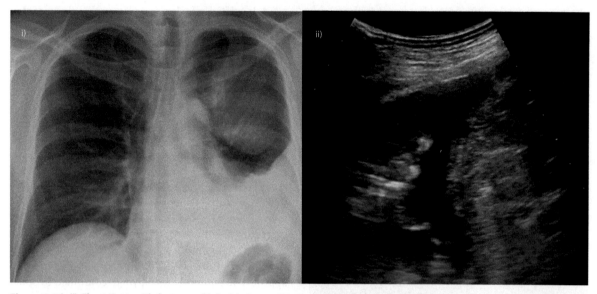

Figure 3.53 (i) Chest X-ray with features of left-sided consolidation with a pleural effusion. (ii) Lung ultrasound confirming consolidation with a simple pleural effusion.

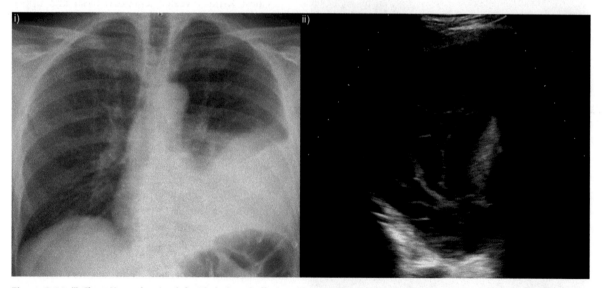

Figure 3.54 (i) Chest X-ray showing left-sided pleural effusion. (ii) Lung ultrasound revealing a complex pleural effusion that is heavily septated and loculated. *A video is available to view in the online video library.*

to successful insertion and fibrinolytic administration. After two days the drain became blocked and the patient was transferred to the cardiothoracic surgical team who performed video-assisted thoracoscopic surgery (VATS) for drainage. Although required in this case, it is important to remember that surgical procedures have significantly higher rates of chronic pain and bleeding compared to conventional methods of drain and fibrinolysis.

Case – Lung Ultrasound Is Superior to Chest X-Ray

A 28-year-old lady from India presented with a 4 month history of weight loss, fevers and productive cough. Her CXR revealed a moderate left-sided effusion (Figure 3.55i) and LUS showed a large, complex, loculated effusion (Figure 3.55ii). The largest loculation was chosen using LUS and drainage was successful.

Her sputum and pleural acid fast Bacilli (AFB) were positive and she was treated with anti-tuberculosis

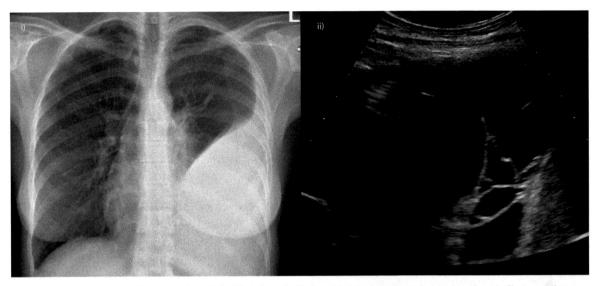

Figure 3.55 (i) Chest X-ray showing a large left-sided pleural effusion. (ii) A large, septated, complex pleural effusion on lung ultrasound. *A video is available to view in the online video library.*

treatment (ATT). She was safely and successfully discharged into the community for close monitoring whilst treatment was completed.

Tuberculosis is one of the top ten causes of death worldwide and is the leading cause of death by a single infectious agent. Multi-drug resistant TB (MDR-TB) remains a public health crisis. TB is curable if presentation is early enough and clinicians in high-risk areas should remain vigilant for symptoms consistent with the disease.

Haemothorax

A haemothorax describes the presence of blood within the pleural space and is usually traumatic. LUS features are variable depending upon when the patient presents. It may appear as an anechoic, hypoechoic or hyperechoic effusion with swirling sediment. With time, the blood will begin to clot and become increasingly hyperechoic. The **plankton sign** may be present and has already been discussed in the earlier text. The **haematocrit sign** refers to the echogenic layering of material within a pleural effusion.

Case – The Plankton Sign on Ultrasound

A 45-year-old male presented to his GP one week after a day of excessive alcohol drinking with his friends. At the time he had recalled an altercation but unfortunately did not remember the details. Over the week, he noted increasing chest discomfort, a persistent, non-productive cough and dyspnoea on exertion.

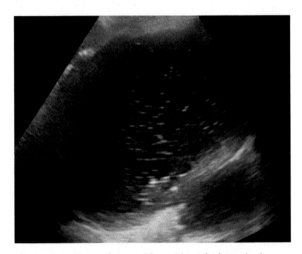

Figure 3.56 Haemothorax with positive 'plankton sign'.

Examination revealed significant bruising over his back and reduced air entry to the left side of his chest. The GP performed a focused LUS that demonstrated a large pleural effusion with a positive plankton sign (Figure 3.56). In view of the assault and bruising this was in keeping with a haemothorax. He was referred urgently to the ED where a large bore intercostal drain (ICD) was inserted which drained blood. The patient was referred promptly to the cardiothoracic team.

Case – Blood in the Chest

An 85-year-old attended the ED two days after falling from a ladder and landing on his right side. He complained of severe right-sided chest pain and presented in extreme respiratory distress. He was on warfarin for atrial fibrillation. Emergency LUS was done which confirmed a haemothorax (Figure 3.57). There was a positive haematocrit sign with a large volume effusion. When aspirated this confirmed blood and an urgent large bore chest drain was inserted and he was referred to the cardiothoracic team. His warfarin was reversed with vitamin K and prothrombin complex concentrate.

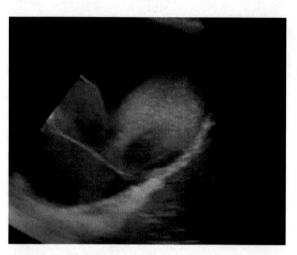

Figure 3.57 Lung ultrasound showing large pleural effusion with mixed echogenicity and a positive haematocrit sign. *A video is available to view in the online video library.*

Both these case studies illustrate the value of LUS in diagnosing haemothorax which if left untreated can be life threatening. LUS enables prompt intervention with an ICD and referral to the cardio thoracic team.

Hydropneumothorax

A hydropneumothorax is a combination of a pleural effusion and pneumothorax. There are many causes including trauma, bronchial or oesophageal fistula, rupture of a lung abscess and gas-forming organisms.

Case – Hydropneumothorax

A 23-year-old homeless male with a background of intravenous drug use was found on the street with respiratory distress. An urgent CXR revealed significant mediastinal shift with a large left-sided pleural effusion and suggestion of pneumothorax (Figure 3.58i). LUS showed a large effusion with the plankton sign (Figure 3.58ii). In addition there was an absence of lung sliding.

Computerised tomography scan revealed a large hydropneumothorax with underlying severe compressive atelectasis of the left lung and mediastinal shift to the right. The patient had an urgent intercostal drain inserted which relieved his symptoms.

The aetiology was due to an underlying lung abscess due to intravenous drug use which had been present for some time. Unfortunately, he self-discharged two days after his admission.

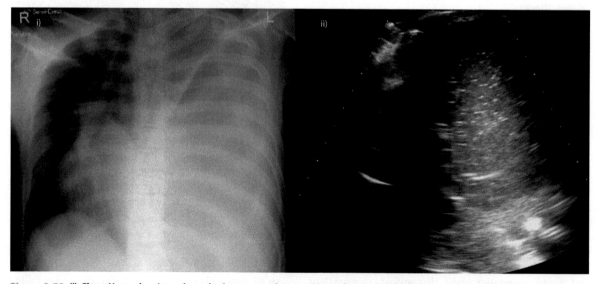

Figure 3.58 (i) Chest X-ray showing a large hydropneumothorax with mediastinal shift. (ii) Lung ultrasound demonstrating plankton sign due to longstanding pleural effusion secondary to lung abscess. *A video is available to view in the online video library.*

Asthma and Chronic Obstructive Pulmonary Disease

Obstructive airway disease will often produce no sonographic signs unless infective exacerbations are associated with consolidation. Normal findings such as lung sliding and A Lines will be present. In severe bronchospasm the lung sliding will be significantly diminished due to poor ventilation.

Lung ultrasound may be useful in excluding alternative diagnoses, e.g. pulmonary oedema or pneumothorax, which will contribute towards a diagnosis of asthma or COPD.

Pulmonary Embolism

Similarly to obstructive airway disease, there are few signs that contribute towards diagnosing pulmonary emboli as a cause of acute shortness of breath. A normal LUS assessment, following the BLUE protocol, increases the probability of pulmonary emboli although this is not specific.

Small peripheral emboli may be identified by well demarcated **'wedge' shapes** although clinically this does not have great significance.

Patients may develop pulmonary infarction which subsequently leads to consolidation. Anterior consolidations can be the first sign of this (Figure 3.59). Further signs which may assist in diagnosing large PE, including echocardiographic interrogation of the right heart and lower leg vascular US for DVT, will be discussed in their respective chapters.

Thoracocentesis

Lung ultrasound is instrumental in performing safe pleural aspiration and intercostal drain insertion with proven evidence of lower risk of pneumothorax and bleeding complications. It may be performed either by US assistance with marking of the region or through direct real-time guidance.

This procedure is frequently performed in the ambulatory setting and training of clinicians in image guidance is important to facilitate an efficient patient journey. Evidence suggests an effusion of >1 cm is safe to aspirate under LUS and under experienced hands.

It is wise to stay within the 'safe triangle' (Figure 3.60) to minimise the risk of damage to local structures. A curvilinear or linear probe may then be used to interrogate the area and identify the best location for needle insertion. Remaining anterior to the posterior axillary line is advised to minimise risk to the neurovascular bundle.

Measurement of distance between the skin and the anterior border of the pleural space provides the clinician with an idea of what depth to expect to penetrate the parietal pleura. The depth of effusion can also be measured to ascertain margin of safety and to select the optimal location for thoracocentesis. This has previously been discussed with examples of effusion size (Figure 3.49).

If using LUS to directly guide needle insertion it is important to insert the needle at 90 degrees to the skin in the identical plane to the US.

Steps must be taken to ensure sterility by using a probe sheath and sterile gel.

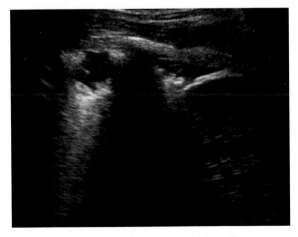

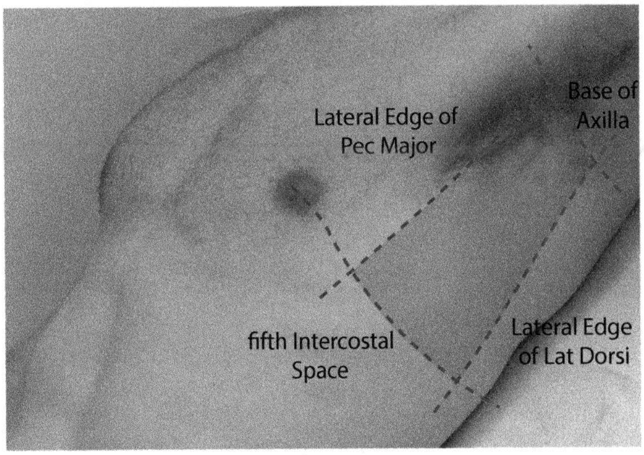

Figure 3.59 Example of anterior consolidation after a pulmonary embolism causing pulmonary infarction and subsequent infection.

Lateral Edge of Pec Major

Base of Axilla

fifth Intercostal Space

Lateral Edge of Lat Dorsi

Figure 3.60 The 'safe triangle' is bordered by the base of the axilla, the lateral edge of pectoralis major, the lateral edge of the latissimus dorsi and the fifth intercostal space.

Summary

- Lung ultrasound is the most simple US application to learn and acquire competence.
- The specificity and sensitivity of LUS is superior to chest radiographs and may circumvent the need to move the patient from their environment or expose them to radiation. The use at the bedside can identify key pathology in both the hospitalised and community patient.
- We advocate the use of the BLUE protocol as a quick tool for assessing key lung fields. This can then be extended to incorporate a more detailed interrogation guided by examination findings.
- In addition to diagnosis, LUS may be used to assess response to long-term treatment. This is particularly useful in the titration of diuretic therapy in patients suffering from congestive cardiac failure.
- Lung ultrasound is mandated for all pleural procedures to ensure safety for patients by improving success rate and decreasing complications.

A full list of references and further reading is available at: www.GeneralistUltrasound.com

Abdominal Ultrasound

Introduction

Abdominal US may appear daunting to the inexperienced user and a full system interrogation is beyond the scope of this book. It is important to approach this assessment with a clear, focused question guided by clinical history and examination to avoid encountering difficulties.

The individual aspects of abdominal point-of-care ultrasound (POCUS) are simplistic but frequently complicated by body habitus, bowel gas and a poorly optimised patient. For example, pelvic ultrasound is challenging without a full bladder, the gallbladder may not be visualised if the patient is not fasted and parts of the aorta are frequently obstructed by bowel gas limiting the ability to exclude aneurysm.

The abdominal systems that are assessed in POCUS include the abdominal aorta, inferior vena cava (IVC), hepatobiliary, renal tract, assessment for free fluid (ascites or blood e.g. focused assessment with sonography in trauma, FAST) and for interventional procedures. This chapter will cover the basic principles of abdominal ultrasound and address each of these regions in turn. We will also consider more advanced abdominal topics including basic liver US, appendicitis and small bowel obstruction.

General Principles

A low frequency (3–5 MHz) curvilinear probe is used to provide visualisation of deep structures (Figure 4.1). A lower frequency (1–5 MHz) may achieve better penetration in larger patients. A phased array or microconvex probe is helpful if the acoustic windows require a smaller footprint. A high frequency linear probe can be used for assessment of the gastrointestinal tract or for direct visualisation of needling during abdominal paracentesis.

It is important to gain familiarity with the echogenicity of key structures to orientate oneself with the intra-abdominal anatomy. Understanding what is 'normal' will aid in identification of key pathological findings. Examples of probe placements with the normal sonoanatomy are demonstrated in Figure 4.2.

Initial approach to point of care abdominal US depends on the indication. The user should ensure the probe marker is directed cranially with a sagittal approach and to the patient's right in a transverse approach. It is important to select an abdominal preset on the machine with the marker on the left side of the screen (Figure 4.3).

Conventionally if assessing for free fluid the right upper quadrant 'flank' view is chosen first. This enables visualisation of the diaphragm, liver, Morison's pouch, right kidney and occasionally the gallbladder. The right flank may be used as an alternative view for major vascular abdominal structures including the IVC and abdominal aorta. The left flank requires a more posterior approach due to the spleen being smaller in size. The diaphragm, spleen, splenorenal recess, and left kidney are seen. Transverse and sagittal views of the pelvis can be acquired in the suprapubic region directly superior to the pubic symphysis. The US beam must be angled inferiorly into the pelvic cavity to identify anatomy. In males, the bladder, prostate, rectum and small bowel loops can be seen here. In females the uterus lies superior to the bladder with the vagina behind the posterior bladder wall.

The major abdominal vessels are assessed with the probe placed in transverse and sagittal views at the epigastrium. The aorta should be tracked inferiorly through identification of key branches including the coeliac axis, superior mesenteric artery (SMA) and the bifurcation into right and left common iliac arteries. The IVC can be located laterally to the aorta on the patient's right-hand side and is seen to drain directly into the right atrium. The hepatic veins drain into the IVC proximally to the right atrium and are a key landmark for differentiating between the aorta and IVC.

Although detailed assessment of the liver is beyond the scope of this book, knowledge of key structures is helpful in orientation and interpretation of pathology. A right oblique subcostal view allows the right and left hepatic lobes to be interrogated and the convergence of the three hepatic veins into the IVC. The gallbladder has a very variable axis and can be seen anywhere from the abdominal midline to mid-axillary line. A transverse view is useful to initially locate the gallbladder and surrounding structures before attempting to rotate the probe for image optimisation.

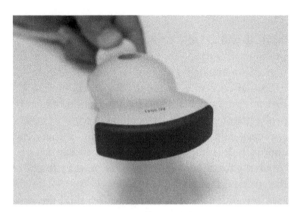

Figure 4.1 The curvilinear probe.

Figure 4.3 For abdominal ultrasound the user should select a curvilinear probe, abdominal preset and ensure the probe marker is located on the left-hand side of the screen (circled).

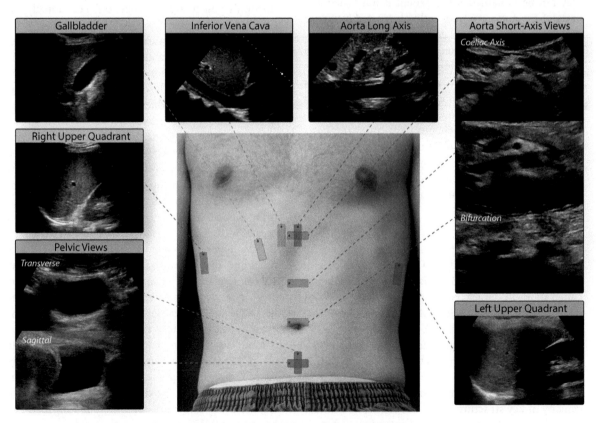

Figure 4.2 Probe placement and notch direction to achieve all basic abdominal windows.

The Abdominal Aorta

Interrogation of the abdominal aorta is one of the most commonly performed POCUS scans in the ED and screening for abdominal aortic aneurysm (AAA) is advised in all males aged over 65 years.

The indication for scanning the abdominal aorta is predominantly to identify the presence of an aneurysm. Although aortic dissection may occasionally be seen extending within the abdominal cavity, CT is required for accurate diagnosis and to identify complications.

Anatomy

The abdominal aorta is a retroperitoneal structure which originates as a continuation of the descending thoracic aorta at the diaphragm. It lies anterior to the vertebral bodies until its bifurcation into the right and left common iliac arteries at approximately the level of the fourth lumbar vertebra (L4). The key branches identified during sonographic assessment are the coeliac axis, superior mesenteric artery (SMA) and its bifurcation (Figure 4.4). The aorta runs parallel to the IVC and differentiation between the structures can be challenging for the inexperienced user. The IVC and its differentiating features will be considered separately within this chapter.

Pathological Findings

Aneurysm

An arterial aneurysm is defined as a focal dilation of a blood vessel. The most common type is a fusiform aneurysm which is a symmetrical expansion of the entire circumference of the vessel. This is also known as a true aneurysm. Saccular aneurysms, also known as pseudoaneurysms, are asymmetrical localised dilations forming a sac-like swelling commonly caused by trauma to the vessel. Lifetime incidence of an AAA is 8.9% in males and 2.2% in females with risk increasing with age. Around 90–95% of AAAs are localised to the infra-renal aorta highlighting the importance of assessing the full aortic tract. Additionally, although the vast majority of intra-abdominal aneurysms are aortic in origin, involvement of the iliac, splenic or renal vessels can occur.

Rupture of an AAA is associated with a 60–80% mortality rate despite advances in treatment and early identification may allow surgical or endovascular

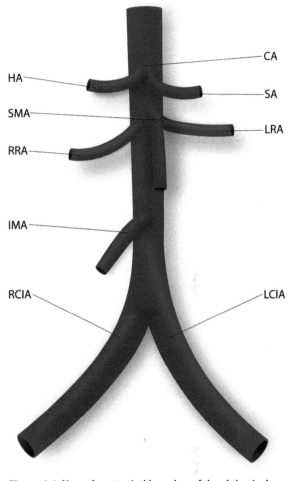

Figure 4.4 Normal anatomical branches of the abdominal aorta. CA, coeliac axis; SA, splenic artery; HA, hepatic artery; SMA, superior mesenteric artery; LRA, left renal artery; RRA, right renal artery; IMA, inferior mesenteric artery; LCIA, left common iliac artery; RCIA, right common iliac artery.

intervention prior to this outcome. The normal diameter of the abdominal aorta is 1.4 cm to 2.5 cm and once it reaches 3 cm it is classed as aneurysmal. The common iliac arteries have a normal calibre of 1.1 cm to 1.4 cm and are aneurysmal when greater than 1.4 cm. The risk of rupture is dependent on the size and expansion rate. An AAA measuring between 4.5 cm and 5.5 cm has an annual risk of rupture of 2–4% with a mortality rate for open surgical repair of 5%. Beyond 5.5 cm the risk of rupture exceeds the risk of surgery and intervention may be offered. Endovascular repair is associated with significantly lower morbidity and mortality rates than elective open surgical repair and may be considered in higher risk patient cohorts.

The NHS offers screening to all male patients aged 65 and over. The Royal College of Emergency Medicine (RCEM) suggest consideration of AAA leak or rupture in all patients over the age of 50 with abdominal, flank or back pain and hypotension. Clinical assessment of the abdominal aorta is unreliable and the use of US by non-radiologists to identify AAA has been suggested to have a high sensitivity (94–100%) and specificity (99–100%).

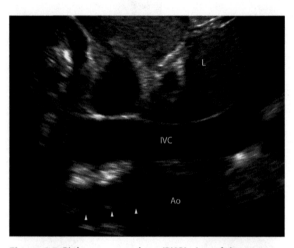

Figure 4.5 Right upper quadrant (RUQ) view of the aorta and IVC demonstrating dissection flap in the abdominal aorta (arrows). This patient sustained an iatrogenic aortic dissection during cannulation for cardiopulmonary bypass. The subcostal windows were unavailable due to post-operative drains and therefore the RUQ window was selected. Ao, aorta; IVC, inferior vena cava; L, liver. *A video is available to view in the online video library.*

Aortic Dissection

Contrast CT is the imaging modality of choice for aortic dissection. US may occasionally reveal an intimal flap within the abdominal aorta and colour flow Doppler or pulse wave Doppler can be used to identify blood flow within the true and false lumens (Figure 4.5).

Although an important incidental finding it is essential not to use US to rule out an aortic dissection.

Transthoracic echocardiogram (TTE) and transoesophageal echocardiogram (TOE) are used to identify any complications associated with aortic dissections including valvular incompetence and cardiac tamponade (Figure 4.6).

Method

Imaging of the aorta begins at the epigastrium with both transverse and sagittal views. A low frequency curvilinear probe (3 MHz) should be used with an abdominal preset (medium to low dynamic range). The aorta will be found overlying the vertebral bodies and image depth should be optimised to limit the field of view beyond this. Tracking distally will reveal the coeliac axis followed by the SMA as the aorta gradually decreases in depth before the bifurcation (Figure 4.7, 4.8, 4.9 and 4.10).

The right or left flank coronal view may be considered as an alternative approach to view the aorta if bowel gas is obscuring the abdominal vessels (Figure 4.11). As previously mentioned, it is essential to image the aorta throughout its entire course in

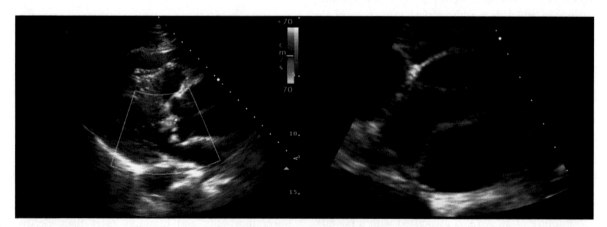

Figure 4.6 Echo of patient with type A aortic dissection. (i) PLAX view showing dilated ascending aorta with visible dissection flap, aortic regurgitation colour jet and a pericardial effusion. (ii) Modified aortic view demonstrating the appearance of a dissection flap on US. *Videos are available to view in the online video library.*

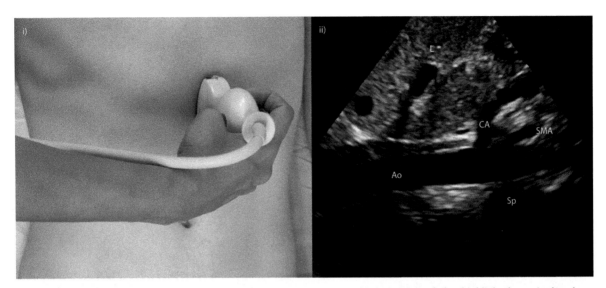

Figure 4.7 (i) Probe location to achieve a long axis view of the aorta. Note this image is angled to highlight the sagittal probe orientation and the probe should be placed perpendicular to the skin in the midline. (ii) Key anatomical structures. The coeliac axis and superior mesenteric artery branches are the major landmarks and can help to differentiate between the aorta and IVC. Ao, aorta; Sp, spine; CA, coeliac axis; SMA, superior mesenteric artery; L, liver.

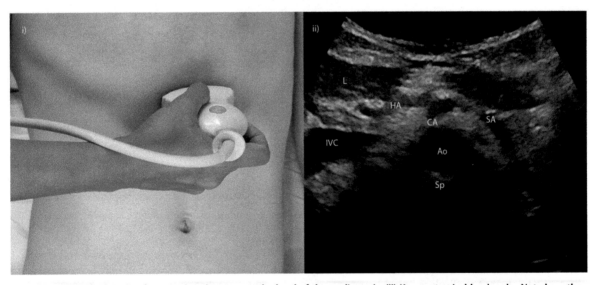

Figure 4.8 (i) Probe location for scanning the aorta at the level of the coeliac axis. (ii) Key anatomical landmarks. Note how the aorta directly overlies the vertebral bodies behind which there is acoustic shadowing. Ao, aorta; Sp, spine; CA, coeliac axis; HA, hepatic artery; SA, splenic artery; IVC, inferior vena cava; L, liver.

both transverse and sagittal planes to ensure an aneurysm is not missed.

If an aneurysm is present, the maximal anteroposterior (AP) diameter is measured from the outer edges of the vessel wall in transverse (out of plane) and sagittal (in plane) views. AP measurement is preferred because the lateral walls may be obscured by bowel gas and US has relatively poor lateral resolution. Longstanding aneurysms may be calcified and contain mural thrombus which may be confused for surrounding tissue causing significant underestimation of size. Care must be taken to ensure a perpendicular slice is measured to avoid under- or overestimation of the vessel calibre (Figure 4.12).

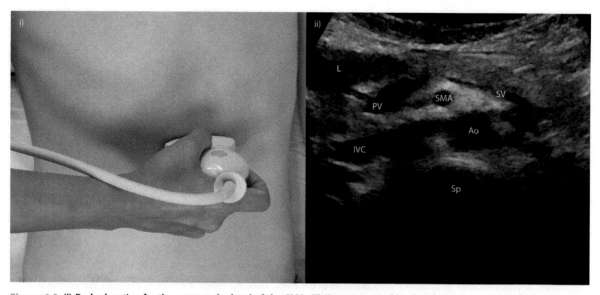

Figure 4.9 (i) Probe location for the aorta at the level of the SMA. (ii) Key anatomical landmarks. Ao, aorta; Sp, spine; SMA, superior mesenteric artery; SV, splenic vein; PV, portal vein; IVC, inferior vena cava; L, liver.

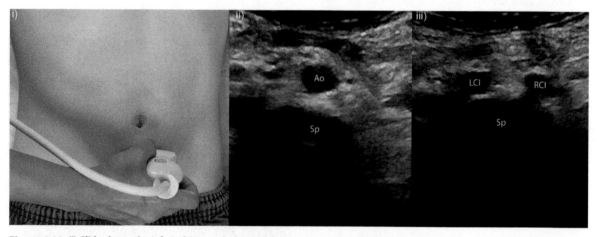

Figure 4.10 (i) Slide the probe inferiorly to track the path of the aorta (ii) until its bifurcation into the common iliac arteries (iii). Ao, aorta; Sp, spine; LCl, left common iliac artery; RCl, right common iliac artery.

If bowel gas is obscuring the view of the aorta the user may apply some firm pressure whilst rocking the probe to attempt to displace bowel loops.

Ultrasound is unreliable in identifying a leak or rupture of an aneurysm and even a very large retroperitoneal haematoma is likely to be missed. If this is suspected in the acute setting it is important to seek further diagnostic imaging (CT) or urgent vascular surgical involvement.

Key Points

- A low frequency curvilinear probe should be used to interrogate the abdominal aorta in transverse and sagittal views along its entire course.

- Abdominal aortic aneuryms are common and should be considered in all male patients over 50 years of age with abdominal, flank or back pain.

- If an aneurysm is present, the maximum anteroposterior (AP) diameter should be measured from the outer edges of the vessel wall.

- Ultrasound cannot reliably rule out a leak as the majority of patients surviving to hospital will have retroperitoneal bleeds. Contrast CT is the imaging modality of choice to confirm leak or rupture.

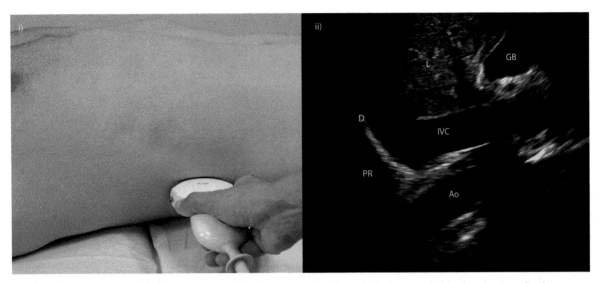

Figure 4.11 (i) Probe placement to acquire a RUQ view of the aorta and IVC. (ii) Key anatomical landmarks. Note the deeper location of the aorta compared to the IVC. Ao, aorta; IVC, inferior vena cava; L, liver; GB, gallbladder; D, diaphragm; PR, pleural recess.

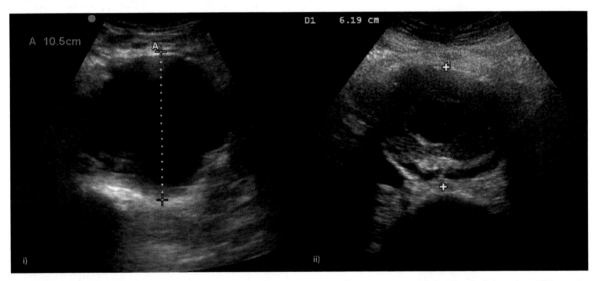

Figure 4.12 (i) Extremely large AAA measuring 10.5 cm. (ii) An example of an aneurysm with intraluminal thrombus. This emphasises the importance of outer edge to outer edge measurement of the calibre to avoid significant underestimation.

The Inferior Vena Cava

The use of the IVC for assessment of volume status and right atrial pressure is discussed in Chapter 2. This chapter will highlight key anatomical differences to identify the IVC and differentiate from other structures within the abdomen.

Anatomy

The IVC is located to the right of the aorta and has a very short thoracic course before draining into the right atrium. As it is the major capacitance vessel within the body it has a very variable size depending on fluid filling status. If a patient is severely hypovolaemic the IVC may be difficult to identify for non-experienced sonographers. It exhibits pulsatility with cardiac beat-to-beat variation and respiratory variation during inspiration. The walls are much thinner than the aorta and the degree of compressibility can be used to indirectly estimate right atrial pressure.

The major landmark to identify is the junction of the hepatic veins which join the IVC just below the

103

diaphragm. Figure 4.13 shows the normal anatomy of the IVC.

Method

Assessment of the IVC follows the same process as for the transverse and sagittal views of the aorta using a low frequency (1–5 MHz) curvilinear or phased array probe (Figure 4.14).

The IVC lies to the right of the aorta and should be seen to drain into the right atrium. Measurements are taken 1–3 cm below the junction with the hepatic veins in either B-mode or M-mode. A longitudinal (sagittal) view with M-mode is the most commonly used view within echocardiography and the patient may be asked to 'sniff' to reduce intrathoracic pressure and aid IVC collapse. As with imaging of the aorta it is

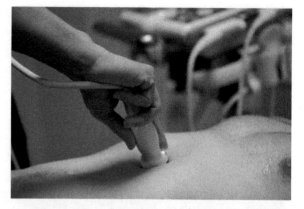

Figure 4.14 Typical probe location for the IVC view. Note the probe marker is pointing upwards towards the patient's head.

important to consider the potential for underestimation of IVC size if the 'in-plane' view is not perpendicular to the vessel highlighting the importance of utilising transverse and sagittal approaches together. Collapsibility index may be calculated to apply a percentage to the degree of IVC collapse during respiration which is used to estimate right atrial pressure (Figure 4.15).

The right flank view may be used to identify the IVC when the view is obscured from the midline approach. This is more technically challenging than imaging from the midline and it may be difficult to distinguish from the aorta.

It is important to appreciate that IVC calibre and collapsibility is influenced by many factors including congestive heart failure, valvular disease, pulmonary hypertension and cardiac tamponade. Hepatic fibrosis and cirrhosis may limit the ability of the IVC to collapse due to structural tethering. Collapsibility is an unreliable surrogate of right atrial pressure and should be used with caution as an isolated measure of volume status. Please see Chapter 2 for more information about haemodynamic assessment.

Key Points

- Both the aorta and IVC should be recognised and differentiated.
- The IVC should be assessed in both transverse and sagittal planes.
- Size and collapsibility of the IVC may be used as a surrogate marker of right atrial pressure and volume status. It is inherently an inaccurate measure and care should be taken to consider factors which may mimic hypo- or hypervolaemia.

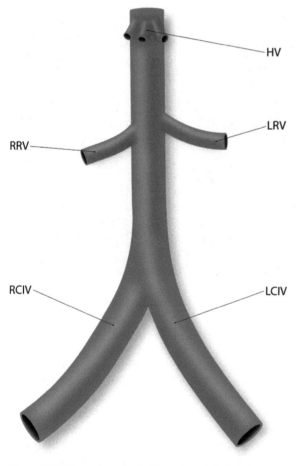

Figure 4.13 Normal anatomical branches of the inferior vena cava. HV, hepatic veins; LRV, left renal vein; RRV, right renal vein; LCIV, left common iliac vein; RCIV, right common iliac vein.

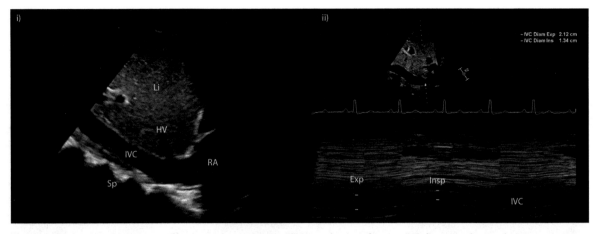

Figure 4.15 (i) Normal IVC view with structural annotations. (ii) M-mode view showing IVC diameter change during respiratory cycle with inspiratory and expiratory measurements. IVC, inferior vena cava; RA, right atrium; HV, hepatic vein; Li, liver; Sp, spinous processes; Exp, expiration; Insp, inspiration. *A video is available to view in the online video library.*

Abdominal Free Fluid and Focused Assessment with Sonography in Trauma

The use of POCUS for identification of free fluid in the abdomen is widely practiced in EDs to identify haemorrhage in trauma. Although the use of trauma CT has largely superseded FAST in major trauma centres, the use of US is popular in the prehospital and district hospital setting. Transfer of an unstable patient to CT is not without risk and the identification of free fluid with US, presumed to be blood in the trauma setting, may expedite a decision to proceed to surgery.

Focused assessment with sonography in trauma aims to identify free fluid in potential spaces within the abdomen and the same principles can be applied to any circumstances where free fluid may be present including ascites or organ rupture (e.g. intestinal, splenic or ectopic pregnancy rupture). This chapter will consider general approaches to identification of free fluid prior to discussing specific indications.

General Principles

Free fluid will accumulate in dependent regions within the abdomen that may be targeted in a focused assessment. Fluid appears black on US and knowledge of the echogenicity of landmark structures with optimised machine settings is essential for image interpretation.

A low frequency (3–5 MHz) curvilinear probe is used with an abdominal preset. Initial depth should be set to around 15 cm and optimised for each

patient. A microconvex or phased array probe may be used if a smaller footprint is required. The major 'windows' with commonly acquired landmarks are as follows:

- Right upper quadrant (RUQ): diaphragm, liver, Morison's pouch, right kidney and occasionally gallbladder. May be extended to the right pleural cavity in trauma to identify haemothorax.
- Left upper quadrant (LUQ): diaphragm, spleen, splenorenal recess and left kidney. May be extended to the left pleural cavity as described above.
- Pelvic/suprapubic view: bladder, rectum, small bowel loops, prostate in males and uterus and vagina in females.
- Right or left iliac fossa: useful as a safe location for US-guided paracentesis.
- Subxiphoid view: an extension to the traditional FAST scan to identify pericardial fluid.

The RUQ is the most common initial window to acquire and may demonstrate free fluid in up to 66% of positive FAST exams. The probe is placed in the right flank in a sagittal plane with the probe marker pointing cranially (Figure 4.16i). From this position the probe may be rotated to lie parallel to the ribs to reduce acoustic shadowing artefact obscuring the image.

In normal subjects the diaphragm resides on the left of the screen with the liver beneath. In the absence of pleural fluid there may be mirror image artefact of the liver on the opposite side of the diaphragm which

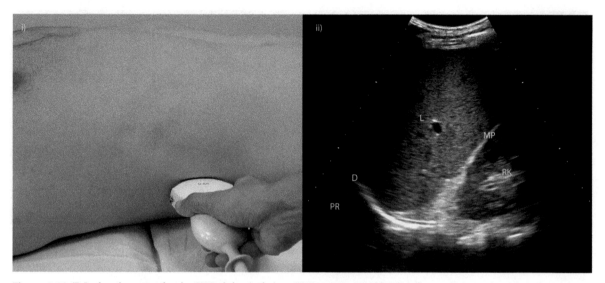

Figure 4.16 **(i) Probe placement for the RUQ abdominal view. (ii) Key anatomical landmarks on ultrasound.** L, liver; RK, right kidney; MP, Morison's pouch; D, diaphragm; PR, pleural recess.

is a normal finding. The liver is a large structure and therefore a reliable landmark to orientate the user within the abdomen. The liver and right kidney should be adjacent and separated by a hyperechoic layer of perinephric fat. This hepatorenal recess is known as Morison's pouch. The user should ensure the inferior pole of the kidney is visualised. It is found adjacent to the psoas muscle. Normal anatomy is demonstrated in Figure 4.16ii.

A static image is unlikely to be sufficient to exclude the presence of free fluid and once the landmarks have been identified the user should 'fan' the probe to fully interrogate the potential spaces. The inferior margin of the liver is frequently missed from an assessment and may be the only location fluid can be identified. Free fluid will accumulate in any tissue plane and therefore will appear angular compared with fluid located within hollow viscera which have smooth edges. Positive RUQ exams are shown in Figure 4.17.

Key potential spaces to interrogate include:

- Right pleural recess (not abdominal free fluid but may guide further management).
- Subphrenic space: between liver and diaphragm.
- Morison's pouch: hepatorenal recess between the liver and right kidney.
- Inferior pole of the kidney: adjacent to colic gutter.

The LUQ window may be more challenging to optimise due to the relatively small size of the spleen and a

more posterior approach is usually required. The probe is placed in the left flank in a sagittal plane with the probe marker pointing cranially (Figure 4.18). The user may be required to place their knuckles onto the bed to identify the landmarks. Once again this may be optimised by rotating the probe to be parallel with the ribs.

In normal subjects the diaphragm appears on the left of the screen with mirror artefact superiorly. Normal anatomy is demonstrated in Figure 4.18. The spleen has a similar echotexture to the liver and should be centred in the image. Potential spaces to be interrogated include:

- Left pleural recess.
- Subphrenic recess: between diaphragm and spleen.
- Splenorenal recess: between spleen and left kidney.
- Inferior pole of left kidney.

These areas require full interrogation as with the right upper quadrant. Fluid has a particular propensity to localise to the subphrenic recess and inferior pole of the spleen and therefore should be closely assessed (Figure 4.19).

The pelvic views are acquired by placing the probe superior to the pubic symphysis and will need to be angled caudally to identify pelvic organs. A transverse view is routinely performed first with the probe marker pointing to the patient's right (Figure 4.20). The longitudinal view will be acquired next in the abdominal midline with the probe marker pointing cranially

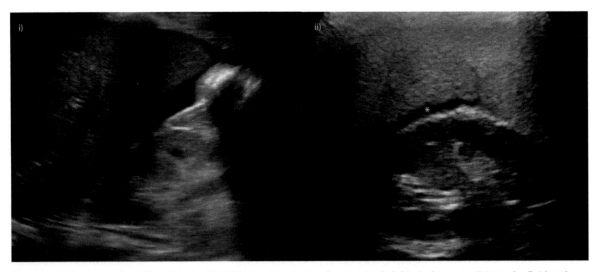

Figure 4.17 Two examples of free fluid in the RUQ view in patients who sustained abdominal trauma. (i) Note the fluid at the inferior margin of the liver. This should always be assessed during a FAST scan. (ii) Small volume of fluid noted in Morison's pouch (*).

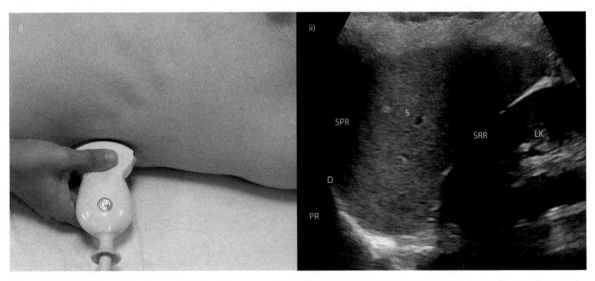

Figure 4.18 (i) Probe position to acquire the left upper quadrant abdominal view. (ii) Key anatomical landmarks on ultrasound. S, spleen; LK, left kidney; SRR, spleno-renal recess; SPR, sub-phrenic recess; D, diaphragm; PR, pleural recess.

(Figure 4.21). It is once again important to understand that a still image of the pelvis is not sufficient to exclude abdominal or pelvic free fluid and therefore detailed assessments of the potential spaces are required by systematically fanning through the image.

The major acoustic window in the pelvic view is the fluid-filled bladder. An empty bladder may make clear delineation of structures challenging. Furthermore, acoustic enhancement posterior to a full bladder may result in deeper structures appearing more echogenic and therefore 'brighter' on the image. The use of time gain compensation (TGC) to reduce the 'far gain' can optimise the image.

Key structures in normal individuals will evidently vary depending on the gender of the patient. In males, the small bowel is often identified superficially with the bladder and rectum posteriorly. The prostate and seminal vesicles may be seen behind the bladder.

In females the uterus lies cranially to the bladder with the vagina behind the posterior bladder wall.

107

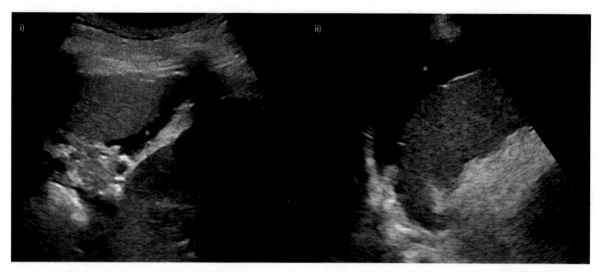

Figure 4.19 Two examples of free fluid (*) seen in the LUQ view. Note how in (i) the fluid is mostly in the spleno-renal recess where in (ii) it is mostly located in the sub-phrenic recess.

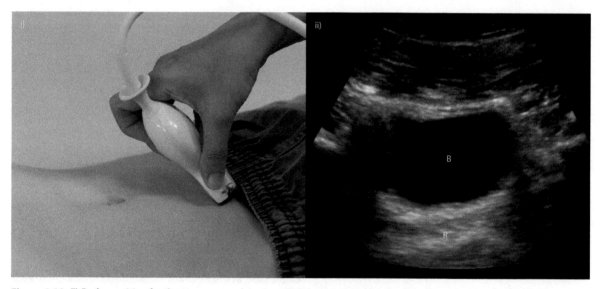

Figure 4.20 (i) Probe position for the transverse pelvic view. (ii) Key anatomical landmarks when assessing for free fluid. B, bladder; R, rectum.

A more detailed summary of basic pelvic US in females is discussed in Chapter 8.

Identification of small volumes of free fluid may be challenging to the inexperienced user. It is important to reinforce that fluid-filled viscera will have rounded edges whereas free fluid leads to formation of angular, 'pointy' hypoechoic collections (Figure 4.22).

Key potential spaces include:

- Surrounding bowel loops.

- Surrounding the bladder: superior, lateral and posterior.
- Rectovesical (male) or rectouterine (female) spaces: the rectouterine space is also commonly known as the Pouch of Douglas (POD).

Identification of bowel loops floating in free fluid is a straightforward finding. Pelvic fluid will typically accumulate first in the rectovesical space or the Pouch of Douglas (POD) and may be challenging to identify in suboptimal conditions. Small volumes

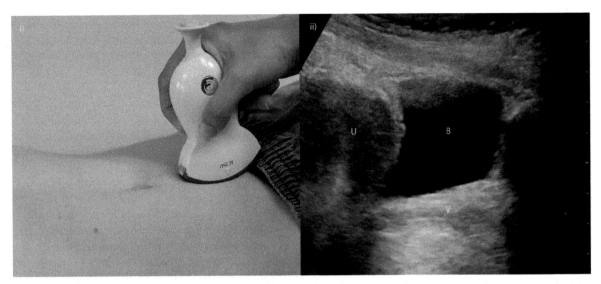

Figure 4.21 (i) Probe position for the sagittal view. (ii) Key anatomical landmarks in a female patient. B, bladder; U, uterus; V, vagina.

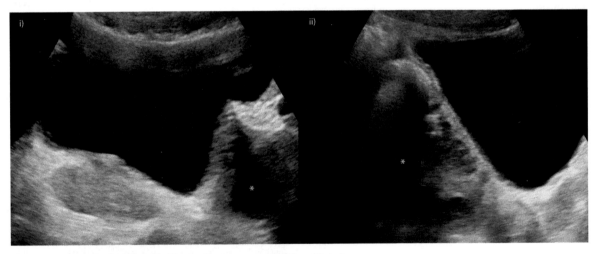

Figure 4.22 Free fluid (*) identified in the (i) transverse and (ii) sagittal views.

of fluid within the POD may be normal following ovulation.

Focused Assessment with Sonography in Trauma

The FAST algorithm is for use at the bedside or in prehospital settings to identify free fluid in the setting of trauma. It is an accelerated protocol which is extended to include the pleural cavity for haemothorax and the subxiphoid view for haemopericardium.

The role of US in major trauma centres has largely been replaced by protocolised trauma CT scanning for all major trauma patients. This allows accurate identification and description of all injuries sustained including visceral, intracranial and bony injuries. However, US is still utilised in many time-critical or low resource settings with the aim of streamlining management of major haemorrhage. Some potential settings are listed below:

- District general hospital or community setting where access to CT is limited.

- Identification of multisystem trauma in district hospitals prompting transfer to major trauma centres.
- Prehospital services (e.g. helicopter medicine) where early identification of bleeding can expedite mobilisation of trauma surgery at the destination hospital to bypass the resuscitation department.
- Serial scanning providing dynamic assessment of pathology in changeable clinical scenarios.
- Identification of bleeding in young patients without exposure to radiation – particularly the paediatric cohort.

In FAST the presence of abdominal free fluid is presumed to be blood. Many additional causes of free fluid must be considered in the context of the patient's past medical history. Furthermore, only acute bleeding will be seen as hypoechoic and clotted, organised blood may have a similar echogenic texture to visceral organs and muscle. This is particularly significant for haemopericardium where clotted blood may appear extremely similar to myocardium.

The FAST protocol is usually started with the RUQ window. If fluid is identified in this view, there is no utility in assessing any further abdominal windows as free fluid has been confirmed. It is still important to interrogate the pericardial and pleural spaces as definitive management of haemorrhage in these regions will often precede laparotomy.

Many criticisms of FAST result from the failure to perform a systematic assessment and is often performed by clinicians with insufficient experience. It must be considered an additional tool in the clinician's arsenal and used with care and consideration in addition to all conventional clinical assessment tools.

Rupture

The assessment of early pregnancy complications is discussed in Chapter 8 and therefore will not be considered in detail here.

The use of focused transabdominal US to identify free fluid in the setting of a suspected ruptured ectopic pregnancy has a significant evidence base as a rule in measure. It is essential to appreciate the limitations of US and maintain a differential diagnosis in the acute setting. Once again, it is a tool to guide investigations and management rather than exclude pathology.

Identification of free fluid may strengthen surgical referrals from the generalist and expedite definitive operative management. Cases of spontaneous rupture

of viscera, such as the stomach or spleen, can be diagnostically challenging and US may reveal time-critical pathology which requires urgent intervention.

Ascites

Ascites is a common clinical finding and will appear as a homogeneous, anechoic collection. Ascitic fluid with a volume of as little as 5–10 mls may be identified using US. Figure 4.23 shows a large quantity of ascites with underlying bowel.

Abdominal paracentesis is a common procedure performed in the acute and ambulatory setting. The use of US to confirm free fluid and to identify a location to aspirate significantly improves the safety of this procedure. Furthermore, colour Doppler may assist in localising superficial vessels to reduce the risk of bleeding from inadvertent puncture of the inferior epigastric arteries. This has resulted in the publication by the Society of Hospital Medicine to release a position statement advocating the use of US for paracentesis (Table 4.1).

The most common location for aspiration/paracentesis is the right or left iliac fossa. Callipers may be used, as in Figure 4.24, to measure the depth of the fluid before undertaking the procedure to provide reassurance that there is significant fluid volume and no underlying organs.

It is important not to move the patient after selection of location as the ascites may move within the abdominal cavity. A low frequency (3–5 MHz) transducer is used to identify and measure depth of the ascitic fluid volume. Measurement of the abdominal wall is useful to estimate the needle insertion depth

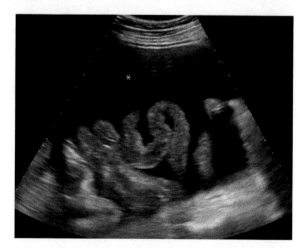

Figure 4.23 Ascites (*) with floating loops of small bowel.

Table 4.1

Society Of Hospital Medicine Recommendations on the use of ultrasound for adult abdominal paracentesis

US guidance should be used to reduce the risk of serious complications, the most common being bleeding.

US should be used to avoid attempting paracentesis in patients with insufficient volume to drain.

US will guide the volume, location and where paracentesis can occur safely.

The needle site should be evaluated by using colour flow Doppler to identify and avoid abdominal blood vessels.

Real time US is advised in patients where fluid collection is small or difficult to access.

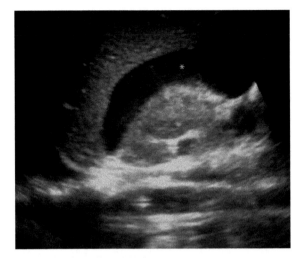

Figure 4.25 **Free fluid (*) noted in the spleno-renal recess secondary to spontaneous splenic rupture.**

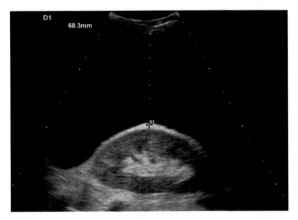

Figure 4.24 **Large volume of ascites with callipers used to measure depth between the abdominal wall and kidney.**

prior to reaching the abdominal cavity. Many centres will mark the skin before preparing for the sterile procedure. The use of a sterile probe cover is an additional option for real-time imaging during the procedure. If the procedure requires aspiration of a shallow pocket of fluid then a high frequency (5–12 MHz) linear probe may be beneficial to provide real time visualisation of the needle akin to in-plane vascular access.

Key Points

- Ultrasound may be used to identify free fluid in key dependent regions within the abdomen.
- Computerised tomography has largely replaced US in the trauma setting but may still have a role in the low resource and prehospital setting or for

non-traumatic pathology e.g. visceral rupture, ascites or to guide procedures.

- The basic 'FAST' views are a good introduction to abdominal scanning for novice users. This skill may familiarise clinicians with abdominal sonoanatomy and be built upon for assessment of other systems.

Case – A Surgical Emergency Diagnosed with Ultrasound

A 22-year-old male presented with epigastric and left upper quadrant abdominal pain. He had no past medical history and observations were unremarkable. He was considered to have gastritis and reassured. Prior to leaving the ED he felt increasingly unwell, became tachycardic and clinical examination demonstrated cool peripheries and worsening abdominal pain.

Bedside abdominal US demonstrated free fluid in all regions – most notably in the left upper quadrant (Figure 4.25).

Computerized tomography abdomen scan was performed at the request of the surgical team which demonstrated a perisplenic haematoma and haemoperitoneum suggestive of spontaneous splenic rupture.

He underwent splenectomy and was discharged from intensive care the following day and hospital five days later.

Although rare, spontaneous rupture of viscera may occur independent of trauma. US may aid in rapid identification of free fluid in acutely unwell patients with abdominal pain and guide further investigation and management.

111

Case – Reassess, Reassess, Reassess

A 34-year-old male presented with epigastric pain on a background of chronic alcohol misuse and chronic pancreatitis. He was confused, vomiting, and intoxicated at the time of assessment. Blood tests revealed mildly raised inflammatory markers and bedside US demonstrated no abdominal free fluid. He was suspected to have acute on chronic pancreatitis and admission was arranged with the surgical team.

After 30 minutes the nursing staff reported a deterioration in his observations and level of consciousness. He appeared increasingly unwell and transiently hypotensive. The abdominal tenderness was more severe and guarding present. US at the bedside was repeated and demonstrated free fluid in the right and left upper quadrants (Figure 4.26).

Computerized tomography was performed and revealed findings consistent with gastric perforation. He underwent surgical repair and was successfully discharged.

This case highlights the importance of serial assessments. Bedside US allows a 'time and place' snapshot of a patient much like clinical examination. If there is a change in the clinical picture then subsequent examination may reveal new findings. US provides a rapid, repeatable bedside assessment without exposing the patient to repeated doses of ionising radiation.

Renal Tract

Bedside assessment of the renal tract is primarily aimed at identifying hydronephrosis in patients presenting with acute kidney injury or abdominal or flank pain. Unilateral hydronephrosis is strongly suggestive of ureterolithiasis and bilateral hydronephrosis must always be identified in unexplained acute kidney injury.

Assessment of the renal tract consists of interrogation of both kidneys, ureters (if visible) and the bladder. The sensitivity of US is lower than that of abdominal and pelvic CT for identifying pathology but is rapidly available at the bedside without exposing the patient to radiation. US may be used to guide the need for further investigations and aid the referral process.

Anatomy

The kidneys are retroperitoneal structures that lie within the paravertebral gutters. They typically extend from T11 to L2–L3 with the right kidney situated more inferiorly due to adjacency to the liver. They lie with a tilted axis with the superior pole lying more posteriorly compared to the inferior pole.

The kidneys consist of three distinct layers: the *cortex, medulla* and *sinus* with a surrounding *capsule* (Figure 4.27):

- **Capsule** – a tough fibrous layer that encapsulates the kidney and adrenal gland.
- **Cortex** – immediately beneath the capsule. *Columns of Bertin* are extensions of the cortex that enter the medulla separating the renal pyramids. The corticomedullary junction requires optimal gain settings to be identified.

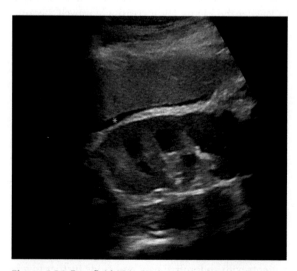

Figure 4.26 Free fluid (*) in Morison's pouch secondary to gastric ulcer perforation.

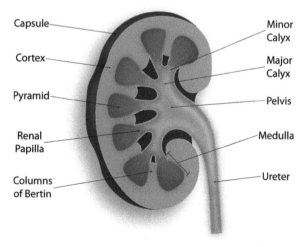

Figure 4.27 Key renal anatomy identified with ultrasound.

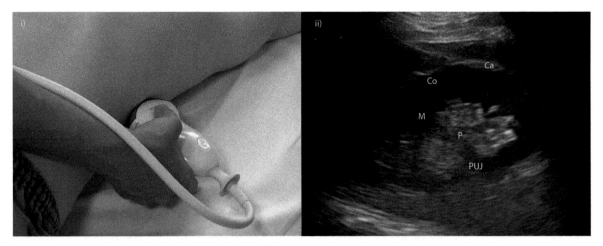

Figure 4.28 (i) Probe position for the long-axis view of the left kidney. (ii) Key anatomic identified on ultrasound. Ca, capsule; Co, cortex; M, medulla; P, pelvis; PUJ, pelviureteric junction.

- **Medulla** – the columns of Bertin segment the medulla into renal or medullary *pyramids* which are characteristically hypoechoic on ultrasound. Each pyramid forms a papilla at its apex where urine is drained into minor calyces.
- **Sinus** – minor calyces coalesce to form major calyces which merge creating the *renal pelvis*. The area surrounding the renal pelvis appears hyperechoic due to the presence of fat in the renal sinus. If seen, the renal pelvis appears hypoechoic as it contains fluid. The pelvis subsequently drains into the *ureter* at the *pelviureteric junction* (PUJ) which is a common site of obstruction by calculi. The major and minor calyces, pelvis, blood vessels, lymphatics and surrounding fatty tissue are collectively termed the *renal sinus*.

The ureters are challenging to identify on US due to frequent emptying by peristalsis. They descend on the medial aspect of the psoas muscle, crossing the common iliacs and drain into the bladder via the *vesicoureteric junctions* (VUJ) - another common site of obstruction.

Method

A low frequency (3–5 MHz) curvilinear probe is used with an abdominal preset and the patient supine. The kidneys should be assessed in a longitudinal and transverse plane.

The right kidney can be imaged by initially placing the probe in a sagittal plane at the anterior axillary line with the probe marker pointing cranially. The liver is used as an acoustic window in this view. Upon image acquisition the user should fan the probe to view the entirety of the kidney (Figure 4.28).

The probe is then rotated 90 degrees and the kidney is imaged in a transverse view. The user must again fan the probe from pole to pole to fully interrogate the kidney.

The left kidney may be more challenging to image as the spleen is a smaller organ and less amenable for use as an acoustic window. The probe is placed in the left flank in a sagittal plane with the probe marker pointing cranially. The user may be required to place their knuckles onto the bed to identify the landmarks. In a well patient it may be beneficial to turn the patient into the right lateral decubitus position to gain a more posterior approach. The left kidney should again be assessed in a longitudinal and transverse plane.

Pathological Findings

Hydronephrosis

Hydronephrosis is the dilatation of the renal pelvis and calyces of the kidney due to obstruction of urine flow. This may be unilateral or bilateral. Unilateral hydronephrosis is most commonly associated with ureterolithiasis and bilateral hydronephrosis is a potentially correctable cause of unexplained acute kidney injury.

Computerised tomography has a much higher sensitivity for identifying hydronephrosis and can demonstrate hydroureter along with the exact size

113

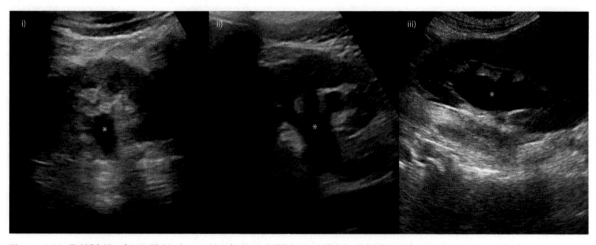

Figure 4.29 (i) Mild (Grade 1), (ii) Moderate (Grade 2) and (iii) Severe (Grade 3) hydronephrosis (*).

and position of a ureteric stone. However, US may be beneficial where diagnostic uncertainty exists and the identification of unilateral hydronephrosis can justify referral for definitive imaging.

Hydronephrosis is classified from stage 1 to stage 4 (Figure 4.29):

- Grade 1 – mild hydronephrosis – mild dilatation of the renal collecting system.
- Grade 2 – moderate hydronephrosis – dilatation of the renal pelvis with no calyceal dilatation.
- Grade 3 – severe hydronephrosis – dilatation of the renal pelvis and calyces.
- Grade 4 – chronic, severe hydronephrosis with thinning of the renal parenchyma.

Additional causes of hydronephrosis include urinary retention, benign prostatic hypertrophy and pregnancy. These will typically lead to bilateral hydronephrosis.

Several structures may mimic hydronephrosis. Renal vessels can be prominent and the use of colour Doppler will distinguish vessels from a dilated collecting system. Renal calyces may appear hypoechoic and be mistaken for hydronephrosis in some individuals. It is important to identify dilatation of the collecting system and renal pelvis to confirm hydronephrosis.

Calculi are most commonly seen at the pelviureteric junction (PUJ) or vesicoureteric junction (VUJ). They will appear as very hyperechoic structures with a post-acoustic shadow. Reduction of gain may be beneficial to distinguish between the renal sinus and the brighter calculi as both structures are hyperechoic. Moving the focal point to the depth of a renal calculus and turning off compound imaging will help

accentuate post-acoustic shadowing. Placing colour Doppler over the stones can demonstrate a 'twinkle artefact' whereby many colours are shown in a disorganised pattern.

Demonstrating ureteric jets can confirm patency of the ureters. Partial obstruction will still yield a jet but this may be smaller than the contralateral jet. Due to differing levels of peristalsis the rate at which this happens is very variable but should be seen several times per minute. A transverse view of the bladder is obtained and the colour Doppler velocity scale reduced. Red jets can be visualised draining urine into the bladder.

Case – An Extra Bedside Test

A 36-year-old female presented with right upper quadrant pain associated with nausea. At the time of assessment, the patient had pain in the right upper quadrant and flank. Urine dip was performed and was negative for haematuria. Blood tests had not yet been performed as were not deemed required by triage staff.

Right upper quadrant US was performed as biliary colic was suspected. This demonstrated no gallstones and a normal gallbladder wall thickness. Due to the unexpected finding a further interrogation of the abdomen was performed. This revealed moderate right-sided unilateral hydronephrosis (Figure 4.30). The patient was referred for computerised tomography of kidneys, ureters and bladder (CT KUB). Ordinarily this would have been a challenging imaging request in a young patient with no haematuria but the presence of unilateral hydronephrosis expedited the referral.

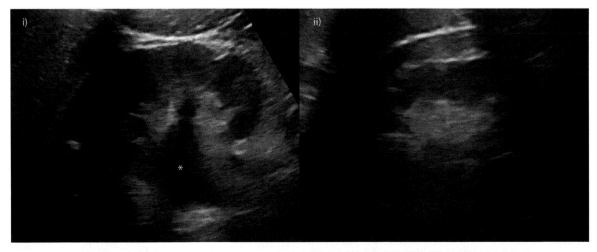

Figure 4.30 (i) Hydronephrosis (*) in the right kidney. (ii) The left kidney appeared normal with no hydronephrosis.

Computerised tomography demonstrated an obstructing mid-ureteric stone and the patient was admitted under the care of the urology team for further assessment.

This case highlights the potential inaccuracy of routine bedside tests and how US may aid the referral process for definitive investigations. In cases with diagnostic uncertainty it may provide additional information to guide the differential diagnosis.

Renal Cysts

Simple renal cysts may be seen in any part of the kidney. They are usually of little significance but should be measured and described in a report. Benign cysts are thin walled, regular structures and warrant no further investigation (Figure 4.31). Cysts with thickened, irregular walls or septations should be referred for specialist assessment.

Polycystic kidney disease may present in young patients with kidney failure. The entire architecture of the kidney may be obscured with the cysts extending far beyond the expected size of a normal kidney. These cysts may be very large and be mistaken for originating from the liver. It is important to highlight that adult polycystic kidney disease may also lead to hepatic cysts. If identified, these should prompt referral for definitive investigation.

Case – The Missing Piece of the Jigsaw

A 20-year-old male presented with general lethargy to the ambulatory care unit. No investigations had been performed. He also reported some intermittent flank

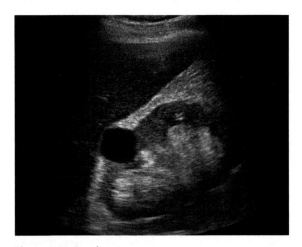

Figure 4.31 Renal cyst.

pain which was not present at the time of assessment. There was a history of type 1 diabetes mellitus and he had been poorly compliant with treatment and follow-up. The referral was made to ambulatory care with the intention of seeking assistance from the diabetic specialist team for education and optimisation of management.

Although blood sugars were poorly controlled this did not appear to be the principal concern and the attending clinician suspected they could palpate abdominal masses bilaterally. Bedside US was performed and demonstrated widespread renal cysts obscuring the renal architecture consistent with polycystic kidney disease (Figure 4.32).

Blood tests returned with a haemoglobin of 60g/dl and an estimated GFR of 5ml/min. Prompt referral to

115

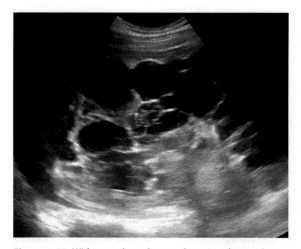

Figure 4.32 Widespread renal cysts obscuring the renal architecture consistent with polycystic kidney disease. *A video is available to view in the online video library.*

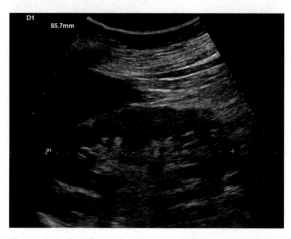

Figure 4.33 Renal atrophy in a patient with chronic kidney disease. The kidney measures 8.5 cm compared with normal values of 10–12 cm. It also appears hyperechoic compared with surrounding structures (note the hypoechoic liver).

the renal team was made and CT confirmed findings with additional features suggesting haemorrhage within several cysts.

Bedside echocardiography was performed and demonstrated left ventricular hypertrophy and a small global pericardial effusion suspected to be uraemic in aetiology.

Chronic Kidney Disease

In chronic kidney disease (CKD) the kidneys appear atrophic and hyperechoic (Figure 4.33). Clinicians must familiarise themselves with the echogenicity of normal kidneys in comparison to surrounding structures to identify this. The cortex of healthy kidneys have a similar echogenicity to the liver and this may act as a simple comparison.

Measuring the kidney at its most maximal point will give further information on whether kidney injury is acute or chronic. Figure 4.33 shows a patient with CKD; note the increased echogenicity and measurement of 8.6 cm indicating chronicity.

Pyelonephritis

Infection has a very inconsistent appearance on US and the assessment by point-of-care clinicians should be aimed at excluding other pathology. Renal or perinephric abscesses may appear as hypoechoic structures in the renal parenchyma or within the perinephric space respectively.

Renal Cancer

Renal cancers have a very variable appearance and the identification of any structure of unknown significance should prompt the point-of-care clinician to understand their limitations and refer for definitive assessment.

Bladder Residual Volume

Identification of urinary retention is a simple clinical diagnosis when severe. US can be used to identify a distended bladder but is not usually required for diagnosis. POCUS may be beneficial when there is uncertainty over bladder volume. Examples include: identifying a blocked catheter; or where conventional 'bladder scanners' suggest there may be significant residual volume – for example where ascites is present.

Quantification of residual volume is commonly required in patients with chronic urinary retention or following prostatic surgery prior to hospital discharge. Significant bladder residual volume renders the patient at risk of urinary tract infection and further acute on chronic retention.

Many methods of estimating residual volume exist and no method has been demonstrated to be superior to another. All measures require multiplication of linear measures and therefore are subject to error if these are inaccurately performed. The most commonly used method is:

$$Volume\ (ml) = Length\ h\ (cm) \times Width\ (cm)$$
$$\times\ Height\ (cm) \times 0.52$$

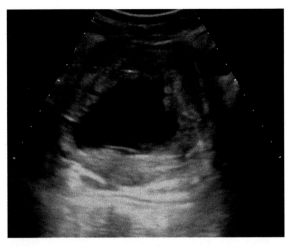

Figure 4.34 Significantly thickened bladder wall in a patient with bladder cancer.

Bladder Cancer

Painless haematuria is usually the sole symptom in patients presenting with bladder cancer. Cystoscopy is the gold standard in evaluation of haematuria. On US you may see a thickened wall, clots, polyps or focal masses (Figure 4.34).

Key Points

- Point-of-care ultrasound assessment of the renal tract is predominantly aimed at identifying hydronephrosis or significant bladder residual volume. This has many clinical applications and must be guided by clinical presentation.
- More detailed assessment of renal architecture is beyond the scope of the generalist but understanding normal sonoanatomy and echotexture allows users to identify abnormal findings and refer for specialist assessment.

Basic Hepatobiliary Ultrasound

Hepatobiliary (HPB) US is more complex than the earlier techniques described and does not appear in the curriculum of many point-of-care accreditation pathways. At the bedside, imaging of the HPB system is predominantly focused on identifying basic gallbladder and biliary tree pathology including gallstones, choledocholithiasis and cholecystitis.

The liver is a difficult organ to assess and requires appreciation of subtle changes in brightness and texture. Basic assessment of the liver and hepatic vascular will be discussed in more detail later.

Method

The gallbladder has a very variable axis and can be seen anywhere from the abdominal midline to mid-axillary line. A sensible approach is to begin in a sagittal plane in the abdominal midline with the probe marker directed cephalad to the patient's right shoulder. This orientation will optimise visualisation of the portal hepatis, common bile duct and gallbladder neck. The costal margin can then be followed until the gallbladder is identified. It is typically seen laterally to the midline on the right-hand side of the patient. If the gallbladder is very superficial it may either require assessment between rib spaces or by asking the patient to take a deep breath which causes contraction of the diaphragm and downward displacement of the biliary system.

If possible, turning the patient left lateral will significantly improve the view. This is particularly important for visualisation of the gallbladder neck which is where small gallstones often sit and are therefore missed if not scanned in this position.

The gallbladder should be assessed in the longitudinal and transverse axes. The variable axis is due to it only being tethered at the gallbladder neck and therefore influenced by surrounding anatomy. Acquiring a subcostal sagittal image usually demonstrates a longitudinal view of the gallbladder. The body, neck and portal triad should be visualised. Colour Doppler may be used to differentiate between structures of the portal triad: the portal vein, hepatic artery and common bile duct (Figure 4.35).

The anterior gallbladder wall should be measured if there is any concern about cholecystitis (Figure 4.36). The posterior wall may be more difficult to distinguish from the peritoneal fat and bowel and therefore is not routinely measured. Normal wall thickness is < 3 mm unless the patient is postprandial where the gallbladder is contracted with thickened walls.

The probe is then rotated 90 degrees to assess the gallbladder in the transverse plane. The probe must be 'fanned' to visualise the entire structure and identify localised pathology.

For all imaging of the upper abdomen the liver is a dominant structure. It can be used as an acoustic window to assess many structures. Although detailed assessment of the liver is beyond the scope of this text, knowledge of key structures is helpful in orientation and interpretation of pathology. A right oblique

117

subcostal view allows the right and left hepatic lobes to be interrogated and the convergence of the three hepatic veins.

Pathological Findings

Cholelithiasis

The most frequent reason for a POCUS assessment of the right upper quadrant is to identify gallstones. Gallstones appear to have a hyperechoic leading edge

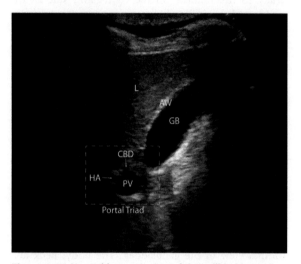

Figure 4.35 Normal long-axis view of the gallbladder and portal triad. Colour Doppler is used to differentiate between the hepatic artery and common bile duct. The anterior wall of the gallbladder is labelled and is the recommended site for wall measurement. GB, gallbladder; AW, anterior wall of the GB; PV, portal vein; CBD, common bile duct; HA, hepatic artery; L, liver.

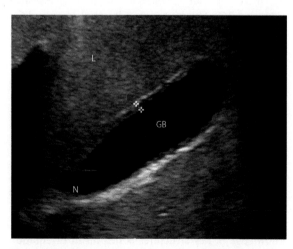

Figure 4.36 Measurement of the anterior gallbladder wall using callipers. GB, gallbladder; N, gallbladder neck; L, liver.

and typically cast a hypoechoic shadow (Figure 4.37). They are seen in dependent regions of the gallbladder (GB) and may move with repositioning. Small stones < 2 mm may not demonstrate an acoustic shadow unless numerous stones are adjacent to one another.

A 'wall echo shadow' (WES) is seen when the gallbladder is densely filled with stones and the anterior gallbladder wall appears hyperechoic with an acoustic shadow (Figure 4.38). Appearance of WES may be confused with porcelain gallbladder (PG) where calcification of the gallbladder occurs due to chronic cholecystitis. WES and PG can be differentiated by the presence of a hypoechoic stripe between the GB wall and the gallstone which is not present in PG. PG is associated with malignancy and therefore further investigation is warranted.

Location of stones within the gallbladder is important as a stone seen to impact the gallbladder neck should prompt surgical review and assessment for cholecystitis.

Biliary 'sludge' is precipitation of bile and the early stages of stone formation. It manifests as an irregularly demarcated dependent, low amplitude echogenic shape that will move with position change.

Acute Cholecystitis

A spectrum of findings may be present in patients presenting with cholecystitis. The presence and severity of each sign will increase with the degree of gallbladder inflammation. These signs include:

- Sonographic Murphy's sign: direct compression of the gallbladder with the US probe incites the patient's symptoms. This is suggested to be more sensitive than clinical Murphy's sign (Figure 4.39).

- Gallbladder wall thickening: measurement of the anterior gallbladder wall demonstrates inflammation (Figure 4.40). A diameter of over 3 mm is abnormal.

- Dilated common bile duct: this suggests choledocholithiasis in the acute setting which will be discussed below.

- Pericholecystic fluid: in severe cholecystitis and necrotising cholecystitis fluid may appear surrounding an inflamed gallbladder.

As with other forms of POCUS it is essential to correlate findings clinically. There are many systemic

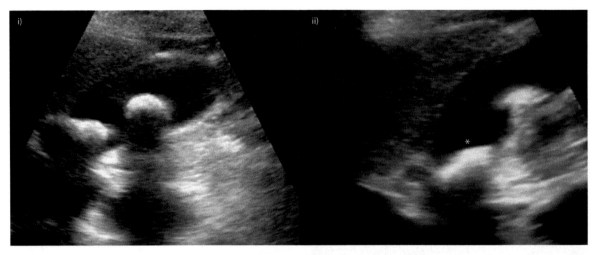

Figure 4.37 Two examples of gallstones within the GB. (i) Note the post acoustic shadow deep to the gallstones. (ii) There are multiple gallstones identified with one located in the gallbladder neck (*).

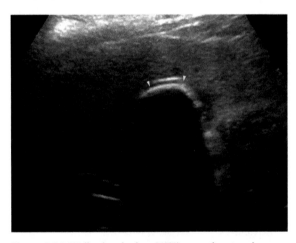

Figure 4.38 Wall echo shadow (WES) secondary to a large gallstone. Note the hypoechoic stripe (arrows) between the GB and the gallstone. This aids differentiating between Porcelain GB and WES.

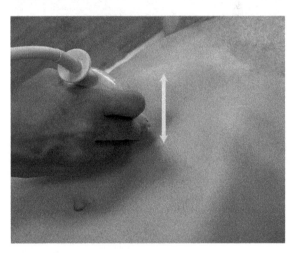

Figure 4.39 Sonographic Murphy's sign.

causes of gallbladder thickening and its identification is not pathognomonic for cholecystitis.

Choledocholithiasis

Dilatation of the biliary tree is an important finding and, within the acute setting, is most suggestive of bile duct obstruction from a gallstone. Painless jaundice will require a more detailed and definitive investigation to assess for liver, biliary tree and pancreatic pathology.

The common bile duct (CBD) is the key structure to identify when assessing for choledocholithiasis.

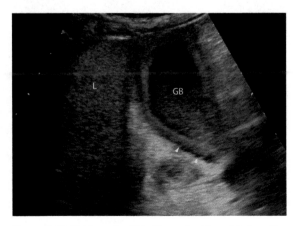

Figure 4.40 Thickened gallbladder wall with pericholecystic fluid (arrows) in patient with cholecystitis. GB, gallbladder; L, liver.

119

Identification of stones within the CBD is challenging and not reliable in the point of care setting.

The portal triad – the portal vein, hepatic artery and CBD – may be seen located next to the neck of the gallbladder (Figure 4.35). With a longitudinal gallbladder view the portal triad is seen in cross section. The large lower vessel with hyperechoic walls is the portal vein with two smaller structures, the hepatic artery and CBD, located superiorly. Colour Doppler may be used to differentiate between the hepatic artery and CBD. This view of the portal triad is sometimes described as the 'Mickey Mouse' sign,

with the portal vein being Mickey's face and the hepatic artery and CBD the ears.

With a transverse gallbladder view, a longitudinal image of the portal vein is seen with a smaller CBD superiorly travelling in parallel (Figure 4.41). The hepatic artery may be seen between these structures in an 'out of plane', transverse view but this is not always visible. The appearance of a dilated CBD in this view is sometimes described as a 'double barrel shotgun' appearance alongside the portal vein (Figure 4.42).

The CBD may be measured in either view from inner edge to inner edge. Normal size varies with age and a common estimate is of 4 mm with an extra 1 mm with every decade beyond 40. For example:

- 18-year-old – 4 mm is normal.
- 60-year-old – 6 mm is normal.

It is important to note that a dilated CBD may be present following cholecystectomy or represent any pathology of the biliary tree. Identification should prompt further investigation guided by conventional history and examination. Figure 4.42 demonstrates two examples of a dilated CBD.

Key Points

- The generalist may wish to assess the gallbladder and biliary tree to identify gallstones, cholecystitis or choledocholithiasis.
- It is a more complex assessment due to the variable size and axis of the gallbladder, obscuring bowel gas and a similar appearance of nearby structures.

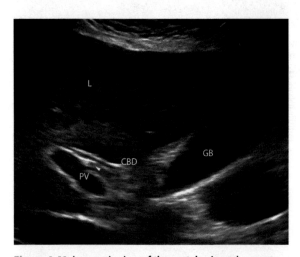

Figure 4.41 Long-axis view of the portal vein and common bile duct. The hepatic artery (arrow) is visible in cross-section between these structures. GB, gallbladder; L, liver; CBD, common bile duct; PV, portal vein.

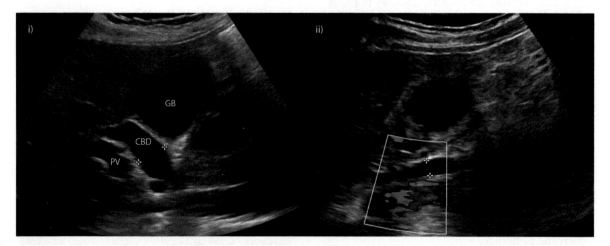

Figure 4.42 Two examples demonstrating a dilated CBD and the 'double barrel shotgun' appearance. Note the calibre compared to the portal vein. Image (ii) demonstrates the use of colour Doppler to differentiate between the CBD and the portal vein. CBD, common bile duct; PV, portal vein; GB, gallbladder.

- Colour and pulse wave Doppler may be useful to differentiate structures and assess flow. This is a more advanced technique that will require experience and practice.

Additional Topics in Abdominal Ultrasound

The major features we have covered in this chapter are core 'point-of-care' topics. Abdominal US is clearly a much larger discipline and clinicians may find themselves identifying pathology with which they are not familiar.

These topics will be discussed as an introduction to other elements of abdominal US that are becoming increasingly popular.

Small Bowel Obstruction

Small bowel obstruction (SBO) accounts for 2% of patients presenting to the ED with abdominal pain and 20% of all surgical admissions. Studies have shown that US is superior to abdominal x-ray (AXR) in diagnosis of SBO with a sensitivity of 90% and specificity of 97%.

The patient should be in the supine position and you should scan using the "lawnmower technique" starting in the paracolic gutter and sweep along the course of the flanks on each side proceeding across the abdomen in a systematic fashion (Figure 4.43).

Normal bowel may be challenging to visualise due to obscuring gas but can appear as a single, circular, hypoechoic layer with hyperechoic contents. If you do encounter bowel loops with air, gentle pressure may be applied to displace the air. Normal diameter of small bowel is < 3 cm and large bowel < 6 cm.

In SBO, the bowel is dilated (> 3 cm) and usually fluid filled with pendulum peristalsis which is the to and fro motion or 'swirling' of bowel contents. The valvulae conniventes (also known as plicae circulares) are often prominent in jejunal loops and this is referred to as the 'keyboard sign' (Figure 4.44). The key findings are summarised in Table 4.2.

Features suggestive of bowel ischaemia include bowel wall thickening (> 3 mm), intra-mural gas (pneumatosis intestinalis), complete loss of peristalsis or extraluminal free fluid or gas. Any of these findings should prompt an urgent request for specialist imaging and surgical referral.

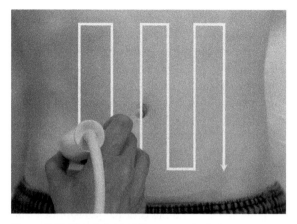

Figure 4.43 **The abdominal lawnmower technique.**

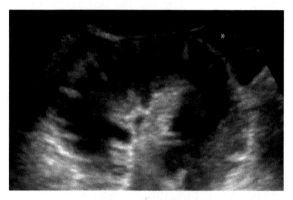

Figure 4.44 **The appearance of small bowel obstruction on ultrasound. Note the fluid-filled bowel with prominent valvulae conniventes (plicae circulares). Free fluid (*) is seen between bowel loops which is the Tanga sign.**

Table 4.2

Small bowel obstruction ultrasound findings
Fluid-filled small bowel
Outer diameter of > 3 cm
Increased bowel wall thickness > 3 mm
Prominent and thickened plicae circulares in jejunum (Keyboard sign)
Well circumscribed fluid collections (Tanga sign)
Pendular peristalsis (to and fro peristalsis)

Appendicitis

The diagnosis of acute appendicitis is frequently challenging due to non-specific symptoms which overlap with other common abdominal pathologies. POCUS has a high specificity of 96% and may be of use in suspected cases.

There are two major approaches to scanning:

- Method 1 – point of maximal tenderness. The probe should be placed where the patient is most tender with the probe marker pointing towards their right-hand side.
- Method 2 – systematic approach. With this method the user should start in the RUQ with the probe marker pointing towards the patient's right-hand side. The ascending colon should be traced downwards until the caecum is reached. At this point the key landmarks of the psoas muscle and iliac vessels may be identified.

The linear probe provides the best resolution for imaging the appendix although the curvilinear may be required in obese patients. The appendix is located between the iliac artery and psoas muscle and should be visualised both in plane and out of plane. Key landmarks are described in Figure 4.45. Out of plane the appendix can be distinguished as a blind-ending 'pouch' with peristalsis.

The appendix has a normal outer wall to outer wall diameter of < 6 mm and is compressible. Any diameter > 6–7 mm is deemed to be abnormal and consistent with acute appendicitis. Additionally, there will be a loss of peristalsis and compressibility.

Ancillary features of acute appendicitis include:

- Increased bowel wall thickness > 3 mm.
- 'Target sign' – in the short-axis view the central region of the appendix is hypoechoic with a hyperechoic wall and surrounding hypoechoic region. This creates a 'target-like' appearance.
- Abdominal free fluid adjacent to the appendix.
- Hyperechoic appendicolith with posterior acoustic shadowing.

The appendix may be challenging to visualise in the obese patient or when there is overlying bowel gas. It may also be obscured by the caecum. Incomplete or inadequate views should prompt referral for specialist imaging.

Liver Ultrasound

Assessment of the liver is beyond the scope of most POCUS practitioners. However, as you progress with your US journey you will become accustomed to seeing the liver in a large proportion of your scans as it is a key landmark. It is not uncommon to identify differences in echogenicity or findings such as cysts or liver masses when imaging for other indications.

The normal liver has a homogenous echogenicity similar to the renal cortex. The smooth capsular contour should also be assessed to exclude any coarseness or nodularity.

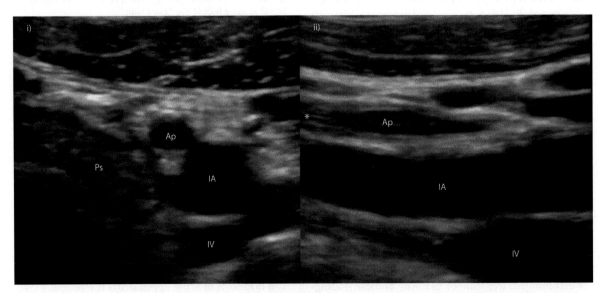

Figure 4.45 Landmark anatomy for identification of the appendix. (i) Out of plane (transverse) view of the appendix nested between the iliac artery and psoas muscle. (ii) In plane view (sagittal) of the appendix. Note the blind end of the appendix (*) and its position overlying the iliac artery. Ap, appendix; IA, iliac artery; IV, iliac vein; Ps, psoas muscle.

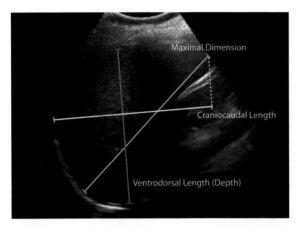

Figure 4.46 Typical measurements for the liver in the sagittal plane through the mid clavicular line. Normal measures: maximal dimension – < 18 cm; craniocaudal length < 16 cm; ventrodorsal length < 13 cm).

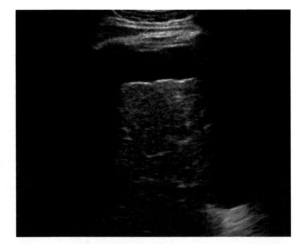

Figure 4.47 Liver cirrhosis. Note the nodularity of the liver surface and the presence of ascites.

The most important measurement is the craniocaudal length (Figure 4.46). Although extremely variable, the liver should be < 16 cm in craniocaudal length. For this measurement the liver should be imaged in the sagittal plane through the mid-clavicular line

Acute Hepatitis

Hepatomegaly is the most sensitive POCUS finding in acute hepatitis defined as craniocaudal length > 16 cm. Due to the accumulation of inflammatory fluid the liver parenchyma may appear hypoechoic and resemble a 'starry sky' appearance although this has been noted to have a poor sensitivity and specificity. The 'stars' are the portal venous walls adjacent to the oedematous hepatocytes.

Cirrhosis

A cirrhotic liver will appear to have a coarse echotexture with surface nodularity and irregularity (Figure 4.47). Hypoechoic nodules may be noted. It is important to remember that in the early stages of cirrhosis the liver will be enlarged and will only become atrophied as the cirrhosis progresses.

Fatty Liver

Fatty liver disease is a common clinical disease and appears on US as increased liver echogenicity due to fat deposits. The liver parenchyma should have a similar echogenicity to the renal cortex and the two structures should be routinely compared.

Liver Cysts

Liver cysts are common and affect 5% of the population and are seen as fluid-filled cavities. They are often incidental and appear as hypoechoic lesions (Figure 4.48i). Polycystic liver disease is a rare genetic condition where cysts form throughout the liver and obscure the liver architecture (Figure 4.48ii).

Liver Abscess

Abscesses have a very variable appearance and can range from well- or ill-defined hypoechoic nodules to a large hypoechoic lesion with septae and debris. CT and MRI are the gold standard modalities in these cases.

Liver Masses

Identification of incidental liver lesions should prompt urgent further assessment. Liver metastases can appear in many ways, most commonly appearing hypoechoic (65%) followed by hyperechoic, 'bullseye lesions', cystic, calcified or a combination of the above. POCUS users may be the first clinicians to identify these lesions and should further interrogate the liver and save images to enable accurate reporting and referral for specialist imaging and service.

Hepatic Vasculature

The hepatic blood vessels are readily identified with US and require assessment with colour and spectral Doppler. This is a more advanced assessment but

123

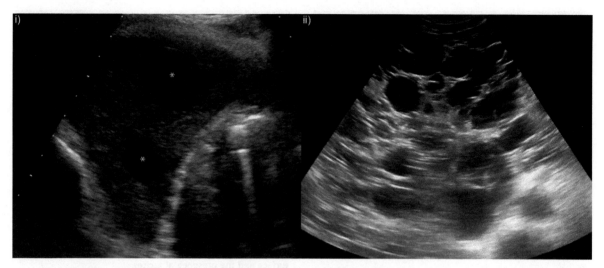

Figure 4.48 (i) Liver cysts (*). (ii) Polycystic liver disease. Note the architecture of the liver has been completely replaced by cysts which are causing acoustic enhancement in the far field.

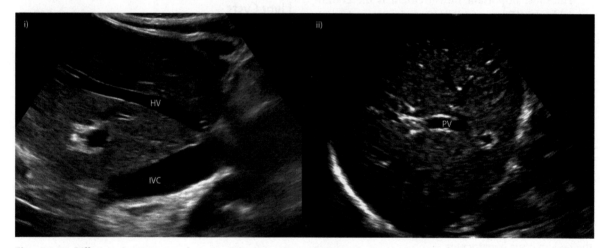

Figure 4.49 **Difference in appearance between (i) hepatic veins and (ii) portal veins.** Note the thin wall of the hepatic vein and its course can be followed into the IVC. The portal vein travels in a different direction and has thick, hyperechoic walls. HV, hepatic vein; IVC, inferior vena cava; PV, portal vein.

is gradually entering the curriculum for POCUS accreditation pathways. The key differences between hepatic veins and portal veins will be considered.

The hepatic veins are thin-walled hypoechoic structures which can be seen to converge and drain into the inferior vena cava (Figure 4.49i). Identifying a patent portal venous system is a common indication for departmental imaging requests. They can be differentiated from the hepatic veins by identifying the thick, hyperechoic walls characteristic of the portal veins (Figure 4.49ii). Although assessment of flow characteristics is an advanced technique, normal findings will be briefly discussed.

Hepatic Vein Flow

Flow within the hepatic vein can be assessed using pulse wave Doppler (Figure 4.50). This is a more advanced technique and can be used to identify fluid congestion and grade severity of tricuspid regurgitation.

Hepatic venous Doppler is described in more detail in the haemodynamic section of the echocardiography chapter.

Portal Vein Flow

Assessment of portal venous flow is a frequent indication for departmental scans as thrombosis may

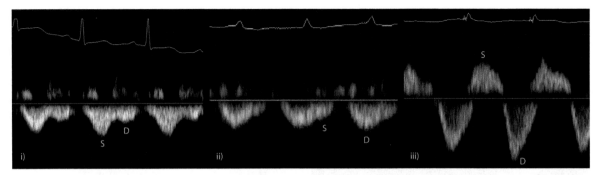

Figure 4.50 Comparison of different hepatic venous Doppler flow profiles: (i) normal systolic dominant flow with a brief A wave reversal that is barely visible in this clip; (ii) blunting of the systolic flow with the largest peak representing the diastolic flow; (iii) complete reversal of the systolic flow as seen by the S wave rising above the baseline. Although experienced users may be able to infer the S and D waves by eye alone, we recommend using the ECG trace to better delineate between systole and diastole.

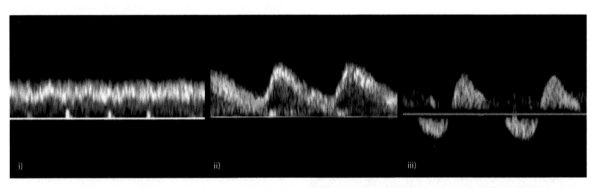

Figure 4.51 Comparison of different portal venous Doppler flow profiles: (i) normal continuous antegrade flow; (ii) reduced systolic flow leading to portal venous pulsatility; (iii) systolic flow reversal.

precipitate acute liver failure. Changes in portal vein flow may be suggestive of portal hypertension when combined with supporting features e.g. splenomegaly.

Pulse wave Doppler in the portal vein should demonstrate a continuous, undulating, non-pulsatile 'hepatopetal flow'. Hepatopetal describes the antegrade flow of blood towards the liver. Venous congestion and severe tricuspid regurgitation may lead to progressive pulsatility or even biphasic reversal of flow within the portal veins (Figure 4.51). Discussion of portal venous flow in haemodynamic assessment is described in more detail in Chapter 2.

Portal hypertension leads to a dilatation of the portal vein (> 13 mm in diameter). Supporting features such as splenomegaly are useful to identify if portal hypertension is suspected. The spleen may be measured from the LUQ view with maximal diameter of > 12 cm suggestive of splenomegaly. In severe portal hypertension, portal venous flow may reverse and become 'hepatofugal' which describes continuous, retrograde flow.

Assessment of portal hypertension is a more advanced US technique and clinical suspicion should prompt referral for definitive imaging.

Other pathology may be noted within the portal venous system. Gas flowing towards the liver through the portal system is a rare example which is suggestive of bowel ischaemia and a case example of this is shown in Figure 4.52.

Case – Ultrasound Diagnoses What Computerised Tomography Cannot

A 62-year-old female was a patient on the ICU for several months following bilateral lung transplantation complicated by right ventricular failure requiring mechanical support. During her admission she required renal replacement therapy (RRT) and had multiple episodes of sepsis with multiorgan dysfunction.

She deteriorated overnight with a fever and increased vasopressor requirement. There was no metabolic derangement with a normal lactate whilst

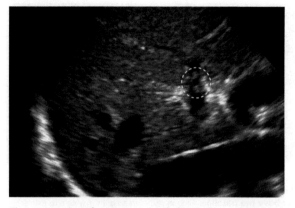

Figure 4.52 Portal venous gas (circled) noted in a patient with a displaced intra-aortic balloon pump. The portal venous gas is readily visible in the online video library. *A video is available to view in the online video library.*

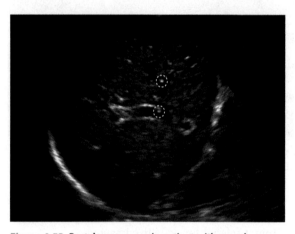

Figure 4.53 Portal venous gas in patient with caecal ischaemia. *A video is available to view in the online video library.*

on RRT. There was some abdominal distension but no discomfort and this had been reported for the preceding three days. NG feed was being absorbed.

Abdominal X-ray demonstrated non-specific bowel dilatation with no free air and no evidence of bowel obstruction.

Bedside echocardiography was performed to assess the patient's haemodynamic status. The IVC could not be visualised in the subcostal view due to bowel dilatation and the right upper quadrant view was selected.

There was an incidental finding of gas within the hepatic portal veins (Figure 4.53). Given the haemodynamic deterioration the patient was transferred for a CT abdomen which was inconclusive for ischaemia. The patient remained in a steady clinical condition for 24 hours prior to further deterioration and the decision for laparotomy. Intraoperatively there was evidence of caecal ischaemia.

This case demonstrates that subtle findings may be present and guide the need for ongoing investigation and management. Portal venous gas is almost exclusively a poor prognostic sign and should prompt clinicians to search for severe intra-abdominal pathology.

Summary

- The aorta is a key structure to differentiate from the IVC and is routinely assessed to exclude aneurysm.
- The identification of intra-abdominal free fluid in dependent regions may provide valuable information for identification of visceral injury or perforation.
- Although 'FAST' is becoming less prevalent within major trauma centres, it remains a useful tool in district hospitals and prehospital or resource-poor settings to identify injuries secondary to trauma.
- Hydronephrosis is a simple finding that may aid in the diagnosis of renal stones and post-renal acute kidney injury.
- Biliary tract ultrasound is a relatively simple technique that is essential in the setting of RUQ pain and obstructive jaundice to identify gallstones, cholecystitis or choledocholithiasis.
- More advanced techniques to identify small bowel obstruction, appendicitis, liver lesions and changes in hepatic vasculature will provide invaluable information at the bedside for generalist clinicians.

A full list of references and further reading are available at www.GeneralistUltrasound.com

Chapter 5

Vascular Ultrasound

Introduction

The assessment of the vascular system with ultrasound (US) is required in many fields from the ambulant out-patient to the most critically unwell intensive care patient. The same fundamental principles may be applied to diagnosing a deep vein thrombosis (DVT) in a General Practice clinic, challenging peripheral cannulation in intravenous drug users and the insertion of arterial lines in patients on mechanical cardiovascular support.

This chapter will provide an overview of the techniques required for the following disciplines:

- DVT assessment – lower limb
- DVT assessment – upper limb
- Venous and arterial access

General Principles

A high frequency (5–12 MHz) linear probe provides high resolution images of the superficial vascular structures (Figure 5.1). Crystals within a linear probe emit sound waves in a straight line producing a rectangular image sector. This is of particular importance for vascular access as the reflected image will more

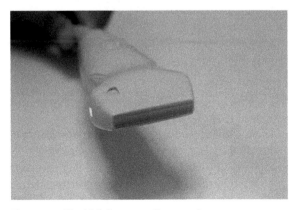

Figure 5.1 The high frequency linear probe.

accurately represent a needle's true location when compared with a curvilinear or phased array probe.

For assessment of deeper vessels or in patients with a higher body mass index the low frequency (3–5 MHz) probe may be required.

Identification and differentiation of key structures is an essential initial step in assessment of the vascular system. Machine settings must be utilised to optimise sector width, depth and gain. As a minimum requirement the user should be able to distinguish between arteries, veins and nerves. Structures surrounding the neurovascular bundle should also be interrogated and proximity to target vessels noted prior to needling e.g. the pleura during US-guided axillary vein cannulation.

Arteries are reliably distinguished from veins by their thick, hyperechoic walls. They have a consistent, round shape and are not easily compressible except in extremely hypovolaemic states (Figure 5.2). Colour Doppler demonstrates the direction of flow (remember: Blue Away Red Towards) although this requires angulation of the probe with interpretation of colour depending on probe direction (Figure 5.3). Spectral Doppler may be used and demonstrate a much higher flow velocity than veins.

In contrast, veins are thin-walled structures that are readily compressible. Their shape will vary significantly depending on the volume status and positioning of the patient but tend to appear more 'oval' than arteries. Although generally non-pulsatile, larger central veins may demonstrate biphasic pulsation consistent with a central venous pressure trace. Spectral Doppler will demonstrate much lower velocity flow when compared with arteries.

Appreciation of the structural differences, beyond simply 'pulsatile versus non-pulsatile', is important in situations whereby flow is altered. An example of this is in a patient with a left ventricular assist system (LVAS), e.g. the Heartmate 3 device, where arterial flow is generated by a pump and is laminar and not

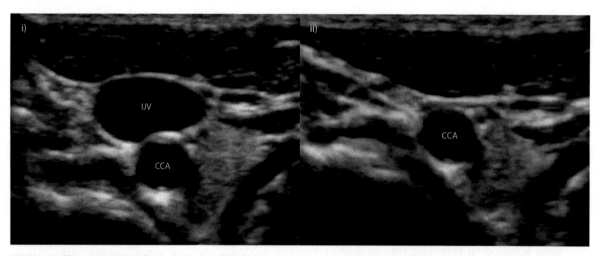

Figure 5.2 The appearance of the major arteries and veins (i) before and (ii) after compression. Note the oval, thin-walled appearance of the internal jugular vein which is readily compressible. The carotid artery is round with thick walls and retains its shape upon compression. IJV: internal jugular vein; CCA: common carotid artery. *A video is available to view in the online video library.*

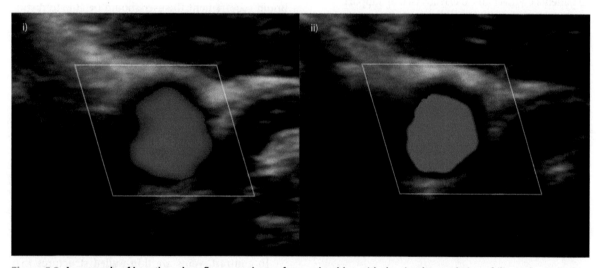

Figure 5.3 An example of how the colour flow may change from red to blue with the simple angulation of the probe. In (i) the blood is flowing towards the probe and therefore appears red. In (ii) the blood flow is away from the probe – hence blue.

pulsatile. There is therefore no palpable pulse and US is required for arterial blood sampling and access. Furthermore, the central venous vessels will often appear *more pulsatile* than the surrounding arteries, potentially complicating vascular access. Although this may seem a highly specialised example, an increasing number of patients have a LVAS as destination therapy (i.e. not proceeding to heart transplantation) resulting in a higher frequency of presentations to generalists in district hospitals when acutely unwell.

Deep Vein Thrombosis Assessment – Lower Limb

Venous thrombosis, including DVT and pulmonary embolism (PE), are a commonly encountered clinical problem with an estimated annual incidence of 1–2 in 1000 adults. Risk factors include increasing age, immobility, hospitalisation, pregnancy, recent surgery, trauma, malignancy, obesity, hypercoagulation disorders and hormone use (e.g. combined oral contraceptive pill, hormone replacement therapy).

A proximal leg vein US scan should be performed for all patients with a high probability of DVT based on the two-level Wells score.

Anatomy

See Figure 5.4. A lower-leg DVT assessment begins with the femoral vein at the level of the inguinal ligament. The femoral vein typically lies medial to the femoral artery (Figure 5.5). This is the image that should be acquired for femoral central venous cannulation.

Sliding the transducer distally will reveal the junction with the long saphenous vein – the sapheno-femoral junction (SFJ). The appearance of these structures is called the 'Mickey Mouse Sign' with Mickey's 'face' representing the common femoral vein and the great saphenous vein and femoral artery the 'ears' (Figure 5.6).

Continuing distally will reveal the bifurcation of the common femoral vein. The superficial femoral vein (SFV) should be followed into the adductor canal at the mid-thigh level until it is no longer visible as its course continues behind the knee (Figure 5.7).

Lastly the popliteal vein should be visualised superficial to the popliteal artery within the popliteal fossa (Figure 5.8). The vein is followed proximally until no longer visualised and then distally until the popliteal trifurcation is located (Figure 5.9).

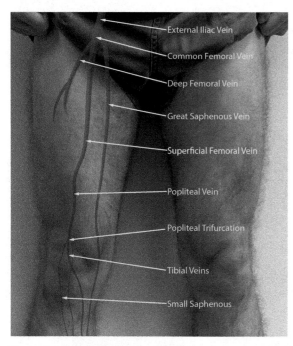

Figure 5.4 **Lower limb venous anatomy.**

Method

Patient positioning should be considered to optimise leg filling e.g. reverse Trendelenburg or head up and externally rotate the hip and flex the knee. The vessels should be assessed in the transverse (out of plane) view (Figure 5.10). Where possible, the longitudinal (in plane) views should also be attained and are of particular use for spectral Doppler assessment.

Identification of a clot requires compression of the venous system. This is achieved by delivering

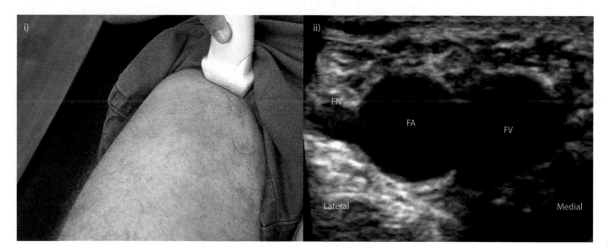

Figure 5.5 **(i) Probe position to commence the DVT scan and to identify the femoral artery and vein. (ii) The appearance of the femoral nerve (FN), artery (FA) and vein (FV) on US.**

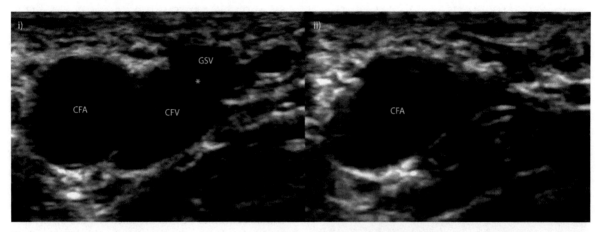

Figure 5.6 The sapheno-femoral junction (*) demonstrated before (i) and after (ii) compression. CFA, common femoral artery; CFV, common femoral vein; GSV, great saphenous vein.

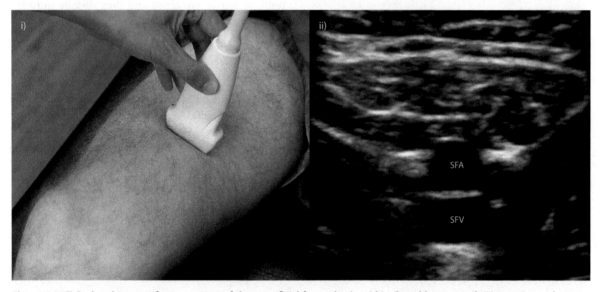

Figure 5.7 (i) Probe placement for assessment of the superficial femoral vein within the adductor canal. (ii) Location and orientation of the superficial femoral artery and superficial femoral vein. SFA, superficial femoral artery; SFV, superficial femoral vein.

downward pressure at 1–2 cm intervals as the venous system is followed. This pressure should be sufficient to cause wall to wall opposition of the venous system and will tend to deform the artery (Figure 5.10). Within the adductor canal there is no bone underlying the superficial femoral vein and therefore the non-scanning hand may be held under the medial aspect of the thigh to optimise compression. If a clot is present a hyperechoic structure will be visualised within the vessel and the user will be unable to compress the opposing venous walls together (Figure 5.11).

There is no evidence to suggest that compression US increases the risk of thromboembolism in patients

with a DVT. Despite this, care should be taken to avoid applying excessive pressure for compression.

The study should be started at the level of the inguinal ligament and the user should slide the probe distally compressing at 1–2 cm intervals until the popliteal trifurcation. Particular attention should be paid to the venous junctions where thrombus may be missed. The region between the distal SFV and popliteal is frequently not possible to follow as described above. Figure 5.12 shows US images of clot within SFV extending into the popliteal vein.

This assessment is limited to the regions being directly visualised and will not identify venous

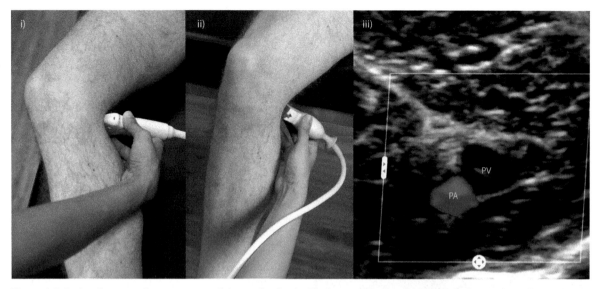

Figure 5.8 Probe placement for assessment of the popliteal vein. The leg may be placed in (i) external rotation or allowed to rest over the edge of the bed (ii). (iii) The typical appearance of the popliteal vein and artery. Colour Doppler has been used to aid identification and differentiation. PA, popliteal artery; PV, popliteal vein.

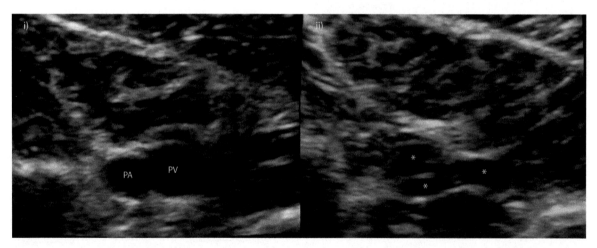

Figure 5.9 From the view of the popliteal vein (i) the user should continue to track the vessel inferiorly until the popliteal trifurcation is seen (ii). The tibial veins are labelled (*). PA, popliteal artery; PV, popliteal vein.

thrombosis in the IVC, iliac veins or in superficial vessels distal to the transducer. Additional techniques may be used to identify signs suggestive of DVT, but these are more advanced techniques and may be beyond the skillset of the generalist:

- Respiratory variation – during the respiratory cycle there is variation within the venous system. This is termed respiratory phasicity and is assessed by placing pulse wave Doppler over the common femoral vein (Figure 5.13i). Lack of

normal respiratory variation is suggestive of a venous thrombosis proximal to the probe (Figure 5.13ii).

- Augmentation – pulse wave Doppler is placed over the popliteal vein and the calf is compressed. There should be a resulting spike in flow within the popliteal vein due to increased venous return. If the vessels distal to the probe are obstructed there will be no flow augmentation. This technique is losing popularity as may be prone to error.

131

Point-of-care ultrasound accreditation pathways advocate a 'three-point approach' as a *rule-in* assessment for DVT. These points are as follows:

1. Common femoral vein at the saphenofemoral junction.
2. Superficial femoral vein at the adductor canal.
3. Popliteal vein to the trifurcation.

Although these pathways are designed to deliver a quick, 'rule-in' test, we would advocate a more detailed assessment due to the incidence of missed DVTs with two- or three-point approach.

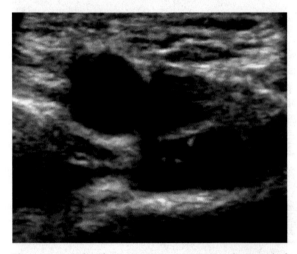

Figure 5.10 Video demonstrating compression ultrasound of the upper leg. *A video is available to view in the online video library.*

Pitfalls

It may be challenging for the generalist to distinguish between acute and chronic thrombi. Chronic thrombi tend to be more echogenic and lead to thickening of the vein walls. Furthermore, as previously mentioned, any thrombi that are outside of the region directly assessed by US may be missed without more advanced techniques. Assessments performed by non-ultrasound specialists should be considered 'rule-in' rather than 'rule-out' and if clinical suspicion of DVT remains, despite a negative focused scan, referral for comprehensive imaging is indicated.

Numerous structures may appear similar to a DVT. These include: lymph nodes, Baker's cyst and distended superficial veins/thrombophlebitis. Some of these topics are discussed in Chapter 6. In cases of diagnostic uncertainty, the patient should be referred for definitive imaging.

Key Points

- Optimising patient position and machine settings will aid clinicians to distinguish between anatomical landmarks and improve the sensitivity of the scan.
- Compression US is used at 1–2 cm intervals from the common femoral vein at the inguinal ligament to the popliteal trifurcation. Lack of wall-to-wall opposition of veins upon compression is indicative of thrombus.

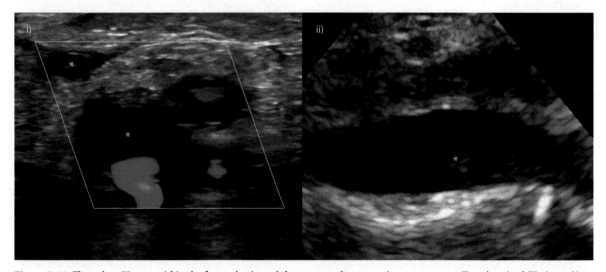

Figure 5.11 Thrombus (*) seen within the femoral vein and the great saphenous vein on transverse (i) and sagittal (ii) views. Note the appearance of the thrombus and absence of colour flow through the majority of the femoral vein. *Videos are available to view in the online video library.*

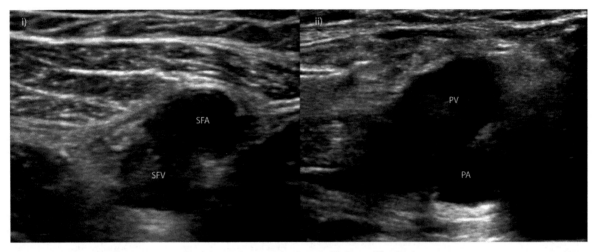

Figure 5.12 Thrombus in (i) the superficial femoral vein extending to (ii) the popliteal vein. SFA, superficial femoral artery; SFV, superficial femoral vein; PV, popliteal vein; PA, popliteal artery.

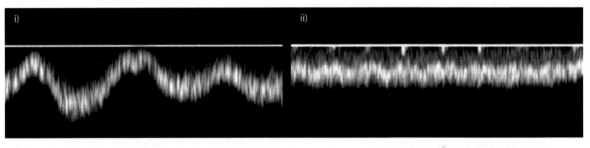

Figure 5.13 (i) Normal phasic flow within the femoral vein. Note the natural variability due to the impact of respiratory and cardiovascular mechanics. (ii) An example of continuous flow due to upstream obstruction such as vena cava or iliac vein thrombosis. Obstruction leads to a lack of upstream flow characteristics to be transmitted.

- Thrombus may be present in vessels outside of the vessels directly visualised. Additional advanced techniques can demonstrate features suggestive of DVT in these areas.
- Referral for definitive imaging should be considered in all patients with high DVT probability and a negative focused scan.

Deep Vein Thrombosis Assessment – Upper Limb

Venous thromboses of the upper limb are significantly less common than in the lower limbs and account for around 4–10% of all DVTs. They may occur within any vein in the upper limb and thoracic inlet including the jugular, brachiocephalic (innominate), subclavian, axillary and brachial veins. Although not technically deep veins, the basilic and cephalic veins warrant assessment for thrombosis due to their size and frequency of cannulation. Commonly affected sites include the subclavian vein (62%), axillary vein (45%) and jugular vein (45%).

Primary upper limb DVTs may be idiopathic or associated with syndromes including thoracic outlet syndrome and Paget-Schroetter syndrome (PSS). Although risk factors for upper limb DVT are largely the same as for lower, central venous access (including peripherally inserted central catheters), cardiac pacemakers/defibrillators, chemotherapeutic agents and tumour-related hypercoagulability are by far the most common precipitants.

Anatomy

See Figure 5.14. The ulnar and radial veins originate from the dorsal aspect of the hand and extend proximally to the elbow becoming the paired brachial veins. Brachial veins then join to form the axillary

133

vein in the upper arm. The axillary vein extends through the upper arm and axilla until it crosses the first rib and forms the subclavian vein.

The subclavian vein lies in front of the subclavian artery and extends between the first rib and clavicle. The clavicle obscures the mid subclavian vein. The internal jugular vein is located running vertically down the neck, overlying or adjacent to the carotid

artery, draining into the brachiocephalic vein that may be visualised deep to the medial aspect of the clavicle. The basilic vein is found lying medially to the brachial vein in the medial upper arm.

Method

When compared with the lower limb, assessment of the upper limb venous system relies more upon pulse wave and colour Doppler due to incomplete visualisation of veins and the chest wall and clavicle limiting compression.

Each vein should be systematically examined with compression US in turn and imaged along its entire course. If the vessel is obscured by overlying structures or is non-compressible (e.g. subclavian and brachiocephalic) then colour Doppler and pulse wave Doppler should be utilised. Colour Doppler allows the user to identify filling defects within a vessel. Pulse wave Doppler should demonstrate venous flow signal with respiratory variability as described earlier in the lower limb text. Augmentation may be performed by compression of the forearm.

The patient should be positioned supine with arms by their side. The jugular vein is assessed in the neck with the patient's head rotated to the contralateral side (Figure 5.15i). Valsalva manoeuvre will aid distension of the vein. The carotid artery is seen adjacent to or underlying the internal jugular

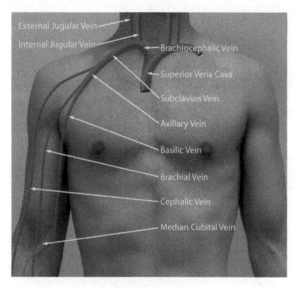

Figure 5.14 Upper limb venous anatomy.

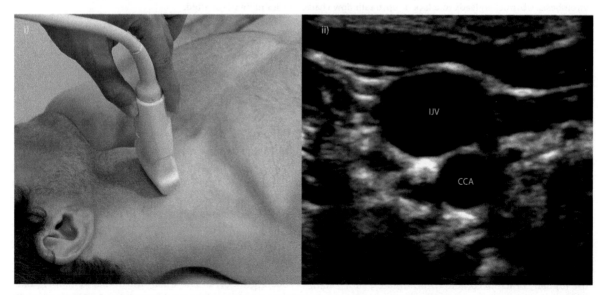

Figure 5.15 (i) Probe placement for assessment of the internal jugular vein. (ii) Appearance of the internal jugular vein overlying the common carotid artery. This is the most common point of central venous access in critical care patients. When performing central access, it is useful to track the wire distally to ensure it has passed into the brachiocephalic vein rather than deviated into the subclavian vein. IJV, internal jugular vein; CCA, common carotid artery.

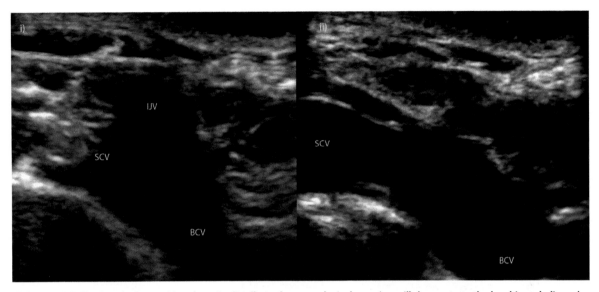

Figure 5.16 Following the internal jugular vein distally to the supraclavicular region will demonstrate the brachiocephalic and subclavian veins. (i) Demonstrates the flow of the internal jugular into the brachiocephalic vein. (ii) An optimised image of the subclavian vein and brachiocephalic vein. It may be necessary to tilt the tail of the probe towards the patient to angle the US beam 'into the thorax' to visualise the BCV. IJV, internal jugular vein; SCV, subclavian vein; BCV, brachiocephalic vein.

vein (Figure 5.15ii). The user should be cautious performing excessive compression in elderly patients who may be particularly sensitive to vagal stimulation from carotid sinus massage.

Follow the internal jugular vein inferiorly to the junction with the subclavian vein and brachiocephalic vein (Figure 5.16). The brachiocephalic may be visualised extending inferiorly towards the superior vena cava (Figure 5.16).

A supraclavicular approach (Figure 5.17) using colour Doppler should be used to follow the subclavian vein in transverse and longitudinal planes until it is no longer visible underneath the clavicle (Figure 5.18).

The patient should then be asked to abduct their arm placing their ipsilateral hand on their head. The junction between the distal subclavian vein and axillary vein may be seen from an infraclavicular approach. The axillary vein is followed into the axilla until the bifurcation into the basilic and brachial veins (Figure 5.19).

Filling of the arm veins is better achieved with the patient sat upright on the side of the bed with their arm supinated. The brachial and basilic veins should be interrogated and are readily compressible. At the antecubital fossa the brachial vein divides into the radial and ulnar veins that may be followed distally.

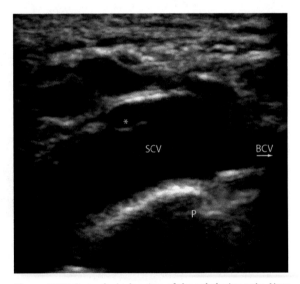

Figure 5.17 Supraclavicular view of the subclavian vein. Note the valve (*) within the SCV and the proximity of the vessel to the pleural line. SCV, subclavian vein; BCV, brachiocephalic vein; P, pleural line.

Key Points

- Interrogation of the lower limb venous system alone may miss up to 10% of DVTs.
- The upper limb venous system is more challenging to assess due to thoracic structures obscuring vessels and limiting compressibility.

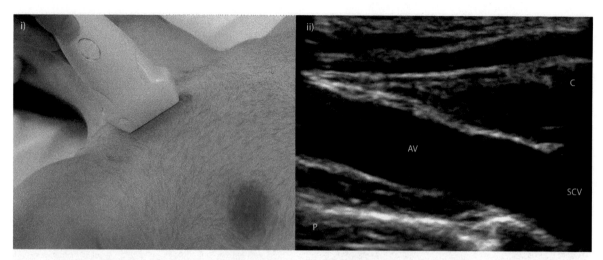

Figure 5.18 The infraclavicular axillary vein in long-axis view. An out of plane view may also be achieved by rotating the probe 90 degrees to appreciate the proximity of the axillary artery to the axillary vein. This view is ideal for performing infraclavicular central venous cannulation of the axillary vein (an US-guided 'subclavian line'). AV, axillary vein; SCV, subclavian vein; C, clavicle; P, pleural line.

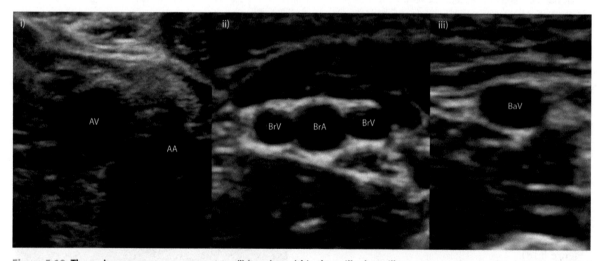

Figure 5.19 The major upper arm venous system. (i) Imaging within the axilla the axillary artery can be visualised. (ii) The brachial artery and paired brachial veins are visible in the middle of the upper arm. (iii) Moving the probe medially with reveal the basilic vein. The axillary vein and artery are potential points of central venous and arterial access in critically unwell patients. The basilic vein is the vein of choice for peripherally inserted central catheters (PICC). AV, axillary vein; AA, axillary artery; BrA, brachial artery; BrV, brachial vein; BaV, basilic vein.

- Colour and spectral Doppler play a key role in the assessment of the upper limb vessels.
- If a study is challenging or incomplete, the patient should be referred for definitive imaging e.g. departmental US or CT venogram.

Venous and Arterial Vascular Access

Ultrasound-guided vascular access is an essential skill for hospital practitioners. It has surpassed landmark technique as the gold standard for central venous cannulation and is invaluable in emergency and ward settings for difficult peripheral venous access.

Ultrasound use reduces the complication rate for central venous access including multiple cannulation attempts, inadvertent arterial puncture and pneumothorax. Cochrane database analysis suggests a reduction in complication rates from 13.5% to 4% when using US for internal jugular vein cannulation. Furthermore, US assessment of the target vessel identifies anatomical variability and confirms patency prior to beginning the procedure.

Challenging vascular access is common and estimated at 30% of all emergency, acute and hospitalised patients. Peripheral access is vital for life-saving treatments and delays can lead to increased morbidity and mortality. US guidance increases the likelihood of successful cannulation in the most challenging of patients in whom early and prompt treatment is likely to confer the greatest benefit. It may also reduce the need for multiple cannulation attempts which will reduce the pain experienced by patients and therefore improve the patient-doctor relationship. The same technique has been shown to yield a higher first-attempt success and lower failure rate in arterial cannulation when compared with palpation alone.

Increasingly medical schools are incorporating US-guided peripheral cannulation as a mandatory part of the curriculum. The same principles may be applied for central venous cannulation, peripheral venous cannulation and arterial blood gas sampling or cannulation.

Method

There are two key methods for performing vascular access: transverse (out of plane, Figure 5.20i) and longitudinal (in plane, Figure 5.20ii). The optimal approach is dependent on the target vessel, surrounding anatomy, user experience and speed in which vascular access must be acquired.

Transverse approach involves obtaining a cross-sectional view of the target vessel. The differences in appearance of an artery and vein are described earlier and differentiation is a key initial step. The user should track the course of the vessel proximally and distally to identify its direction of travel and optimal point of puncture. The probe marker should be pointing to the same side as the screen indicator meaning a medial or lateral correction in needle angle will occur in the same direction on the US screen.

Figure 5.21 is an example of probe position for out of plane vascular access with a short-axis view of the target vessel. The target vessel is placed in the middle of the screen with the image optimised. Excessive image depth should be particularly avoided. The needle is introduced just distal to the middle marker of the probe at a 30–45 degree angle and will be seen as a bright, echogenic dot on the screen. The probe should be advanced beyond the needle incrementally to ensure the structure seen is the needle tip. The most significant pitfall with the transverse approach is the user incorrectly believing the needle tip to be shallower than it is because they have failed to sweep the probe proximally during insertion. Visualisation of the tip may be improved by fanning the probe backwards and forwards or gently bouncing the needle tip to see movement of the tissue planes.

The longitudinal approach is a more challenging technique but enables visualisation of the entirety of the needle throughout its course of insertion (Figure 5.22). Many users will preferentially acquire an image of the vessel in a transverse (out of plane) view and rotate the probe 90 degrees to acquire a longitudinal view. The needle is then inserted just distally to the probe and visualised entering the image

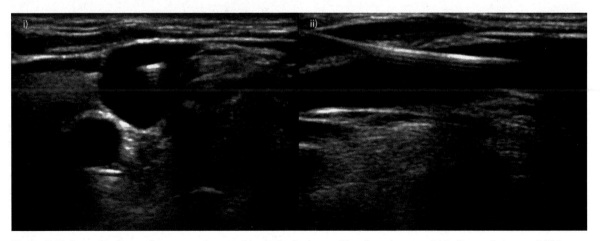

Figure 5.20 Example of central venous catheter guidewire in the internal jugular vein seen within (i) out of plane and (ii) in plane views.

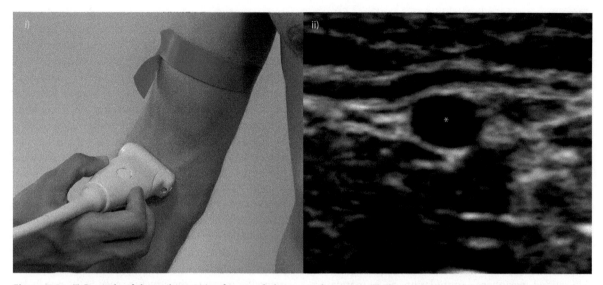

Figure 5.21 (i) Example of the probe position for out of plane vascular access. (ii) Short-axis view of the target vessel (*).

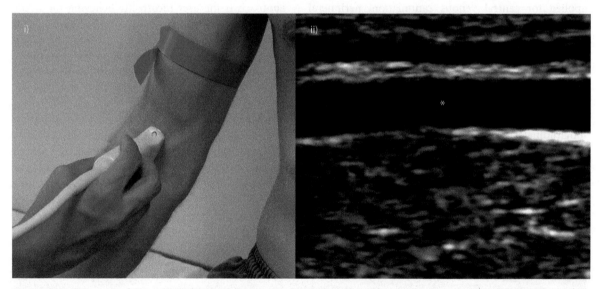

Figure 5.22 (i) Example of the probe position to achieve a view for in plane vascular access. (ii) Long-axis view of the target vessel (*).

from the side of the screen. During insertion, the needle tip can be followed until entry into the vessel and, if applicable, the cannula advanced and position confirmed. The major difficulty with this approach is due to the thin beam width of only ~1 mm. A small lateral deviation in either US probe or needle will result in a complete loss of needle visualisation. The user must be disciplined in only moving the needle when it is clearly visualised on the US screen to prevent inadvertent puncture of structures lateral to the target.

Choosing the Right Approach

There is no correct answer for which is the correct method for performing vascular access. Although both techniques may be successfully implemented for any vessel there are certain factors that may guide selection. An example of needle placement for out of plane and in plane arterial access is shown in Figure 5.23.

Firstly, the longitudinal approach is a more challenging technique with a steeper learning curve. Novice users may be more comfortable with the

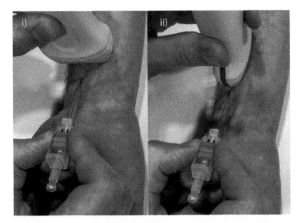

Figure 5.23 (i) Out of plane or transverse approach versus (ii) in plane or longitudinal approach for radial artery cannulation.

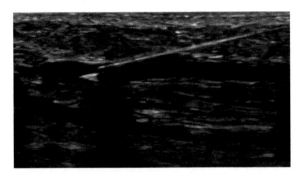

Figure 5.24 In plane or longitudinal technique for cannulation of a peripheral vein. Note the needle may be followed throughout its entire course and be seen to enter the vein.
A video is available to view in the online video library.

transverse technique as it allows for easier lateral correction of needle placement. Additionally, if there is a vessel in close lateral proximity to the target vessel then a transverse approach may reduce the risk of inadvertent puncture of the wrong structure.

Conversely, any circumstance where there is a structure directly beneath the target vessel, e.g. artery or pleura, may benefit from the longitudinal approach due to a more accurate visualisation of the needle tip throughout insertion. Figure 5.24 demonstrates how the entire needle can be visualised throughout its course when using an in plane, longitudinal approach.

The longitudinal technique tends to require more time and careful positioning of the patient. In situations whereby vascular access needs to be obtained rapidly the transverse approach may be preferred.

Similarly, suboptimal patient positioning or patient agitation will increase the difficulty of maintaining an optimal longitudinal view.

Some users will prefer to employ a hybrid approach. The initial insertion will be performed with a transverse approach until the vessel is punctured. After this the clinician will rotate the probe to acquire a longitudinal view and confirm that the cannula is correctly advancing into the vessel.

Key Points

- Transverse and longitudinal techniques may be utilised for vascular access. Selection is dependent upon user experience, target vessel, surrounding anatomy and speed in which vascular access is required.
- Mastering of both techniques is advantageous to provide the user with a versatile skill set.
- Regardless of approach, visualisation of the needle tip is key to preventing adverse events.

Summary

- Deep vein thrombosis is a commonly encountered clinical scenario and may be diagnosed using compression US.
- The 'three-point approach' is a simple, rule-in method for identifying DVT that is advocated by most POCUS training pathways. This may be extended to track the key vessels throughout their visible course.
- Up to 10% of DVTs occur within the upper limb venous system. This should particularly be assessed in patients with risk factors for upper limb DVT.
- Ultrasound-guided vascular access is the gold standard for central venous cannulation. It increases the likelihood of first-attempt success and reduces the risk of significant complications.
- Ultrasound-guided peripheral venous and arterial access is a mandatory skill for all clinicians. Whether in plane or out of plane techniques are used, US enhances the first-attempt success rate in the most challenging of patient populations.
- Ultrasound-guided peripheral venous access is being introduced at undergraduate-level training.

A full list of references and further reading is available at www.GeneralistUltrasound.com

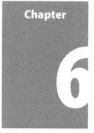

Soft Tissue and Musculoskeletal Ultrasound

Chapter 6

Ultrasound (US) is used extensively in the management of soft tissue and musculoskeletal (MSK) conditions and its clinical utility has evolved with the development of portable, cheaper and high-quality US machines. In Primary Care and the Emergency Department it is an invaluable tool for all generalists in reaching timely diagnoses and determining appropriate management. This may include simple reassurance through to oral antibiotics or the need for urgent surgical intervention. MSK injuries may be diagnosed rapidly and accurately at the 'pitch side' and guide immediate management and intervention for elite athletes.

In this chapter we will explore the role of US within basic soft tissue conditions and expand to the assessment of MSK structures. It will include five main sections:

1. Probes, methods, settings and basic structures.
2. Soft tissue pathology.
3. Lumps and bumps.
4. Introduction to muscle, bones and tendons.
5. Basic musculoskeletal ultrasound (MSKUS).

Method

Probes

The high frequency linear probe is the most commonly utilised probe for soft tissue and MSKUS and is appropriate for the majority of structures. The hockey stick probe may be used for smaller structures, such as the hand and wrist, where a smaller footprint is required. The curvilinear probe is sometimes used to assess deeper structures such as the hip joint.

Some machines have the software capability to simulate the image of a curvilinear probe, allowing a larger field of view of the deeper structures. This 'virtual convex' ability makes the machines more portable and affordable without the need for an additional probe.

Settings

The capacity to modify machine settings will vary between US machines. Settings such as depth and frequency can be modified by the user to best suit the structure being examined and optimise resolution. Most machines have programmed presets that are available for key structures to streamline the examination process. These settings are discussed in more detail in Chapter 1. Table 6.1 summarises the recommended imaging frequencies for commonly imaged structures.

Callipers are commonly used to measure the length or diameter of structures and are particularly valuable for diagnosing injuries.

Technique

The probe should be positioned overlying the anatomical structure under examination. It is important to adopt a light touch with soft tissue and MSKUS. Excessive pressure may result in compression of the structure under investigation and influence the diagnostic utility of images (Figure 6.1). Structures may be followed throughout their course and should be examined using multiple imaging planes (Figure 6.2).

Tissue harmonic imaging (THI) and compound imaging are modern signal processing techniques that provide enhanced image clarity. These settings will optimise the detection of fluid-filled structures and are typically switched on by default by modern US machines. Colour Doppler and power Doppler are important adjuncts of most examinations. Colour

Table 6.1 Recommended frequency for commonly imaged musculoskeletal structures

Region	Frequency
Shoulder/hip	8–12 MHz
Elbow/knee/ankle	10–12 MHz
Wrist/hand/foot	12–18 MHz

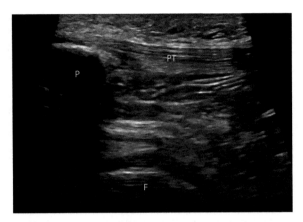

Figure 6.1 **Ultrasound scan of a patellar tendon using the virtual convex setting and a linear probe. The deeper structures are seen in a larger field of view.** P, patella; PT, patellar tendon; F, femur.

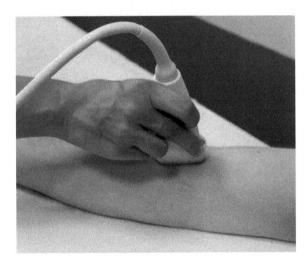

Figure 6.2 **Scanning in a longitudinal or sagittal plane.**

Doppler is described in detail in Chapter 1 and power Doppler will be discussed below.

Anatomy of small structures, such as the hands and feet, can be challenging to image due to the surface irregularity. In acute injuries, pain may also limit the examination. The use of a water bath can significantly improve the quality of image as the water replaces the gel as an acoustic window. The area of interest is placed in a clean container filled with warm water. Resting the body part on the base of the container helps to avoid movement (Figure 6.3i). The probe is waterproof and placed directly over the structure being examined with a slight gap between the skin and the probe to improve the resolution. Machine setting can be modified to further improve this (Figure 6.3ii). Although this is a useful technique in challenging patients it relies on the availability of a water bath and will not be practical in settings with more limited resources.

Power Doppler

Power Doppler (PD) follows the same principles as colour Doppler but generates a signal that is independent to the velocity and direction of flow. As such, it is more sensitive for detecting low velocity signal when compared with colour Doppler. PD is an integral aspect of diagnosing MSK pathology, such as synovitis, tenosynovitis and enthesitis, where an increased Doppler signal is suggestive of inflammation and neovascularity (Figure 6.4).

Neovascularisation is a hallmark feature of tendinopathy and the severity, assessed using US and PD, is integral to the grading of tendinopathy using the 'Modified Ohberg Score'.

To improve sensitivity, the user must use plenty of gel, hold the probe steady and with light pressure to avoid compression of the vascular structures embedded in the pathology. Compression US may help to distinguish between various anechoic structures. Areas of neovascularisation are often targeted during US-guided interventional procedures such as corticosteroid injections.

Normal Structures

All superficial anatomical structures may be potentially interrogated using US and a thorough understanding of normal anatomy is vital for identifying pathology. Key characteristics of superficial anatomical structures are listed below (Figure 6.5).

- *Epidermis* – the most superficial structure appearing as a hyperechoic layer closest to the probe.
- *Hypodermis* – the second layer containing mostly subcutaneous fat and is generally hypoechoic compared to epidermis or fascia. There is significant variability in thickness depending on the patient's body habitus. The hypodermis is the usual location for development of cellulitis.
- *Fascia* – fascial planes appear as hyperechoic lines bordering muscle compartments.
- *Muscle* – hypoechoic compared to fascia or epidermis and has a typical striated appearance. Blood vessels and nerves may be identified throughout this layer.

141

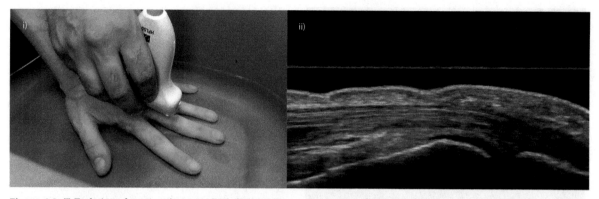

Figure 6.3 (i) Technique for using the water bath for imaging small structures. (ii) Corresponding image of the finger. Note the hypoechoic region below the probe tip (horizontal line) which is the water allowing easy transmission of ultrasound waves. *A video is available to view in the online video library.*

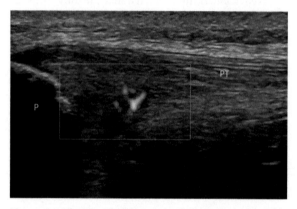

Figure 6.4 Ultrasound of the proximal patellar tendon origin at the distal pole of the patella. Note the neovascularity with the application of power Doppler. P, patella; PT, patellar tendon.

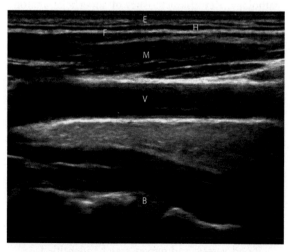

Figure 6.5 Normal soft tissue anatomy. E, epidermis; H, hypodermis; M, muscle; V, blood vessel; B, bone.

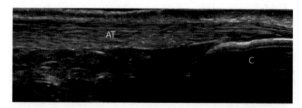

Figure 6.6 The linear pattern of a normal Achilles tendon from the insertion on to the calcaneus. The fibres run parallel and show no irregularity, no thickening and no calcification. AT, achilles tendon; C, calcaneus.

- *Tendon* – linear fibrillar structure of tendons is reflected with an US image as parallel hyperechoic lines best seen in the longitudinal axis (Figure 6.6). In cross-section the tendons are represented by hyperechoic dots. Fluid within the tendon sheath is seen as an anechoic area surrounding the tendon.
- *Ligament* – ligaments are not as readily visible as tendons and can appear hypoechoic due to anisotropy (Figure 6.7). Ligaments are commonly tested for dynamic stability using US.
- *Bone* – appears as a hyperechoic line with post-acoustic shadowing due to US impedance. Appreciating normal bone appearance is helpful in determining the presence of cortical irregularities such as osteophytes, enthesophytes or fractures.
- *Joints* – readily identified using US but visualisation is limited with deeper structures such as the hip. Joint fluid contained within the capsule can be identified as an anechoic area between two hyperechoic lines of the bony surface. Care must be taken to ensure the anechoic articular cartilage is not mistaken for fluid contained within the joint.

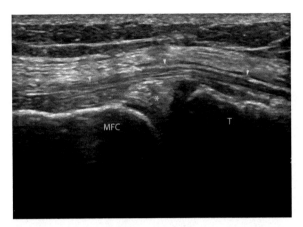

Figure 6.7 Ultrasound of the medial knee demonstrating the peripheral edge of the medial meniscus (*) and the overlying medial collateral ligament (arrows). MFC, medial femoral condyle; T, tibia.

- *Cartilage* – hyaline cartilage overlying the osteochondral margins is homogeneously hypoechoic on US. Fibrocartilaginous structures such as the meniscus appear hyperechoic.
- *Nerves* – In a longitudinal plane, nerves are visualised by alternating hypoechoic and hyperechoic lines and are occasionally confused with tendons. A cross-sectional axis of the nerve bundle is used to differentiate the nerve and represents a 'honeycomb' appearance, seen as the hypoechoic nerve surrounded by the hyperechoic nerve sheath.
- Blood vessels – Vessels appear anechoic on US and can be confirmed with the application of colour Doppler. Key features differentiating arteries from veins are discussed in Chapter 5.

Introduction to Soft Tissue Ultrasound

The role of point-of-care ultrasound (POCUS) for soft tissue conditions is aimed at answering specific, binary diagnostic questions. It may guide frontline clinicians to deliver procedural intervention or establish a diagnosis to avoid hospital referral or admission. Many soft tissue lumps may require formal US evaluation.

A thorough history and examination is vital to determine the size of a lesion and how long it has been present. Recent trauma, history of malignancy, and anticoagulant use are all important factors. Rapidly growing lesions should be considered suspicious and managed as such.

Soft Tissue Pathology

Cellulitis

Ultrasound is an ideal modality to diagnose skin and soft tissue infections. It has been reported to result in a change of management in 56% of patients through the detection of occult abscesses, preventing unnecessary intervention or to guide further imaging or management referrals.

Cellulitis is a common condition seen across multiple medical settings. It is a soft tissue infection involving the hypodermis where activation of an inflammatory cascade leads to the hypodermic space filling with serous fluid. On clinical examination, this will appear as an oedematous, warm, erythematous area.

Early cellulitis on POCUS appears as a delineation or blurring of previously sharp borders of normal soft tissue planes. Scanning proximally or distally to the affected region or the contralateral asymptomatic side is recommended to compare the integrity and characteristic of tissue.

Fat stranding may progress to mature cellulitis which is represented by oedema in the interstitial space between adipocytes. With US, this is seen as hypoechoic strands between hyperechoic fat lobules with hypervascularity. This is described as the *'cobblestone'* appearance (Figure 6.8i).

Cobblestone appearance may be due to any causes of interstitial fluid such as congestive cardiac failure, nephrotic syndrome and renal failure. Clinical examination should allow differentiation between cellulitis and these aetiologies. Figure 6.8ii is taken from a patient with congestive cardiac failure and significant peripheral oedema. In regions with a higher proportion of adipose tissue, such as the upper leg or abdomen, the cobblestone appearance may be more marked.

Abscess

An abscess is a collection of pus in response to a skin and soft tissue infection with a walled-off collection of necrotic tissue, inflammatory cells and bacteria. US is 98% sensitive and 88% specific for diagnosis of abscesses compared with clinical examination which is 86% sensitive and 70% specific.

The typical appearance of an abscess is an anechoic collection of fluid. Hypoechoic debris or loculations may be present within the abscess (Figure 6.9).

Occasionally, debris or pus may cause the abscess to appear similar in echogenicity to soft tissue. Applying

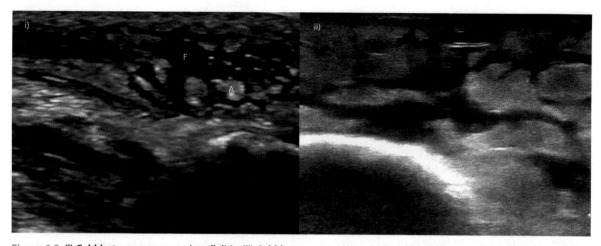

Figure 6.8 (i) Cobblestone appearance in cellulitis. (ii) Cobblestone appearance in lower leg due to severe peripheral oedema.
Note the hyperechoic round globules of subcutaneous adipose tissue are separated by a slightly irregular lattice of anechoic or hypoechoic fluid. F, fluid; A, adipose tissue. *Videos are available to view in the online video library.*

Table 6.2 Abscess mimics on ultrasound

Characteristics on ultrasound image	
Abscess	Anechoic to hypoechoic background, ± 'swirl sign'. Responsive to graded compression.
Baker's cyst	Smooth well circumscribed anechoic ovoid area with thin hyperechoic margins.
Infected cyst	Hypoechoic to isoechoic, uniform heterogeneity. Minimal graded compression.
Hematoma	Anechoic to hyperechoic with variability over time.
Herniated bowel	Organized circular tissue planes with thicker hyperechoic walls and visible peristalsis.
Lymph node	Well circumscribed, may present with a hypoechoic halo, vasculature within seen on colour Doppler.

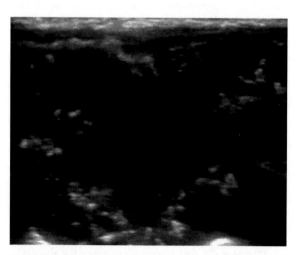

Figure 6.9 Appearance and aspiration of an abscess. *A video is available to view in the online video library.*

downward pressure to the US will cause the pus to move and 'graded compression' is a specific technique of probe manipulation used to differentiate between abscess mimics (Table 6.2). Intermittently delivering pressure through the probe over the suspected abscess will demonstrate motion of fluid. This is the 'swirl sign'. This is an important finding as antibiotics alone are unlikely to be curative and aspiration or incision and drainage of the abscess is likely to be required (Figure 6.10).

Colour Doppler may be used to identify adjacent blood vessels to avoid iatrogenic injury during drainage or aspiration. Neovascularity is likely to be seen within the abscess itself. In deeper structures, such as the thigh, the low frequency transducer is used and the muscle needs to be closely interrogated to avoid missing an intramuscular abscess.

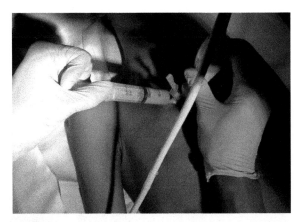

Figure 6.10 **Aspiration of chest wall abscess under ultrasound guidance.**

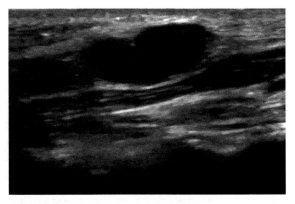

Figure 6.12 **Lymph node. Note the kidney-shaped appearance.** *A video is available to view in the online video library.*

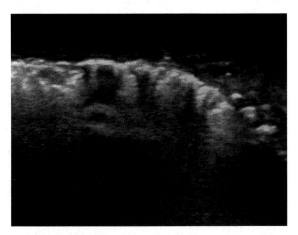

Figure 6.11 **The appearance of nectrotising fasciitis on US.**

Necrotising Fasciitis

Necrotising fasciitis (NF) is a surgical emergency requiring prompt surgical debridement. It is characterised by severe infection of the fascial planes affecting predominantly the immunocompromised, diabetic, obese or patients with a history of intravenous drug use. On US, NF typically demonstrates fascial thickening with adjacent anechoic fluid (Figure 6.11). Gas-forming organisms produce air which appears hyperechoic with reverberation artefact or 'dirty shadowing' deep to the air. Although not sensitive, this is a very specific finding in NF.

Lumps and Bumps

Lymph Nodes

Lymph nodes are solitary structures composed of lymphoid tissue and are distributed along the course

of lymphatic vessels. On US, lymph nodes appear as small, contained, oval-shaped structures that have a relatively hyperechoic centre and hypoechoic periphery. They are typically referred to as having the appearance of 'mini kidneys' (Figure 6.12).

A lymph node is divided anatomically into an outer cortex, inner medulla and a surrounding outer fibrous capsule. The central medulla is hyperechoic due to a dense network of lymphatic cords and sinuses and will be the site of primary vascularity when using colour Doppler in normal or reactive lymph nodes.

In general, lymph nodes are not larger than 7–10 mm. Nodes greater than 15 mm are typically detectable by palpation. US allows accurate assessment of the lymph node site, size, shape, border, internal architecture, adjacent soft tissue oedema, and characterisation of the vascular flow pattern.

Metastatic lymph nodes are markedly hypoechoic with a heterogeneous echotexture and a rounder shape. They may also contain macrocalcification, cystic changes and irregular borders. There is often an increase in *peripheral* vascularity seen with colour Doppler unlike normal lymph nodes where the flow is *central*. These patients should be urgently referred for definitive investigation.

Case – Lumps and Bumps

A 45-year-old male presented with a painful groin swelling following cellulitis in the affected leg. The differential diagnosis included an abscess or an inguinal lymph node. US demonstrated central colour flow with the reassuring characteristic appearance of a enlarged, reactive lymph node (Figure 6.13).

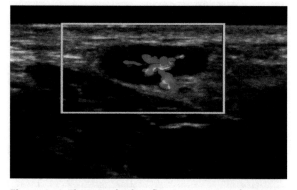

Figure 6.13 **The central colour flow is suggestive of a reactive lymph node.** *A video is available to view in the online video library.*

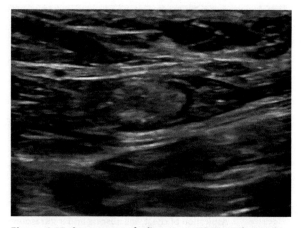

Figure 6.15 **Appearance of a lipoma on US. Note the similar echogenicity to nearby adipose tissue.** *A video is available to view in the online video library.*

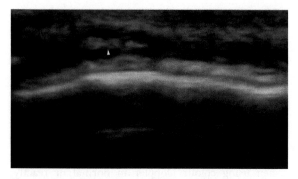

Figure 6.14 **Sebaceous cyst with internal debris (arrow).**

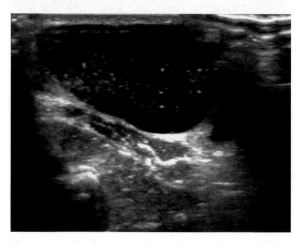

Figure 6.16 **Ganglion cyst with appearance of internal debris.** *A video is available to view in the online video library.*

Sebaceous Cyst

Sebaceous cysts are displaced epithelial cells that outline a cyst filled with keratin and lipid debris. They clinically present as slow-growing, non-painful and mobile structures with well-defined borders.

Ultrasound demonstrates well-defined margins with posterior acoustic enhancement and no internal blood flow (Figure 6.14). There may be a punctum visible on US which tethers the cyst to the overlying epidermis which is diagnostic of a sebaceous cyst.

Infected cysts may cause cellulitic changes in the surrounding tissue. US may be used to guide aspiration or drainage of surrounding pus.

Lipoma

Lipomas are the commonest form of benign skin tumour occurring in the subcutaneous skin layer and typically present as a rubbery mass. Although their appearance may be variable, the echogenicity tends to be similar to the surrounding fat and are oval or elliptical in shape (Figure 6.15). Lipomas are non-vascular and have no edge artefact or colour Doppler signal. Internal septations may be present.

Ganglion Cyst

Ganglion cysts are common, synovial cysts filled with mucoid material that may be identified in any region with joints and tendon sheaths. They most commonly occur in young and middle-aged females. The scapholunate region of the dorsal wrist is the most frequent location for a ganglion cyst to form.

Ultrasound will demonstrate an anechoic structure with posterior acoustic enhancement and no internal blood flow. Smaller ganglions may have internal debris (Figure 6.16) and can develop septations as they increase in size. The cyst may also be seen to be connecting to the joint or tendon sheath.

Introduction to Bones, Muscle and Tendons

Fractures

Ultrasound offers a simple and accurate way to diagnose fractures at the bedside in time-sensitive situations. Additionally, it has a high diagnostic accuracy for frequently occult fractures, such as rib and sternal fractures.

The outer cortex of bone will appear as a hyperechoic line with post-acoustic shadowing. Disruption of the hyperechoic cortical line represents a fracture and is best visualised in a longitudinal plane. US has been reported to be 94–100% sensitive and 56–100% specific in the diagnosis of long bone fractures when used by Emergency Clinicians. In the ED, this is particularly useful when assessing the alignment of long bone fractures, such as Colles' fractures, following reduction and manipulation (Figure 6.17). US may also increase the accuracy and efficacy of guided haematoma blocks which obviates the need for procedural sedation.

Case – Sternal Fracture Diagnosed on Ultrasound

A 35-year-old patient was involved in a road traffic accident where the airbag was deployed. The patient complained of some sternal tenderness and was awaiting a CT scan of the chest. US demonstrated discontinuity in the echogenic cortex suggestive of a sternal fracture that was not visible on the chest X-ray (CXR) (Figure 6.18).

Identifying a sternal fracture in the context of trauma is suggestive of a significant mechanism of injury and increases the incidence of pulmonary and myocardial contusion injuries, pneumothoraces, haemothoraces, pericardial effusion/haemotoma, rib fractures and spinal compression fractures.

Haematoma

Haematoma may develop following any form of trauma with a significant increase in prevalence in anticoagulated patients. Many haematomas are managed conservatively but may require drainage if of sufficient size or develop secondary infection.

Ultrasound features of haematoma are varied and depend on the time elapsed. In the acute stage, haematomas appear anechoic or heterogeneously hypoechoic (Figure 6.19) and may have surrounding oedema. As blood progressively clots, the haematoma will become increasingly hyperechoic, irregular, septated and can develop a thick hyperechoic wall. The

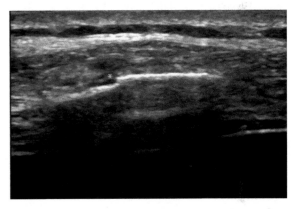

Figure 6.18 Sternal fracture (star) that was not visible on chest X-ray. Note the discontinuity in the echogenic cortex. *A video is available to view in the online video library.*

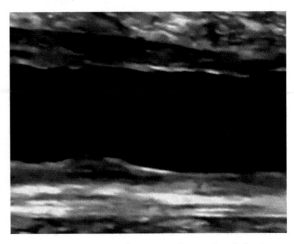

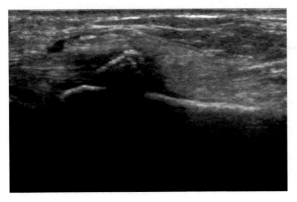

Figure 6.17 Colles' fracture with dorsal displacement of the distal fragment. *A video is available to view in the online video library.*

Figure 6.19 Large acute haematoma in a patient following a sporting injury. Note the hypoechoic fluid.

appearance of chronic haematomas are equally varied and may be anechoic, hypoechoic or hyperechoic. Features such as the plankton or haematocrit sign may be present. These are described in more detail in the haemothorax section in Chapter 3.

Colour Doppler with an appropriately adjusted scale may provide some clues regarding underlying pathology such as an abscess or pseudoaneurysm.

Tendonitis and Tenosynovitis

Tendinopathy is a common MSK presentation and is readily assessed using US. Care must be taken when imaging tendons due to 'anisotropy' which is an angle-generated artefact causing a loss of echogenicity when using an oblique insonating angle (Figure 6.20). This may be falsely suggestive of a tendinopathy or structural tear particularly at tendon insertion points. Hypoechoic areas created by anisotropy disappear by tilting the transducer and therefore changing the angle of insonation. Tendons should always be imaged in orthogonal planes to discriminate between a tendinopathy and artefact.

Tendinopathy can be identified on US by visualising a hypoechoic thickening of the tendon caused by oedema. Power Doppler may reveal an increased signal representing hypervascularity. A tear may be seen as a disruption in the normal fibrillar pattern of the tendon. Tendonitis and tenosynovitis are discussed in more detail in the section below on basic MSKUS.

Baker's Cyst

Bursae are paratendinous fluid-filled sacs which are synovial lined and aid with shock absorption and friction reduction. Normally bursae only contain a small volume of fluid but this may increase following irritation, trauma or infection.

A Baker's cyst is a distended bursa between the medial head of semimembranosus and gastrocnemius muscles on the medial posterior aspect of the knee. They do not occur laterally in the popliteal fossa. Baker's cysts are an important differential diagnosis in any patient presenting with suspected deep vein thrombosis (DVT) and may be readily identified using US.

Ultrasound will reveal an anechoic or hypoechoic cyst and may contain osteochondral loose bodies. They have a classic 'hook' appearance on a lateral view and may be irregular in shape with synovial thickening and surrounding cellulitis (Figure 6.21). Colour flow will help differentiate a Baker's cyst from a DVT.

Foreign Body

Suspected foreign bodies (FBs) are a common presentation to primary care and the ED. Although metal and glass are readily identified on X-ray, radiolucent FBs such as wood and plastic may be missed. Patient history may be misleading and missed FBs can be a cause of significant pain and source of infection.

Ultrasound may be useful in identifying FBs as small as 2.5 mm. The appearance is very variable depending on the type of material. Structures with a high acoustic impedance, such as metal and glass, are typically hyperechoic with post-acoustic shadowing and reverberation artefact. Wood and plastic cause less significant shadowing but will have an atypical shape that is not consistent with any anatomical structure (Figure 6.22).

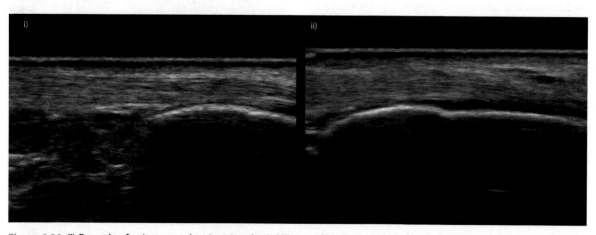

Figure 6.20 (i) Example of anisotropy when imaging the Achilles tendon. (ii) Correction of anisotropy by altering the angle of insonation. *Videos are available to view in the online video library.*

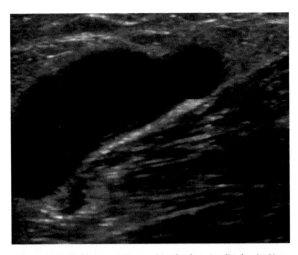

Figure 6.21 Baker's cyst imaged in the longitudinal axis. Note the hypoechoic fluid. Lying the patient on their front will make scanning the popliteal fossa significantly easier. *A video is available to view in the online video library.*

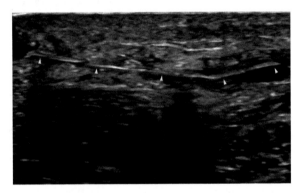

Figure 6.22 Wooden foreign body (arrows). *A video is available to view in the online video library.*

Blind attempts at removal can lead to iatrogenic injury and have poor success rates unless large incisions are created for direct visualisation. Challenging body regions such as web spaces of the feet or concomitant traumatic injury can make foreign body extraction difficult. Localising a FB in a region that requires surgical removal is equally as important as FBs that may be removed within primary care or the ED.

Ultrasound-guided removal of FBs utilises a technique similar to other US-guided procedures. Once the FB is located, the probe should be manipulated to assess the size, extent and relationship to surrounding structures such as blood vessels and anatomical landmarks. After sufficient anaesthesia is infiltrated and an incision has been made, the forcep tip is followed in a manner similar to following the needle tip in

other US-guided procedures until the forceps reach the foreign body. Positioning a separate needle may help as a marker before extraction.

Basic Musculoskeletal Ultrasound

Musculoskeletal ultrasound has evolved significantly since the first published report in 1958. Its application has significantly increased in recent years and is no longer limited to radiologists and sonographers. The use of POCUS has enabled other clinicians to become proficient in MSKUS including, but not limited to, sport and exercise medicine consultants, rheumatologists, orthopaedic surgeons, podiatrists and physiotherapists.

Developments in software and hardware technology have improved portability, accessibility and reduced cost. These factors have cemented US as an invaluable tool used widely across a variety of settings, from routine community MSK clinics to pitch-side trauma. It offers a number of advantages over MRI and CT when applied by a skilled user in the appropriate clinical scenario. The portability and immediate application are particularly valuable in elite sport, where a timely diagnosis, immediate management and appropriate intervention can be pertinent. Unlike other imaging modalities, US has the added advantage of allowing dynamic scanning. The region under investigation can be moved simultaneously under the probe to assess the structures as they are mobilised. An example of this are the lateral ankle ligaments and joint integrity following an inversion ankle sprain.

As with most diagnostic tools there are limitations to the use of US within MSK. The quality of image is reflected by the user's clinical proficiency, experience and scope of regular practice. Even in skilful hands, some MSK structures are challenging to visualise due to excessive depth, are obscured by other bony structures or anisotropy. The meniscus is a prime example as only the peripheral edge is visible with US due to the acoustic impedance of bone. In some cases, acute and low-grade muscle injuries may not be detected on US which falsely reassures the clinician that the injury is non-pathological. Incidental findings are frequently encountered within MSKUS and the user must correlate the images with the conventional history and examination. MSKUS is a complex and broad discipline and any uncertainty with interpretation should prompt specialist referral.

This chapter will discuss a basic approach to MSKUS followed by listing the common sites of injury that the clinician should be familiar with. Probe locations, corresponding images and pathological examples will help the reader to orientate and understand the key landmarks for each anatomical area.

Interventions

A major advantage of US is its ability to direct both diagnostic and therapeutic interventions. In an MSK setting, this can include administration of local anaesthetic for diagnostic purposes, aspiration of structures such as joints, and interventional high-volume injections or injection of sclerosing agents such as corticosteroid injections, hyaluronic acid and platelet-rich plasma.

Although other imaging modalities are available, US is a safe, cost effective and immediately accessible modality within the routine clinical setting.

There are a number of studies discussing the improved accuracy and efficacy of injections when guided with US. An example of this is literature to support injections into the glenohumeral, hip and knee joints using US. Accuracy with US ranged from 91–100% compared with landmark injections with a 64–81% accuracy.

The Beginner's Approach to Musculoskeletal Ultrasound

1. Use the patient history and examination to direct regional scanning based upon the possible differential diagnoses.
2. Place the patient in a comfortable position that enables the clinician to easily control the machine.
3. Use plenty of gel. Thicker US gel can provide better surface contact in areas requiring gentle scanning pressure.
4. Use a high frequency linear transducer and a specific MSK preset.
5. Identify common landmarks.
6. Scan each structure in longitudinal and transverse planes.
7. Scan the entire structure to avoid missing any pathology – medial to lateral and proximal to distal.
8. Use dynamic manoeuvres if appropriate.
9. Use power Doppler if appropriate.
10. Obtain measurements as appropriate.
11. Label the images.

12. If unsure scan the asymptomatic side for comparison.
13. Formally report images for quality assurance purposes.

Upper Limb

Shoulder

Shoulder complaints are the third most common MSK problem presenting to primary care and also one of the most commonly scanned joints. Unlike other joints, the entire shoulder is almost always examined during the course of an US scan.

The majority of clinicians will follow the same pattern when conducting the examination. The patient is typically seated for the scan, with the clinician positioned either in front or behind of the patient, depending on preference.

Firstly, the shoulder is supported in the neutral position, with the elbow at 90 degrees of flexion and supinated.

The long head of the biceps tendon is assessed in the bicipital groove of the humerus and is scanned in short- and long-axis (Figures 6.23 and 6.24). The tendon of the pectoralis major can be visualised moving distally and medially (Figure 6.25).

The long head of the biceps tendon in short-axis view can be followed proximally to the rotator cuff interval. In this view one can visualise the long head of biceps situated between subscapularis and supraspinatus (Figure 6.26). It is in this area that the biceps tendon is an intra-articular structure and is thought to have a role in the depression of the humeral head.

With the patient's hand supported and the arm externally rotated, the probe is moved medially to visualise subscapularis and its tendon. In short-axis view this has a classic 'tiger stripe' appearance (Figure 6.27). The tendon can also be visualised dynamically in long-axis view for evidence of bunching under the coracoid process.

The patient is then asked to place their hand on the posterior aspect of their hip while keeping the elbow tucked in (the modified Crass position). The probe is again placed in the bicipital groove and moved superiorly. In this position the long- and short-axis views of supraspinatus can be found (Figures 6.28 and 6.29). In the long-axis view the tendon can be viewed from its footprint on the greater tuberosity and followed medially until it disappears under the acromium.

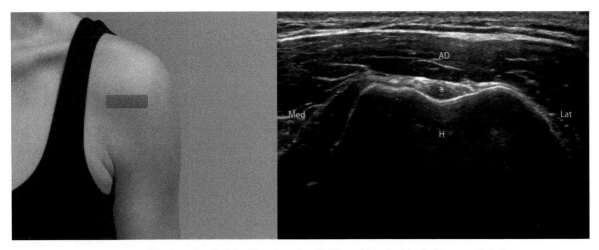

Figure 6.23 Short-axis view of the long head of the biceps tendon (*) lying within the bicipital groove of the humerus. H, humerus; AD, anterior deltoid; Med, medial; Lat, lateral.

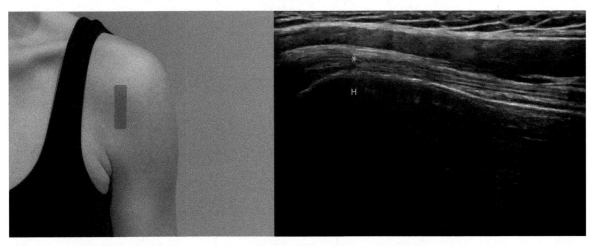

Figure 6.24 Long-axis view of the long head biceps tendon (*) showing the normal fibrillar structure. H, humerus.

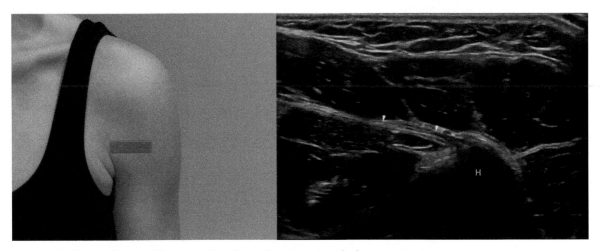

Figure 6.25 The attachment of the pectoralis major tendon (arrows) on the humerus. H, humerus.

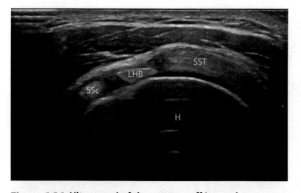

Figure 6.26 **Ultrasound of the rotator cuff interval.** H, humerus; LHB, long head of the biceps tendon; SSc, subscapularis tendon; SST, supraspinatus tendon.

The subacromial bursa can also be visualised in this view and by asking the patient to gently perform abduction movements the tendon and bursa can be seen to bunch underneath the acromium.

The patient is then asked to place their hand on their opposite shoulder for the posterior joint to be scanned. The muscle and tendon of infraspinatus is followed to its attachment on to the posterior aspect of the greater tuberosity. Adjusting depth and focus if needed, the posterior view of the glenohumeral joint is seen (Figure 6.30). It is this view that is used for injections to the glenohumeral joint. The peripheral edge of the labrum is seen here and in the case of posterior labral cysts, these can be visualised and injected if indicated. The permanent management of

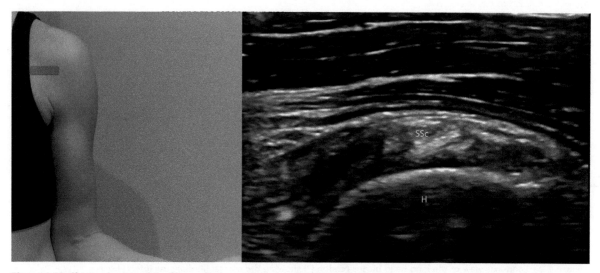

Figure 6.27 **Short-axis view of the fibres of subscapularis showing the tendon bundles.** H, humerus; SSc, subscapularis tendon.

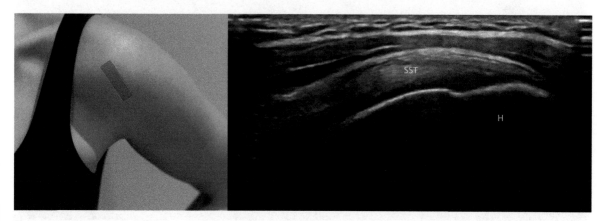

Figure 6.28 **Long-axis view of the supraspinatus tendon showing the footprint at the greater tuberosity of the humerus.** H, humerus; SST, supraspinatus tendon.

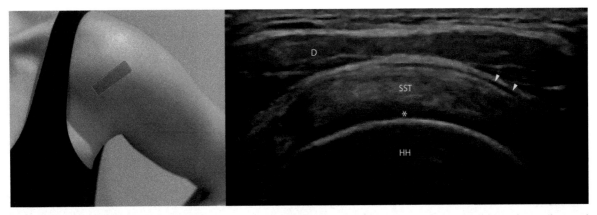

Figure 6.29 Short-axis view of the supraspinatus tendon overlying the humeral head. The * represents the articular cartilage and arrows are the subacromial bursal space. HH, humeral head; SST, supraspinatus tendon; D, deltoid.

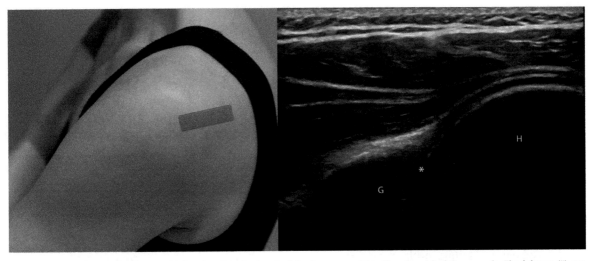

Figure 6.30 Posterior glenohumeral joint showing the head of the humerus within the glenoid of the scapula. The labrum (*) can be seen as a small hypoechoic rim. H, humerus; G, glenoid.

a posterior labral cyst is surgical repair of the labral defect. Posteriorly the spine of scapula is seen and the suprascapular nerve within the notch can be visualised.

The acromioclavicular joint is often injured in contact sports and pitch-side US is useful in the assessment of acute injury and in injecting therapeutic substances to improve pain and function in both the short- and long-term. In an acromioclavicular injury, US findings can include an effusion, a widened joint and cortical irregularities (Figure 6.31). The joint width is easily compared to the normal side, assuming no previous injury and the acromioclavicular index can be calculated. Stability of the joint using cross-adduction can

also be assessed. This joint is small and so MSKUS provides an opportunity for increased accuracy of injected interventions where indicated.

The final joint to consider in a pathological shoulder is the sternoclavicular joint. This joint is susceptible to injury through contact sports like rugby and high-speed sports such as horse-racing. Posterior dislocations require further imaging due to the risk of entrapment to surrounding important neurovascular structures. However, an anterior dislocation is easily assessed both clinically and confirmed with US (Figure 6.32). CT imaging remains the gold standard when investigating sternoclavicular injuries.

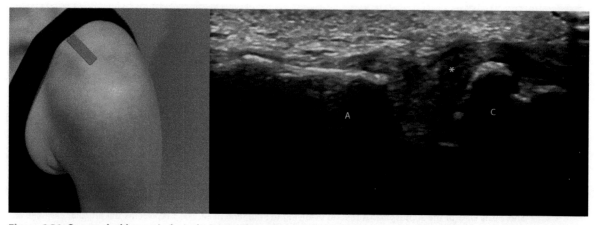

Figure 6.31 One-week old acromioclavicular injury. The end of the clavicle is displaced superiorly. Also note the distended capsule with hypoechoic fluid in the joint (*) and the cortical irregularity of the clavicle. C, clavicle; A, acromium.

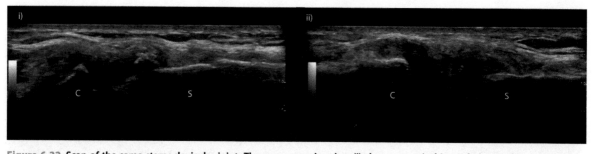

Figure 6.32 Scan of the same sternoclavicular joint. The more superior view (i) shows a cortical irregularity on the sternal side of the joint. Distal to the irregularity (ii) the traumatic effusion and anterior displacement of the clavicle is more readily appreciated. S, sternal side of the joint; C, clavicle.

Elbow

The anterior elbow is commonly scanned for distal biceps pathology. Starting with the elbow fully extended and rested on a surface, transverse and longitudinal images are obtained. In the transverse view the anterior humerus, the neurovascular structures including the median nerve and brachial artery, and a number of muscles including brachialis, biceps and pronator muscles can be seen. The distal biceps tendon can be very difficult to assess particularly in someone with increased muscle bulk. Several methods exist to assess the distal biceps. Using the anterior method, the probe is held in the longitudinal view, slightly obliquely and the distal end of the probe often needs to be 'toed-in' to get the probe parallel to the fibers of the tendon (Figure 6.33). Additional approaches include the lateral approach and cobra views.

Scanning proximally the biceps muscle can be evaluated. Although rare, contusions can occur (Figure 6.34).

The posterior interosseous nerve can be identified anterolaterally and considered as an important differential diagnosis for lateral elbow pain. This is evaluated by moving the probe laterally; in short-axis identifying the radial nerve between brachioradialis and brachialis and following the nerve distally. Here, the posterior interosseous nerve branches off the radial nerve and appears within the belly of the supinator muscle before passing to the arcade of Fröhse.

Lateral elbow pain is one of the most common complaints around the elbow. The common extensor tendon is best evaluated with the elbow in flexion and the probe placed on the lateral epicondyle (Figure 6.35). Long-axis views are most useful and common findings can include tendon thickening, loss of normal fibrillar structure and calcifications can be present. The use of power Doppler can evaluate for presence of enthesitis. Beneath the common extensor the lateral elbow joint can be seen, moving to a short-axis view and distally,

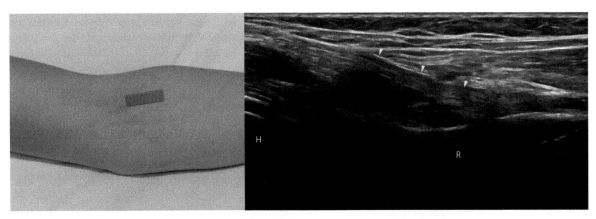

Figure 6.33 Anterior view of the distal biceps tendon (arrows) inserting onto the radial tuberosity. H, humerus; R, radius.

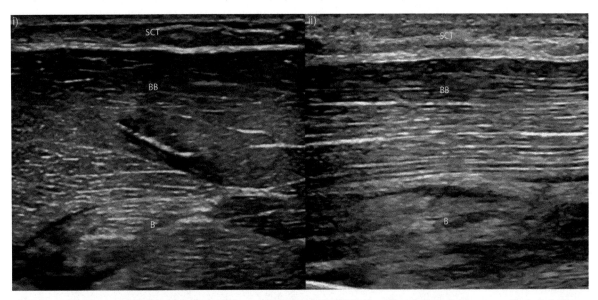

Figure 6.34 (i) Short- and (ii) long-axis views of the anterior upper arm. Note the diffuse hyperechoic areas particularly in the brachialis muscle where the muscle pattern is distorted. This significant contusion was the result of a direct blunt trauma to the front of the arm. SCT, subcutaneous tissue; BB, biceps brachii; B, brachialis muscle.

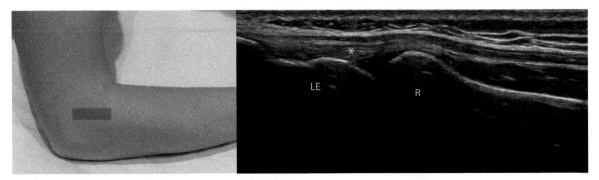

Figure 6.35 The lateral epicondyle serves as the landmark to identify the common extensor tendons (*). LE, lateral epicondyle; R, radial head.

the radial head can be seen with the overlying radial collateral ligament.

The posterior elbow joint is scanned to evaluate the triceps tendon and its insertion on the olecranon; this is best viewed with the patient's elbow held at 90 degrees (Figure 6.36). Triceps tendinopathy, rupture and enthesitis can all be examined here. By moving the joint in and out of flexion gently any posterior joint fluid will be appreciated. This is also the site for the appreciation of loose bodies in the posterior joint.

In the short-axis view and moving medially, the cubital tunnel can be seen between the medial epicondyle and the olecranon. This position is useful to evaluate for compressive lesions of the ulnar nerve. Less commonly, the ulnar nerve can sublux over the medial epicondyle and this is demonstrated with dynamic US scanning.

Two important structures can be assessed with US in the medial elbow. The common flexor origin is most commonly assessed for tendinopathy, while the ulnar collateral ligament at the elbow is described as a common source of elbow instability in baseball pitchers as a result of overuse. This can also be assessed dynamically while applying a valgus stress and comparing it to the asymptomatic side.

Hand and Wrist

The small joints of the hand and wrist are easily evaluated, diagnosed and in some cases treated with US-guided interventions. Assessment of nerves in MSKUS is considered a more advanced skill set. The median nerve examined over the volar aspect of the wrist is one of the easier nerves to assess. Located directly below the flexor retinaculum, it can be traced proximally and distally in short and long sections. In longitudinal view the compression of the median nerve can be demonstrated by thickening distally to the retinaculum and is commonly described as looking similar to a 'kink in a hosepipe'. The sonographic measurement of the cross-sectional area of the median nerve is also used to diagnose carpal tunnel syndrome, a condition where guided US intervention is regularly implemented (Figure 6.37). Normal median nerve cross-sectional area is 9–11 mm^2 and when enlarged may support a suspected diagnosis of carpal tunnel syndrome.

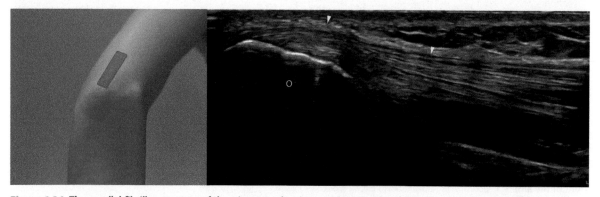

Figure 6.36 The parallel fibrillar structure of the triceps tendon (arrows) is appreciated inserting onto the olecranon. O, olecranon.

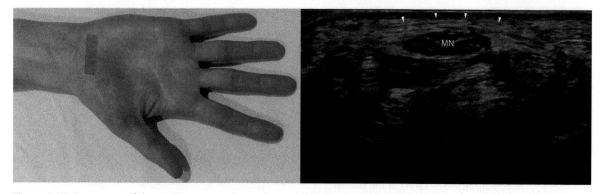

Figure 6.37 Assessment of the median nerve and carpal tunnel. The arrows demonstrate the flexor retinaculum. MN, median nerve.

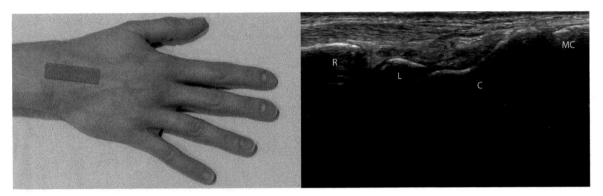

Figure 6.38 The dorsal longitudinal scan of the wrist. R, radius; L, lunate; C, capitate; MC, metacarpal.

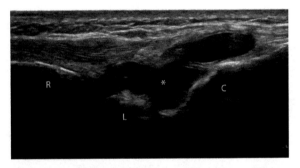

Figure 6.39 Dorsal longitudinal scan of the wrist revealing a multi-loculated cystic structure filled with mostly anechoic fluid. The ganglion (*) is seen to communicate with the carpal joints. R, radius; L, lunate; C, capitate.

The second and smaller nerve is the ulnar nerve, which travels through Guyon's canal and is best identified by locating the pisiform and ulnar artery on either side. Compression of the ulnar nerve at Guyon's canal is also known as handlebar palsy and is seen in cyclists.

The dorsal wrist scan involves assessing the distal radio-ulnar joint, the radiocarpal joint and the scapholunate joint. With the probe in the longitudinal view the joint can be assessed for effusion and it is often that this view reveals the origin of a dorsal ganglion (Figure 6.38).

As previously mentioned, ganglions are cystic structures which can be multiloculated, filled with hypoechoic or anechoic fluid and are compressible. The surrounding capsule may demonstrate power Doppler uptake. Figure 6.39 is an example of a ganglion that communicates with the carpal joints. The use of US-guided aspiration and injection of steroids is common.

In the short axis the distal radio-ulnar joint is seen and moving distally the scapho-lunate ligament is

seen (Figure 6.40). This can also be tested dynamically and compared to the uninjured side in the event of suspected ligament disruption.

The extensor tendons of the hand are held within six compartments. Using Lister's tubercle on the radius and holding the probe in short axis, identify the compartments from the radial to ulnar side. A pathological compartment should be traced proximally and distally in both short and long axis. The first dorsal compartment contains the tendons of abductor pollicus longus and extensor pollicis brevis – a common compartment for tenosynovitis and tendinopathy. In the presence of a hypoechoic rim surrounding the tendons with the uptake of power Doppler, an US-guided corticosteroid injection into the sheath may be effective. An example of this is for De'Quervain's tenosynovitis.

The second to sixth compartments are also easily visualised to examine for pathology in the tendon, by moving the probe proximally and distally along the structure (Figure 6.41). Intersection syndrome can be identified in the proximal intersection between the tendons of the first and second intersection compartment, with the presence of hypoechoic fluid within the tendons and tendon sheath, more commonly seen in rowers and motocross athletes. The distal intersection syndrome is the crossover between the second and third compartment and occurs below Lister's tubercle.

The metacarpophalangeal joints are frequently assessed in rheumatology and can show evidence of effusions, synovitis and superficial bony erosions. This can be used diagnostically to monitor the efficacy of biological agents and disease progression.

Degenerative and osteoarthritic changes can also be assessed particularly in the base of the thumb

157

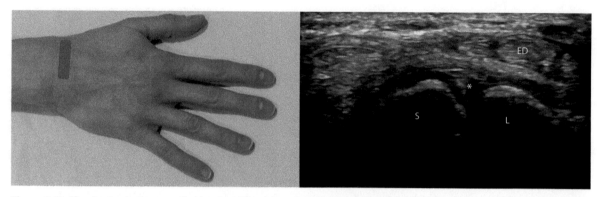

Figure 6.40 **The short-axis view over the dorsum of the wrist revealing the scapholunate ligament (*).** S, scaphoid; L, lunate; ED, extensor digitorum tendon.

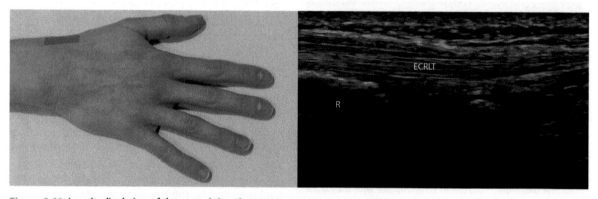

Figure 6.41 **Longitudinal view of the second dorsal compartment.** R, radius; ECRLT, extensor carpi radialis longus tendon.

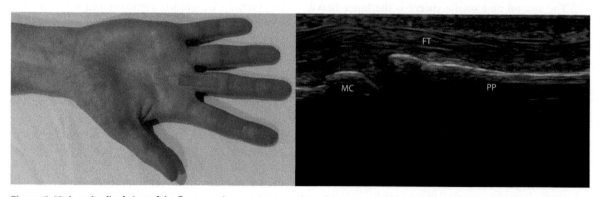

Figure 6.42 **Longitudinal view of the flexor tendon passing over the palmar aspect of the metacarpophalangeal joint.** MC, metacarpal; PP, proximal phalanx; FT, flexor tendon.

where cortical irregularities in the presence of osteophytes can be seen. The ulnar collateral ligament and its stability can be assessed with US and compared to the asymptomatic side, particularly applicable to winter sport injuries of the wrist.

The flexor tendons of the fingers are most effectively scanned with a hockey stick probe; with the small probe identifying the annular pulleys which can appear as a hypoechoic region overlying the tendon (Figure 6.42). In the event of a pulley rupture, the 'bowstringing' of the tendon can be examined dynamically using US. In the case of trigger finger, US may demonstrate a thickened tendon and guide corticosteroid injection.

Lower Limb

Hip

Examination of deep structures such as the hip may be challenging with US and a lower frequency is needed to achieve sufficient resolution. The skillset of the clinician, machine resolution and anatomical variability will directly affect the quality of the image. Depending on the site of suspected pathology, the hip can be scanned using multiple views.

Anteriorly, placing the probe in a longitudinal plane with the patient in a supine position demonstrates the neurovascular bundle immediately lateral the hip joint. This may require an oblique angulation to optimise the image. In this view the femoral head and anterior margin of acetabulum, the joint capsule extending to the femoral neck and occasionally the echogenic labrum are visualised (Figure 6.43).

As illustrated in Figure 6.43 the muscles and tendons overlie the anterior joint. Iliopsoas muscle is clearly seen overlying the joint. The iliopsoas bursa is only visualised in a pathological state. In this position one can also easily see an effusion and use of power Doppler may determine the presence of synovitis. In cases of femoral acetabular impingement, US can sometimes demonstrate the cam and pincer lesions.

Other structures visualised in longitudinal view, as the probe is moved laterally, include the anterior superior iliac spine, anterior inferior iliac spine and the proximal tendon attachment of the head of rectus femoris. US is a safe and effective imaging option for a suspected avulsion fracture in an adolescent athlete involved in kicking sports.

The probe may be rotated to a transverse view to demonstrate the muscle belly and tendon of the iliopsoas. This is useful to dynamically demonstrate anterior hip snapping which is commonly experienced by athletes, dancers and adolescent females.

The quadriceps muscles and their tendons are clearly appreciated scanning proximal to distal and in both long- and short-axis views (Figure 6.44). Vastus intermedius is viewed below rectus femoris and between lateralis and medialis. US is useful in this instance in the event of muscular injuries, including diagnosis and surveillance of intramuscular haematomas.

Returning to the landmark of the anterior superior iliac spine and moving the probe laterally in a short axis, US can identify the tendon origins of the sartorius and tensor fascia lata. Pathology of these two structures at this site is uncommon, however the lateral femoral cutaneous nerve can be visualised below the inguinal ligament just medial to the anterior superior iliac spine and is a source of pathology and potential US-guided intervention site.

Medial pathology such as greater trochanteric pain syndrome, which can include gluteal medius tendinopathy and trochanteric bursitis, is commonly evaluated using MSKUS. With the patient positioned on the unaffected side and a flexed hip, the greater trochanter can be used as a landmark to evaluate this region in both long and short axis (Figure 6.45). In gluteus medius tendinopathy the tendon attachment

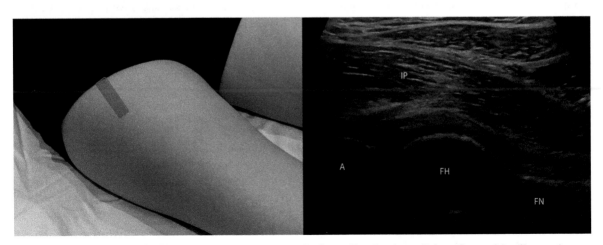

Figure 6.43 Longitudinal view of the anterior hip joint showing the femoral head and acetabulum. The overlying iliopsoas is seen. A, acetabulum; FH, femoral head; FN, femoral neck; IP, iliopsoas.

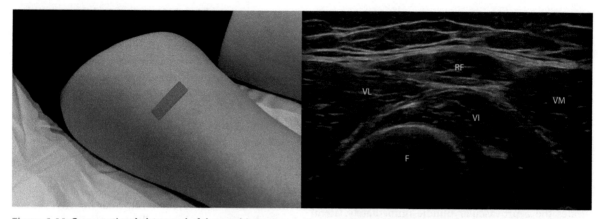

Figure 6.44 Cross-sectional ultrasound of the quadriceps group. RF, rectus femoris; VI, vastus intermedius; VL, vastus lateralis; VM, vastus medialis; F, femur.

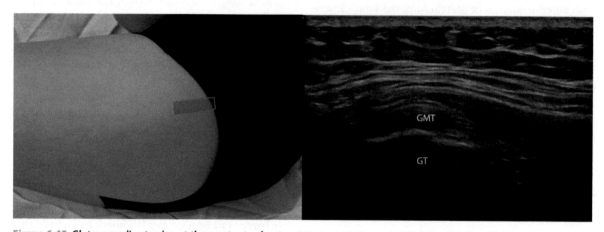

Figure 6.45 Gluteus medius tendon at the greater trochanter. GMT, gluteus medius tendon; GT, greater trochanter.

into anterior and posterior facet of greater trochanter has a loss of normal fibrillar structure. In trochanteric bursitis, the inflamed bursa is illustrated by an anechoic area overlying gluteal medius.

The lateral hip can also be scanned with a dynamic manoeuvre to illustrate lateral hip snapping of the tensor fascia lata over the greater trochanter. In the case of a traumatic event, the lateral hip and upper thigh is also the site of a Morel Lavallee lesion.

The medial and posterior hip is affected less frequently. Hamstring tendinopathy can be identified as a thickened tendon with loss of fibrillar structure and irregularity where the conjoined proximal hamstring tendon inserts into the ischium. Ischial bursitis can be identified with US as an anechoic area overlying the conjoint hamstring tendon (Figure 6.46).

The medial hip is scanned to evaluate the adductor tendons and their attachment on the inferior pubic ramus and more centrally the pubic symphysis joint. This region is better visualised with MRI, particularly in the event of pubic symphysis overload, as pathology can be challenging to differentiate and management principles can overlap.

Knee

Ultrasound of the knee is commonly and effectively used to identify pathology and facilitates knee intervention.

Anterior examination starts with the knee held in 20–30 degrees of flexion and then in 90 degrees to assess the course of the quadriceps and patellar tendon (Figure 6.47). A combination of both the long- and short-axis views are preferred to assess a joint effusion within the suprapatellar pouch, and the approach used for an intra-articular US-guided

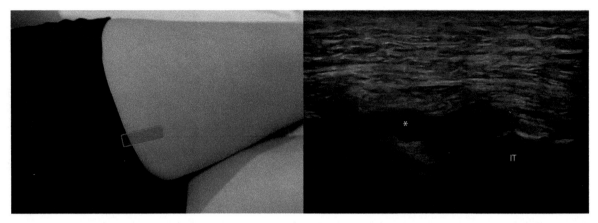

Figure 6.46 Ultrasound showing the ischial tuberosity and a large anechoic area representing a large ischial bursitis (*). IT, ischial tuberosity.

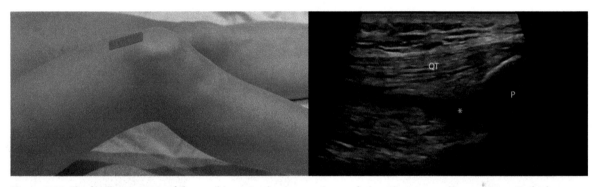

Figure 6.47 The fibrillar structure of the quadriceps tendon is seen. An anechoic region representing an intra-articular knee effusion is evident (*). QT, quadriceps tendon; P, patella.

injection. Increasing the degree of flexion of the knee, the femoral trochlear is seen and assessed for osteophytes or other pathology.

Common pathology encountered at the knee in jumping sports is patella tendinopathy. It is clearly demonstrated by an increase in tendon thickness, loss of fibrillar structure, hypoechoic and anechoic regions with neovascularisation. US can also identify traumatic or overuse bursitis at the anterior knee in addition to tendon rupture and Hoffa's fat pad irritation (Figure 6.48). US can assist in the clinical diagnosis of Osgood Schlatter's which is a common growth-related pathology in adolescents with anterior knee pain. US is a safe and radiation free option for imaging in children, confirming the pathology at the tibial tuberosity.

Medial knee views are best evaluated with the knee held in 80–90 degrees, using the medial femoral condyle as a landmark. The medial collateral ligament is evaluated in a longitudinal view from its proximal insertion to the distal attachment on the tibia (Figure 6.49). This ligament can also be assessed dynamically for stability while applying a valgus force to the knee. The peripheral edge of the medial meniscus is seen as a triangular echogenic structure within the joint and, if extruded in a static position and with increasing flexion, this can suggest medial meniscal pathology (Figure 6.50). In the osteoarthritic knee, cortical irregularities can be seen to represent osteophytes. The probe can be moved obliquely and laterally to assess the pes anserine and any associated pathological bursa which again can easily be injected using US guidance.

Likewise, the lateral knee is best scanned in approximately 30 degrees of flexion using the lateral femoral condyle as a landmark. The lateral collateral ligament is visualised running longitudinally from the lateral femoral condyle to fibular head and can also be

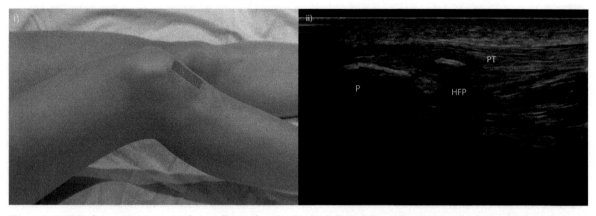

Figure 6.48 **(i) Probe position to assess the patellar tendon. Proximal patellar tendinopathy is evident by thickening, loss of normal fibrillar structure and hypoechoic areas.** P, patella; HFP; Hoffa's fat pad; PT, patellar tendon.

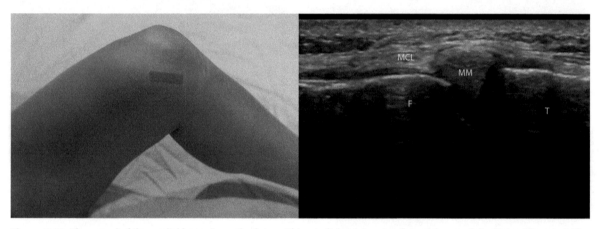

Figure 6.49 **Ultrasound of the medial knee shows the femur, tibia, medial meniscus and overlying medial collateral ligament. The meniscus is mildly extruded.** F, femur; T, tibia; MM, medial meniscus; MCL, medial collateral ligament.

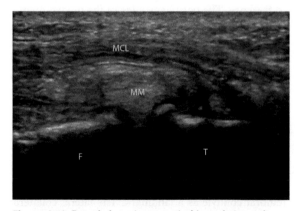

Figure 6.50 **Extruded meniscus, cortical irregularity at the joint line and changes to the medial collateral ligament.** F, femur; T, tibia; MM, medial meniscus; MCL, medial collateral ligament.

tested dynamically under knee varus force. Migrating the probe just anteriorly, the distal iliotibial band can be identified at the lateral tibia condyle (Figure 6.51). In iliotibial band friction syndrome, anechoic areas seen underneath the band can be confused with a joint effusion.

The posterior knee is most commonly scanned when a Baker's cyst is suspected. The appearance of a Baker's cyst has been discussed earlier in this chapter.

Foot and Ankle

Proficient US skills of the posterior leg are important in a MSK setting as injuries of the calf complex and Achilles tendon are prevalent. US enables a thorough examination along the entire length of the

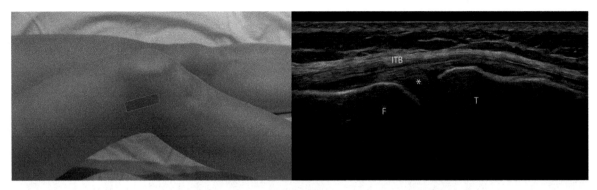

Figure 6.51 Lateral knee joint. Image demonstrating the lateral meniscus (*) and overlying iliotibial band. F, femur; T, tibia; ITB, iliotibial band.

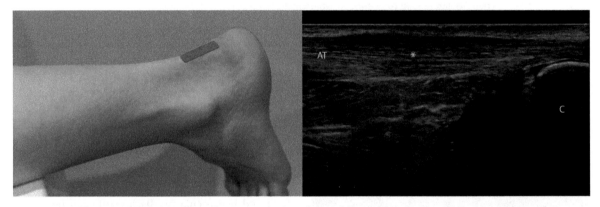

Figure 6.52 Mid-portion Achilles tendinopathy. Long-axis view of the Achilles tendon showing thickening and hypoechoic changes (*). AT, Achilles tendon; C, calcaneus.

gastrocnemius, soleus, adjacent flexor muscles and Achilles tendon to identify the region of pathology. Both the long- and short-axis should be used for a complete assessment. Injury to the calf complex is identified as a hypoechoic or anechoic region at the site of intramuscular haematoma. This is commonly seen in the muscle belly in classic calf muscle strains and between the aponeurosis of the medial gastrocnemius and soleus muscle in 'tennis leg'. US may be used for interventional aspiration and serial imaging.

Ultrasound can assist in the diagnosis of an Achilles injury to identify a partial tear or complete rupture. In regions of injury, normal fibrillar tendon and muscle structure will be replaced by haematoma which appears hypoechoic. In this instance it is crucial for the entire musculotendinous unit to be interrogated.

Ultrasound is considered the gold standard for Achilles tendinopathy as it clearly demonstrates tendon integrity and can differentiate between insertional or mid-portion tendinopathy (Figure 6.52).

Common characteristics include tendon thickening, neovascularity, loss of fibrillar structure, hyperechoic calcifications and tendon hypoechogenicity. The thickness of the pathological tendon is typically measured and compared to normal ranges or measurements of the asymptomatic contralateral leg (Figure 6.53). Pathology at the insertion should raise awareness for enthesopathy and rheumatological conditions including seronegative or reactive arthropathy (Figure 6.54). Pathology within the Achilles paratenon can be identified on US as thickening and reactive changes with power Doppler.

The deeper structures of the posterior ankle can also be examined under US. Pathologies secondary to bony prominences can be identified, including posterior ankle impingement, Os trigonum, cysts and a 'pump bump' or Haglund's deformity. Irritated soft-tissue structures such as the Kager's fat pad and retrocalcaneal bursa may appear hypoechoic with neovascularity. Stress fractures can appear as anechoic

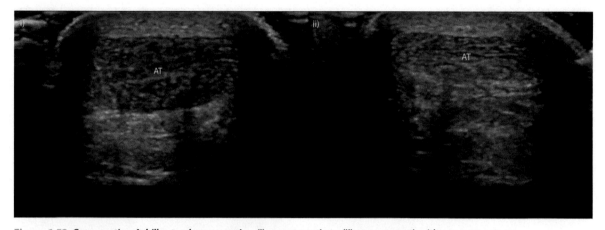

Figure 6.53 Cross-section Achilles tendon comparing (i) symptomatic to (ii) asymptomatic side. AT, Achilles tendon.

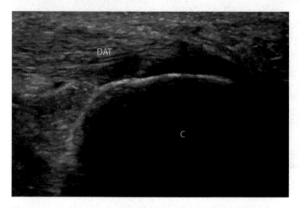

Figure 6.54 Long-axis view showing disruption to the normal structure of the Achilles. The image is taken with the foot in a neutral position and the tendon is seen to buckle at the insertion. DAT, Distal Achilles tendon; C, calcaneus.

cortical irregularities but US imaging is not always conclusive, therefore other imaging modalities may be required. Lastly, US is a safe and reassuring option for imaging adolescent patients with symptoms secondary to calcaneal apophysitis.

Scanning the plantar surface of the foot is routinely used to help confirm the diagnosis of plantar fasciopathy (Figure 6.55). The plantar fascia can be isolated by placing the foot and hallux in a slightly dorsiflexed position. The entire length of the fascia can be scanned using the long-axis to measure the thickness of the structure. Thickening above approximately 4 mm in the presence of pain is consistent with a diagnosis of plantar fasciopathy. Neovascularity, hypoechoic regions and tears can also be visualised in both planes and more commonly seen at the proximal medial insertion. Additional pathology to

consider in the differential diagnosis of plantar heel pain, such as calcaneal bursitis, heel spur or Baxter's nerve entrapment, may also be assessed using US.

Lateral ankle sprains may be readily examined in the acute setting using US. The anterior talofibular ligament is most commonly injured and is examined with the probe placed longitudinally and obliquely from the distal fibula towards the talus neck (Figure 6.56). Injured ligament will have irregular or frayed fibres, hypoechoic regions, evidence of joint fluid and neovascularity. Its integrity can be further evaluated by dynamic testing to identify instability by applying an inversion stress.

Following an inversion sprain the calcaneofibular ligament should also be examined. Plenty of gel is required, with a long-axis probe placement between the distal tip of the fibula and adjacent calcaneus. A small ligament can be identified and described as a 'hammock' supporting the tendons of peroneal brevis and longus. Dynamic testing with ankle inversion will lift the tendons. Finally, the anterior inferior tibiofibular ligament can be examined with the probe placed transversely between the distal tibia and fibula, with application of dorsiflexion. If suspecting laxity at the syndesmosis, an MRI should be obtained.

The peroneal tendons should also be examined following acute or chronic ankle symptoms. The peroneus brevis is a low-lying muscle and should be examined in its entirety in the long- and short-axis for evidence of tears. It runs closest to the lateral malleolus, adjacent to the peroneus longus and inserts into the styloid process on the fifth metatarsal (Figure 6.57). This is a common site of avulsion

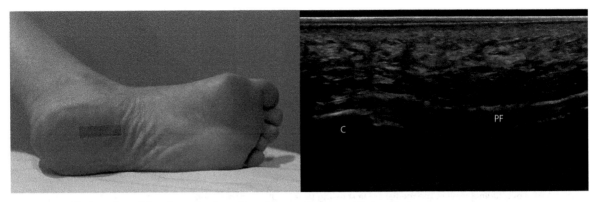

Figure 6.55 The insertion of the plantar fascia on the calcaneus. C, calcaneus; PF, plantar fascia.

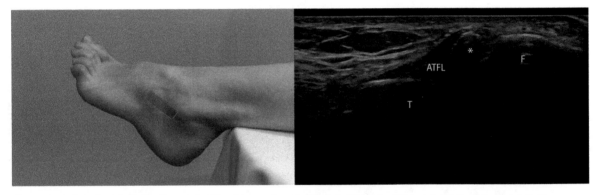

Figure 6.56 Anterior talofibular ligament with evidence of an Os fibularis (*). T, talus; ATFL, anterior talofibular ligament; F, fibula.

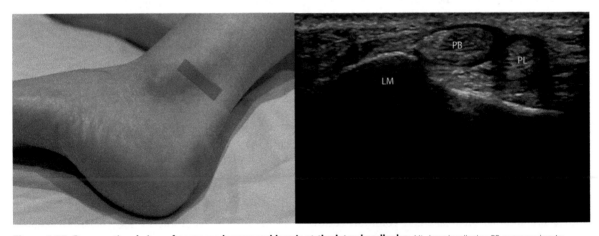

Figure 6.57 Cross-sectional view of peroneus longus and brevis at the lateral malleolus. ML, lateral malleolus; PB, peroneus brevis; PL, peroneus longus.

fractures or rupture. Peroneal tendinopathy can arise in the longus and brevis tendons with the classic tendinopathic features identified on US.

The medial ankle is an anatomically complex but well-defined region on MSKUS. The classic features of tendinopathy are often identified along the tibialis posterior tendon as it wraps around the medial malleolus and into its main insertion at the navicular. Here an Os navicularis may be identified as a source of localised pain and bony prominence.

165

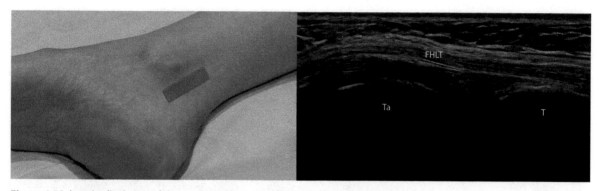

Figure 6.58 Longitudinal view of the medial ankle showing flexor hallucis longus tendon. T, tibia; Ta, talus; FHLT, flexor hallucis longus tendon.

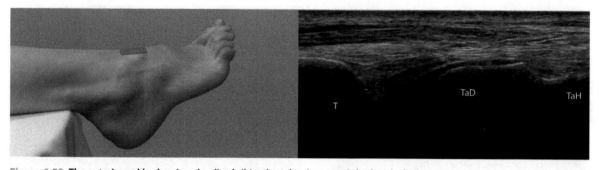

Figure 6.59 The anterior ankle showing the distal tibia, the talar dome and the head of talus. T, tibia; TaD, talar dome; TaH, talar head.

A short-axis assessment superior to the malleolus may be used to examine the structure of the tarsal tunnel including the tibialis posterior, flexor digitorum longus, vascular structures, tibial nerve, and flexor hallucis longus. These long structures should also be fully examined in a long-axis view to identify features of tendinopathy or sheath thickening with neovascularity in tenosynovitis (Figure 6.58).

The integrity of the anterior ankle can be efficiently viewed using both a long- and short-axis view (Figure 6.59). Anterior ankle impingement, degenerative changes and joint effusions can be best visualised across the tibiotalar and talofibular joints with a longitudinal view and is a common region for guided injections. Examination of the tibialis anterior can demonstrate classic tendinopathic and tenosynovitic features. This may also be seen in the extensor hallucis and digitorum longus tendons but is less common.

Ultrasound can be particularly valuable in the examination of the smaller joints of the feet. Plenty of gel should be used to improve visibility as probe contact can be challenging. Hypoechoic structures distally between the metatarsophalangeal (MTP) joints can be examined using a plantar approach and transverse view (Figure 6.60). Compression of the metatarsal heads will compress an intermetatarsal bursal lesion which will likely have increased neovascularity on power Doppler. Conversely, a Morton's neuroma will not compress with dynamic stress testing and may appear as a thickened neural structure between the metatarsals in a longitudinal view. US is a preferred method for administrating guided injections for these small areas.

The first MTP joint is commonly imaged dorsally to identify joint effusions, synovitis and capsulitis as hypoechoic in addition to superficial degenerative joint changes. These characteristics are often observed in rheumatological presentations. A plantar view is used to assess the two sesamoids for bony inflammation or tendinopathic changes of the flexor hallucis tendons, frequently seen in runners (Figure 6.61). Evidence of bony stress to the sesamoid or any of the metatarsal or small foot joints warrants further imaging for a more accurate diagnosis.

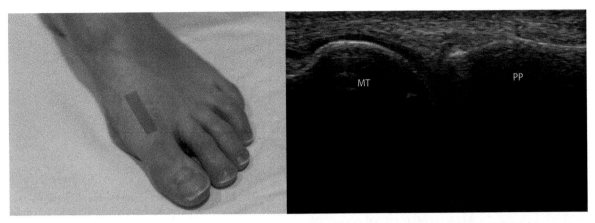

Figure 6.60 Cross-sectional view of the lateral and medial sesamoids with the interposed tendon of flexor hallucis longus. Se, sesamoid; FHLT, flexor hallucis longus tendon.

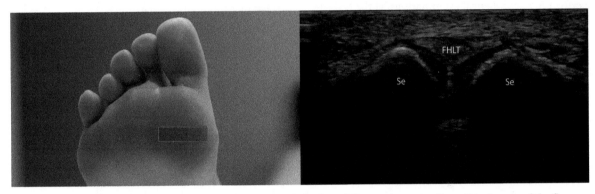

Figure 6.61 A plantar view is used to assess the two sesamoids for bony inflammation or tendinopathic changes of the flexor halluces tendons, frequently seen in runners.

Summary

- Ultrasound is an invaluable tool in the assessment of soft tissue and MSK pathology.
- As the cost decreases and portability of US machines improves, the potential to use soft tissue and MSK US in increasingly diverse clinical settings will increase.
- Ultrasound increases the accuracy of diagnosis and the success rate of intervention for soft tissue and MSK pathology in the routine clinical setting.
- In sports and exercise medicine, the majority of elite teams will travel with a portable US to aid with diagnosis of injuries and enable guided intervention.
- Ultrasound is used across multiple specialties involved in soft tissue, MSK and joint pathology including rheumatology specialists, sports and exercise physicians, podiatrists, physiotherapists and nurse specialists.

A full list of references and further reading is available at www.GeneralistUltrasound.com

Ultrasound for Neurology

Introduction to Neurology

Neurology is a challenging medical specialty and has been rated by undergraduates and postgraduates to be more difficult than any other discipline from a theoretical context. Many doctors have poor confidence performing neurological examinations 'at the bedside' leading to clinical skills being neglected and patients receiving poor assessments. This may potentially lead to delayed or misdiagnosis, patient harm or costly and unnecessary investigations.

Ultrasound (US) can be a useful aid in assessment, diagnosis and management within certain clinical scenarios and is being increasingly utilised. The key areas that will be discussed in this chapter are listed in Table 7.1.

Papilloedema

Papilloedema is defined as raised intracranial pressure (ICP), which leads to optic disc swelling. It is caused by a multitude of conditions which are broadly listed in Table 7.2.

Fundoscopy is a key element of the neurological examination that is used to detect papilloedema. Despite this, it is rarely completed on admission due to complexity, lack of experience, poor conditions and minimal access to mydriatic agents to optimise visualisation of the optic disc. The duration of ophthalmology placements in countries such as the USA and UK at undergraduate level has dwindled over the past 30 years resulting in poor clinical skills in fundoscopy.

Key features of papilloedema on fundoscopy include:

- Absent venous pulsation.
- Optic disc swelling (unclear margins).
- Pallor of the optic nerve.
- Haemorrhages.
- Radial retinal lines extending from the optic nerve (Paton's lines).

Figure 7.1 shows a normal optic disc on fundoscopy in comparison with an abnormal fundus demonstrating papilloedema with optic nerve swelling, radial retinal lines and haemorrhages.

In cases of raised ICP there is dilatation of the optic nerve sheath due to the subarachnoid space extending between the optic nerve and sheath. Using US to recognise increases in the optic nerve sheath diameter (ONSD) is a simple and quick method for diagnosing papilloedema. It has been proven to be a reliable and reproducible method and does not require pupillary dilatation making it particularly useful in acute and emergency settings.

Table 7.1

Use of point-of-care ultrasound within neurology
1. Diagnosis of papilloedema
2. As an aid to performing a lumbar puncture
3. Diagnosis of giant cell arteritis
4. Transcranial Doppler (TCD)

Table 7.2

Causes of papilloedema
Mass or compressing lesion
Malignant hypertension
Idiopathic intracranial hypertension
Intracranial hypertension due to:
– Meningitis/encephalitis
– Arteriovenous malformation
– Chiari 1 malformation
– Cerebral venous thrombosis

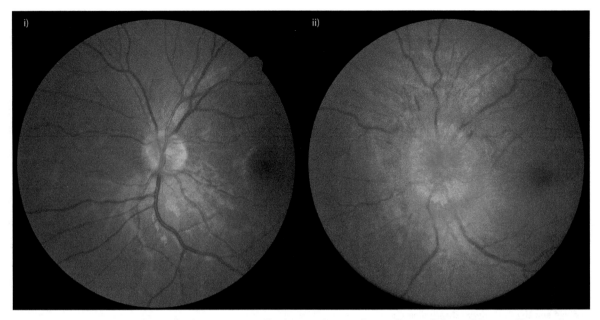

i) ii)

Figure 7.1 (i) Normal optic disc on fundoscopy. (ii) Papilloedema with optic disc swelling, radial retinal lines and haemorrhages.

Method

The high frequency linear probe is used with the patient's eye closed. Dressings or gauze may be used to cover the eye but this is not necessary.

The patient should be supine and the procedure explained. It is not a painful assessment but some pressure may be placed upon the eyelid. US gel is water-based and does not cause damage or irritation to the eye but the clinician should use sterile sachets of gel rather than from a reusable bottle. The patient should keep their eye closed at all times and look directly ahead.

Starting in the transverse plane, the probe should be gently applied to the eyelid whilst anchoring your fingers upon the nose or bony orbit for image stability (Figure 7.2). The user may need to rock or tilt the probe to optimise the view of the optic nerve. Normal anatomy is demonstrated in Fig 7.2ii. The probe should then be rotated to the sagittal plane and all measurements averaged.

Papilloedema causes two specific findings as shown in Figure 7.3:

- Optic nerve sheath diameter >5 mm.
- Optic disc elevation of >0.6 mm.

Studies have suggested that optic disc elevation identified with US can be 82% sensitive and 76% specific for papilloedema. This can be acquired by measuring the distance between the anterior peak of the disc and its intersection to the posterior surface of the globe.

Evaluation of the ONSD has been suggested to have a sensitivity of 100% and specificity of 95% for raised ICP when compared with CT. An ONSD of >5 mm bilaterally correlates with an ICP >20 mmHg.

The ONSD is measured 3 mm posterior from the globe. The position of 3 mm is recommended as the image contrast is greatest and provides a standard for reproducible measurements. Clinicians must ensure the measurements are only attempted if the image quality is sufficient to delineate the optic nerve from the optic nerve sheath. Measurements are performed from outer edge to outer edge of the ONS in transverse and sagittal views and then averaged.

Case – Persistent Headache with Visual Disturbance

A 26-year-old lady presented to her GP with a persistent headache for 2 weeks and visual disturbance. She had previously suffered with migraines and she felt that this headache was similar with features of nausea and photophobia but did not subside with analgesia. This was her third presentation in the past two weeks. The GP carried out a full neurological examination which was normal but struggled to rule out papilloedema on fundoscopy. He carried out an ON US which revealed features of papilloedema

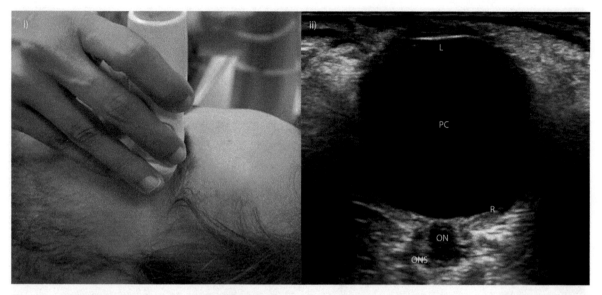

Figure 7.2 (i) Probe position for the measurement of the Optic nerve sheath diameter in the axial or transverse view. (ii) View of the eye and the Optic nerve sheath diameter on ultrasound. L, lens; PC, posterior chamber; R, retina; ON, optic nerve; ONS, optic nerve sheath.

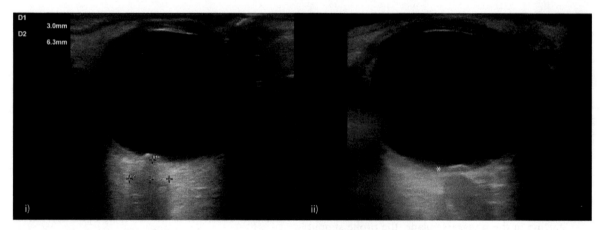

Figure 7.3 The features of papilloedema. (i) Raised optic nerve sheath diameter. (ii) Elevated optic disc (*).

within both eyes with a raised optic disc and an increased ONSD of 7 mm (Figure 7.4).

She was promptly transferred to hospital where urgent CT imaging of the brain demonstrated an intracerebral mass.

This case illustrates many of the previously highlighted issues. Clinicians struggle with confidence and competence in ruling out papilloedema with the use of fundoscopy and an ON US can provide a relatively easy alternative diagnostic tool. Given her history of migraines and multiple previous consults this outcome could have potentially been disastrous.

Lumbar Puncture

The Society of Hospital Medicine have published a statement in which they recommend the use of US guidance for adult lumbar punctures. US may aid with site selection, measurement of subarachnoid space depth and can reduce the number of needle insertion attempts. This is particularly useful in patients who are obese or have difficult-to-palpate landmarks.

This technique is also gaining popularity in obstetric anaesthesia to identify midline spinal landmarks and measure the expected depth for epidural and subarachnoid spaces.

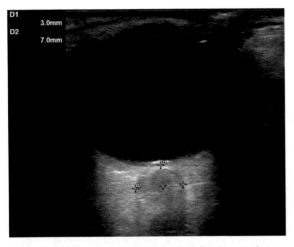

Figure 7.4 **Optic nerve sheath diameter of 7.0 mm with an elevated optic disc.**

Ultrasound-assisted lumbar puncture is easy to learn with a recent study suggesting that even after a brief training session, clinicians can reliably and rapidly obtain high quality images.

Method

The left lateral decubitus position or sitting position may be used (Figure 7.5). The sitting position tends to increase the lumbar puncture (LP) success rate for inexperienced users as the midline is more readily identified. In the left lateral position, the vertebral column may twist and the midline is more challenging to follow. However, in diagnostic cases of idiopathic intracranial hypertension the lateral position

provides a more accurate measurement of ICP and it may be better tolerated in patients with severe headache. The patient should be placed with forward flexion of the lumbar spine to eliminate the lumbar lordosis and open the interspinous spaces.

Once the spinal landmarks have been located and drawn onto the patient it is important that the position is not changed as these markings will no longer be accurate. In pre-operative clinics for obstetric anaesthesia, US is occasionally performed to provide the obstetric anaesthetist with information about the expected depth of landmarks in patients who are overweight.

The curvilinear probe is most commonly used to assess spinal anatomy. In those with a low BMI the high frequency linear probe may be used but this may not provide sufficient depth for many patients.

Lumbar spine US relies on the paramedian views for identification of the key structures. Using the sagittal approach, the spinous processes will obscure the anatomy due to their caudal angulation.

To begin, the back should be palpated to identify L4–L5. The probe is placed in the presumed midline and the spinous processes should be visible as superficial hyperechoic structures with post-acoustic shadowing. The US will be unable to pass any further due to the high acoustic impedance of bone and no other anatomy will be identified.

The next step is to move the probe 1–2 cm laterally. Either side of the midline may be selected. This will reveal the articular processes which appear like hyperechoic 'camel humps' casting acoustic shadows (Figure 7.6).

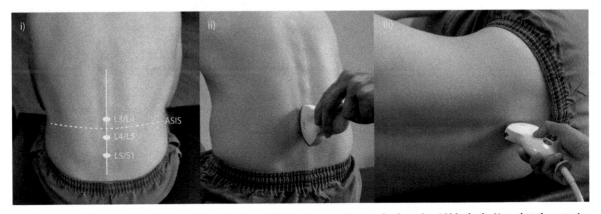

Figure 7.5 **(i) Surface anatomy for interspinous levels used for lumbar puncture and subarachnoid blockade. Note that the anterior superior iliac spine (ASIS) is assumed to be at the L4 level. (ii) Midline probe placement for sitting position. (iii) Midline probe placement for left lateral position.**

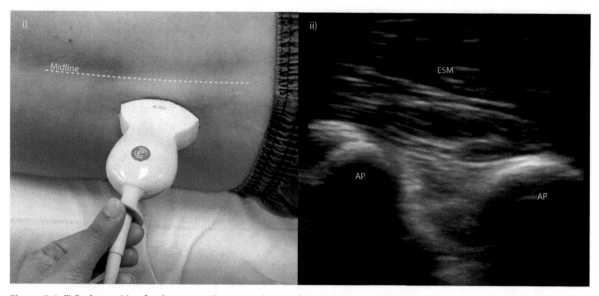

Figure 7.6 (i) Probe position for the paramedian sagittal view of the articular processes. (ii) Sonoanatomy demonstrating the erector spinae muscles and the rounded, 'camel hump' articular processes. ESM, erector spinae muscle; AP, articular process.

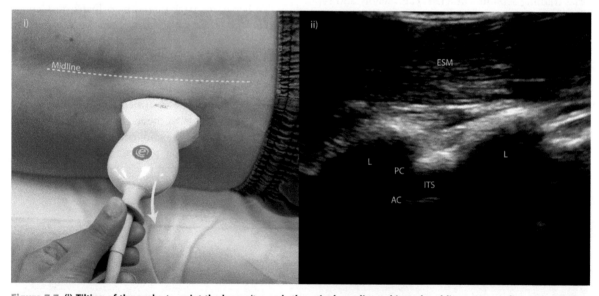

Figure 7.7 (i) Tilting of the probe to point the beam 'towards the spinal canal' to achieve the oblique paramedian view. (ii) The 'camel hump' articular processes now appear as a 'sawtooth' pattern which represent the laminae. The intrathecal space is located between the posterior and anterior complexes. The posterior complex is a collective term used for the ligamentum flavum, epidural space and posterior dura. The anterior complex encompasses the anterior dura, posterior longitudinal ligament and posterior border of the vertebral body and discs. ESM, erector spinae muscle; L, lamina; PC, posterior complex; ITS, intrathecal space; AC, anterior complex.

The probe may then be tilted to point the US beam towards the midline – an oblique paramedian view – and the 'camel humps' will appear more like a 'sawtooth pattern' which represent the down sloping lamina with interlaminar spaces (Figure 7.7). US waves may pass readily through the interlaminar spaces to provide a view of the intrathecal space which is bordered in the far field by the anterior complex. This view may be used for real time US-guided LP or subarachnoid injection.

Ultrasound may also aid the user to correctly identify the vertebral level. Gradually sliding the probe caudally will eventually reveal a longer, horizontal bone which is the sacrum (Figure 7.8). From the sacrum, vertebral levels may be sequentially counted by sliding the probe cranially.

Once the desired level has been reached and midline marked, the probe may be rotated 90 degrees clockwise to the axial or transverse plane. The spinous process will be visible and by making small movements cephalad and caudad the interspinous ligament is identified with erector spinae muscles visible either side (Figure 7.9). The intrathecal space should be seen between the two anterior processes and depth measured using calipers.

Standard practice is to mark the skin at the midline and key vertebral levels and then perform the procedure as per landmark technique. Real-time guidance may be used to directly visualise the needle passing into the intrathecal space using the oblique paramedian approach. If employing this technique, a probe cover must be used to ensure sterility.

Case – Papilloedema and Headache

A 28-year-old female was referred to the ambulatory medical team with ongoing headaches and confirmed papilloedema by her opticians.

Her only past medical history was obesity with a BMI of 38 and she took the combined oral contraceptive pill. She underwent CT brain and CT venogram which were unremarkable, and the working diagnosis was idiopathic intracranial hypertension (IIH). She was counselled and consented for a LP. The trainee doctor attempted the LP with little success and requested assistance from the senior doctor who utilised US for accurate identification of the midline and spinous processes. She was successful on the first attempt and opening pressures were

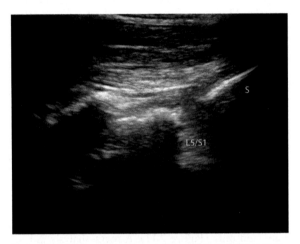

Figure 7.8 Sliding the probe caudally will reveal the sacrum (S) bordered superiorly by the L5/S1 interspinous level.

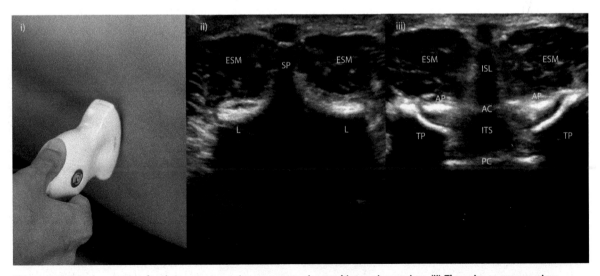

Figure 7.9 (i) Probe position for the transverse spinous process view and interspinous view. (ii) The spinous process view demonstrates the spinous process with a post-acoustic shadow and laminae visible. It is bordered by the erector spinae muscles. (iii) Making small tilting adjustments the user can scan between the spinous processes demonstrating the interspinous ligament, anterior complex, intrathecal space and the posterior complex. Calipers may then be used to measure the distance between the skin and the intrathecal space. SP, spinous process; ESM, erector spinae muscle; L, lamina; ISL, interspinous ligament; AP, articular process; AC, anterior complex; ITS, intrathecal space; PC, posterior complex; TP, transverse process.

measured at 35 mmHg which confirmed the diagnosis of IIH.

Ultrasound in this case avoided the need for referral to anaesthesia for assistance and potential delays in her hospital journey. She was discharged later that day with improved symptoms and follow-up was arranged with the neuro-ophthalmology team.

Giant Cell Arteritis

Giant Cell Arteritis (GCA) is defined as arteritis of large vessels, systemic inflammatory signs and polymyalgia rheumatica. Despite being a *rheumatological* *rather* than *neurological condition*, it is an important differential diagnosis for headache and has therefore been included within this chapter. GCA is a challenging diagnosis and typically presents with persistent severe temporal headaches, scalp tenderness, jaw pain on eating or talking, fevers and visual disturbance. It requires prompt diagnosis to prevent significant deterioration including loss of vision. History, clinical examination and pathology can be non-specific and unnecessarily committing patients to long-term high-dose steroids may lead to significant side effects.

Diagnosis can be made using various modalities. Temporal artery biopsy (TAB) may be inconclusive and challenging to organise in many centres. MR imaging is highly accurate, however accessibility and availability are a challenge. Temporal artery ultrasound (TAUS) is non-invasive, cost effective and enables prompt assessment of the temporal artery. It is reported to have a sensitivity of 77% and specificity of 96% for the diagnosis of GCA and found to be superior to TAB which only evaluates a very limited anatomical area in a systemic disease.

Method

The high frequency linear probe should be used for temporal artery US and colour flow is useful for additional diagnostic features.

Temporal and axillary arteries should be routinely examined for GCA as the temporal arteries are spared in 40% of patients. The probe position for ultrasound of the temporal artery is demonstrated in Figure 7.10. Figures 7.10iii and 7.10iv show a normal transverse and longitudinal view of the temporal artery respectively. If these scans are negative you may need to consider imaging other arteries such as occipital, carotid, vertebral and subclavian.

Early imaging is important as the features disappear within days of commencing steroid therapy. Typical US findings in GCA are summarized in Table 7.3.

Not all features need to be present on TAUS to confirm a diagnosis of GCA and the majority of published studies have addressed the detection of the halo sign only (Figure 7.11). A meta-analysis did not report an increase in specificity or sensitivity for GCA when stenosis and/or occlusion were included in diagnostic criteria in addition to the halo sign alone.

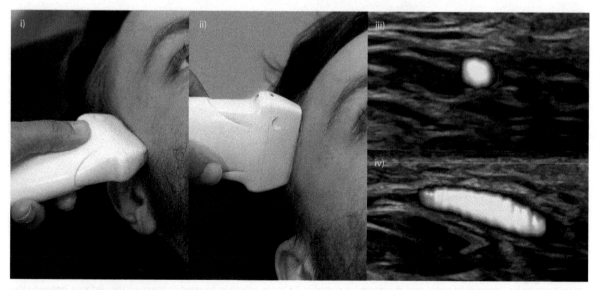

Figure 7.10 Normal probe positions for (i) transverse and (ii) longitudinal views of the temporal artery. (iii) Normal transverse (out of plane) view of the temporal artery with power Doppler demonstrating flow. (iv) Normal longitudinal (in plane) view of the temporal artery with power Doppler.

Table 7.3

Ultrasound characteristics on temporal artery ultrasoundfor giant cell arteritis

Wall thickening (halo sign)

Non-compressible arteries (compression sign)

Stenosis

Vessel occlusion

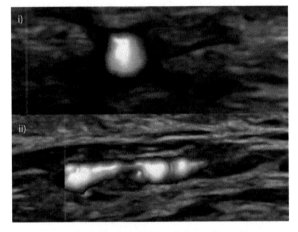

Figure 7.11 The halo sign. (i) Out of plane view with a thickened hypoechoic vessel wall. (ii) Thickened, irregular appearance of the temporal artery with variable lumen size demonstrated by power Doppler.

The halo sign is due to oedema of the artery wall and appears as a hypoechoic thickened wall with flow only visible in the middle of the vessel (Figure 7.11).

As inflammation increases the artery lumen may become occluded or stenosed. This will be characterised by absence of colour flow within the lumen and lack of compressibility. An occluded artery is pathological (Figure 7.12). Figure 7.12i shows a normal artery which is compressible (Figure 7.12ii). Figure 7.12iii shows an example of temporal arteritis with the halo sign and is non-compressible (Figure 7.12iv).

Case – A Unilateral Headache

A 72-year-old man with diabetes and hypertension presented with a right-sided headache and generalised myalgia. The GP had performed blood tests which demonstrated an erythrocyte sedimentation rate (ESR) of 50 mm/hour and a referral was made to the acute medical team querying GCA. The history of headaches was vague with no visual symptoms. He denied jaw claudication but did describe a right-sided headache which worsened as the day progressed with electric-shock-type pains across his face. He had a history of steroid psychosis and was not keen to start them. On examination there were no visual issues and no evidence of proximal myopathy.

The acute medical team carried out a TAUS and this showed a normal temporal artery with

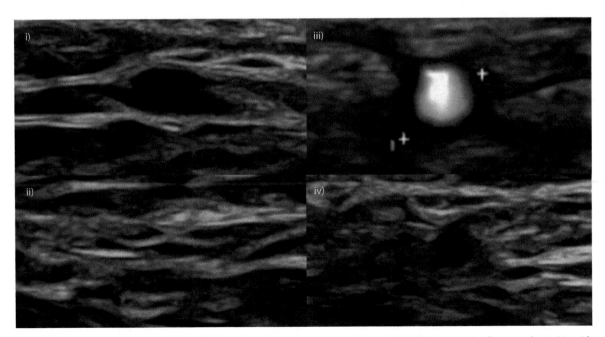

Figure 7.12 (i) Normal temporal artery which is able to be compressed as shown in (ii). (iii) An example of temporal arteritis with the halo sign. (iv) The vessel was unable to be compressed.

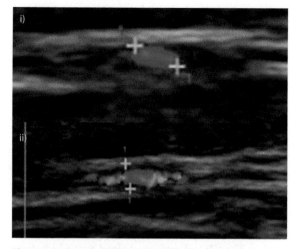

Figure 7.13 Normal (i) transverse (out of plane) and (ii) longitudinal (in plane) view of the temporal artery.

normal compression, no wall thickening or stenosis (Figure 7.13).

The clinical history was more suggestive of trigeminal neuralgia and the point-of-care imaging was reassuring. The patient was commenced on neuropathic analgesia which led to resolution of his symptoms.

This case demonstrates prompt diagnosis in a challenging history with the use of TAUS. Blind initiation of steroid therapy may have been associated with significant complications given the history of steroid psychosis.

Transcranial Doppler

Transcranial Doppler (TCD) is a rapid, reliable and non-invasive method of assessing the velocity of intracranial blood flow using US. Modern US machines utilise colour Doppler for identification of the basal cerebral vessels in the Circle of Willis and pulse wave (PW) spectral Doppler for assessment of flow characteristics.

The major indications for TCD that will be discussed are:

- Recognising an absence of flow in ischaemic stroke.
- Diagnosing intracranial vasospasm post subarachnoid haemorrhage.

Method

A low frequency phased array probe is selected with a TCD preset and the patient is positioned supine. The display marker should be located on the left-hand side

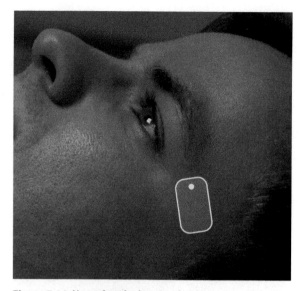

Figure 7.14 Normal probe location for the transcranial Doppler trans-temporal window.

of the screen and the depth set at 10 cm. The probe is placed upon the temporal bone window anterior to the tragus with the probe marker pointing upwards. The probe should be tilted to achieve roughly a 20-degree upward tilt (Figure 7.14). Around 10% of the population will have temporal bone that is too thick to allow US waves to penetrate to the brain. This is particularly problematic in older patients.

The predominant window to acquire is the 'mesencephalic plane' which demonstrates the brainstem (basal cisterns and cerebral peduncles). Colour Doppler is selected with a large colour box and the user should be able to identify the major basal vessels of the Circle of Willis adjacent to the brainstem.

In formal TCD studies the suboccipital, transorbital and submandibular windows will also be interrogated to assess the distal vessels and posterior circulation. This is beyond the scope of this text.

The dominant vascular structure that will be identified is the middle cerebral artery (MCA) which should contain high velocity red colour flow (red = towards the probe). Following the MCA proximally will reveal colour flow in the opposite direction (blue). This is the anterior cerebral artery (ACA). The posterior cerebral artery (PCA) may be seen to wrap around the brainstem with early red flow and late blue flow as its course continues (Figure 7.15).

Pulse wave Doppler is a form of spectral Doppler that may be used to assess the flow characteristics

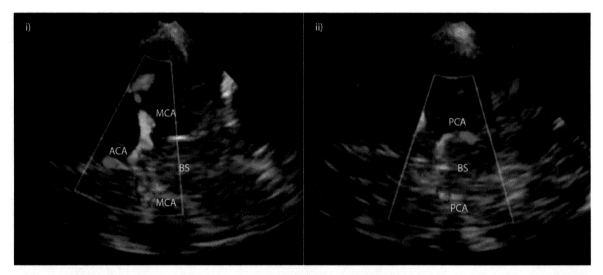

Figure 7.15 Trans-temporal view of the major basal cerebral vessels. **(i) The middle cerebral artery is the dominant structure and may be seen to flow into the anterior cerebral artery where the colour flow changes to blue. Note the contralateral middle cerebral artery visible on the opposite side of the brainstem. (ii) The posterior cerebral artery can be seen to flow around the brainstem with the colour flow changing from red to blue as it changes direction relative to the probe.** MCA, middle cerebral artery; ACA, anterior cerebral artery; BS, brainstem; PCA, posterior cerebral artery.

within these arteries. It is described in more detail in Chapter 1. The flow demonstrated on spectral Doppler may be traced (velocity time integral (VTI) measurement) allowing the machine to calculate the maximum, minimum and mean velocity flow rates. Many machines will have 'TCD packages' that will automatically trace the signal without any user intervention.

Pathology

Ischaemic Stroke

Major territory infarction will lead to an absence of colour flow within the vessel. Although this may be challenging to confidently identify for the novice, comparison of both sides of the cerebral circulation may demonstrate evidence of asymmetry.

Ischaemic findings on plain CT imaging may take hours to days to become evident. The benefit of TCD is to clearly demonstrate absence of flow that can confirm clinical suspicion. This may add weight to the decision to administer thrombolytic agents in a patient with new neurological deficits and a clear initial CT scan.

A case of TCD being used to diagnose an ischaemic stroke in the Himalayas is described in Chapter 11.

Vasospasm

Vasospasm is an extremely common complication occurring in up to 70% of aneurysmal subarachnoid haemorrhages (SAH). Digital subtraction angiography is the gold standard for diagnosis of vasospasm, but this is frequently not performed and blood pressure augmentation therapy empirically initiated. TCD has the ability to diagnose vasospasm in large cerebral vessels by detecting the presence of increased blood flow velocity. This may be performed at the bedside with equipment that is readily available on most high-dependency units.

In this text we will focus on TCD for vasospasm in the MCA although this technique may be used for the ACA, PCA, basilar, vertebral and ophthalmic arteries with adequate experience.

The PW Doppler trace should be placed within the MCA at 1–2 cm intervals. The resulting Doppler signal should be traced using the TCD measurement package to calculate the mean flow velocity (Figure 7.16).

Normal and abnormal *mean velocities* are:

- Normal: 55 cm/second
- Mild vasospasm: >120 cm/second
- Moderate vasospasm: >160 cm/second
- Severe vasospasm: >200 cm/second

Flow velocity within the MCA may be elevated due to any cause of hyperaemia such as severe anaemia and in these instances the elevated velocity will be unrelated to vasospasm. To mitigate for this the **Lindegaard Ratio** may be used. This requires the user

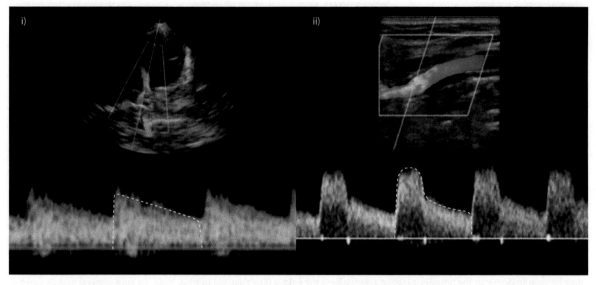

Figure 7.16 (i) Transcranial Doppler with PW Doppler placed within the MCA. An example of how to trace the Doppler signal to calculate the mean velocity is demonstrated. (ii) PW Doppler of the internal carotid artery. The velocity time integral measurement is also depicted in this image.

to perform a long-axis view of the ipsilateral extracranial internal carotid artery (ICA) and use PW Doppler to calculate the mean flow velocity using the same method as for the MCA (Figure 7.16). The mean velocity in the MCA is divided by the mean velocity in the ICA to calculate the ratio:

- <3: hyperaemia
- >3: vasospasm
- 3–6: mild vasospasm
- >6: severe vasospasm

Although this method should not be used to *rule out* vasospasm it may provide excellent objective evidence that vasospasm is present. Potential limitations of this technique are that it is poor for distal vessels and is subject to confounding factors such as cerebral oedema, hypo- or hypercapnoea and changes in blood pressure.

Additional Features in Transcranial Doppler

If using a TCD preset within the ultrasound machine, tracing the 'VTI measurement' for mean velocity will provide an additional value: the *pulsatility index* (PI). The PI is calculated using the following equation:

$$\text{Pulsatility Index} = \frac{\text{Systolic Velocity} - \text{Diastolic Velocity}}{\text{Mean Velocity}}$$

A normal value for PI is 0.8–1.2.

As intracranial pressure rises and cerebral perfusion pressure falls, the pressure will impede the forward diastolic blood flow. This will appear on the spectral Doppler as a progressive fall in the diastolic flow trace and subsequent increase in the PI. This may be preceded by an isolated rise in the systolic peak velocity.

The PI is a marker of impaired cerebral perfusion and the absolute value may be used to infer the estimated intracranial pressure (ICP) by using the following formula:

$$\text{ICP} = (10.93 \times \text{PI}) - 1.28$$

Using this equation, a PI of >2.13 equates to an ICP of >22 which is significantly elevated.

As the intracranial pressure rises, there is progressive deterioration in the diastolic flow rate and may progress to diastolic flow reversal. This is an exceptionally poor prognostic sign and is described as 'cerebral circulatory arrest'. This may be incorporated into the bedside assessment of patients with suspected severe intracranial injury.

Summary

- Ultrasound within the field of neurology can be a useful aid in the assessment, diagnosis and management within certain clinical scenarios.

- The use of US for the diagnosis of papilloedema is gaining popularity and has demonstrated an increased sensitivity and specificity when compared with fundoscopy.
- Ultrasound-assisted LP has increased success rate, reduces complications and can improve patient satisfaction.
- Temporal artery ultrasound is superior to TAB in diagnosis of GCA.

- Transcranial Doppler is being increasingly utilised in the assessment of intracranial blood flow in pathologies such as ischaemic stroke, vasospasm and in cases of raised intracranial pressure.

A full list of references and further reading is available at www.GeneralistUltrasound.com

Gynaecology and Early Pregnancy Ultrasound

Ultrasound (US) is used as the first-line imaging modality for many obstetric and gynaecological (O&G) conditions. It is the perfect tool for general clinicians to narrow down broad differential diagnoses and can identify key pathology in emergency situations. This is a critical skill for clinicians in all fields including general practitioners, remote medical providers, paramedics and emergency or acute care clinicians.

The use of point-of-care ultrasound (POCUS) for O&G presentations has been found to shorten the time taken to see a specialist clinician and reduce the patient's length of hospital stay. This suggests an improvement in the initial quality of care provided as well as the patient's journey during their hospital stay. It is an essential tool in the developing world and low resource countries where early pregnancy-related complications convey a large burden of morbidity and mortality.

Obstetric and gynaecological ultrasound is an extremely detailed subspeciality requiring extensive experience. This chapter will predominantly consider normal anatomy and basic findings that will be required by the generalist. There will be a basic introduction to more advanced topics but these will not be considered in detail. A summary of the key topics are as follows:

- Normal pelvic anatomy.
- Pelvic and abdominal free fluid.
- Confirmation of intrauterine pregnancy.
- Ectopic pregnancy.
- Molar pregnancy.
- Uterine and ovarian masses.
- Intrauterine device malposition and displacement.
- Ovarian cyst, torsion and abscess.
- Pelvic inflammatory disease and hydrosalpinx.

Transabdominal Pelvic Ultrasound

Transabdominal pelvic US is capable of identifying and diagnosing most O&G conditions including life-threatening emergencies such as ectopic pregnancy and ovarian cyst rupture. Furthermore, this is the

modality that is available in most departments and the one generalist clinicians are most familiar with. Transabdominal imaging is potentially limited by the presence of abdominal bowel gas or an empty bladder and, if poor views are obtained, referral should be made for alternative investigation.

Transvaginal ultrasound (TVUS) provides the best visualisation of the female pelvic organs and is being increasingly utilised during the first trimester of pregnancy. However, this is a more invasive tool that is reserved for specialist clinicians and will not be discussed in this text.

Method

For transabdominal pelvic US the patient should ideally have a full bladder as this acts as an acoustic window for the uterus and adnexal structures. The patient is scanned in a supine position and the curvilinear probe selected with a pelvic, abdominal or O&G preset.

The probe is placed in the suprapubic region in a sagittal plane and angled inferiorly into the pelvic cavity with the probe marker pointing cephalad (Figure 8.1i). The bladder will be located in the near field adjacent to the uterus. The uterine fundus and body can be seen to extend to the cervix and vaginal stripe which underlie the bladder. The recto-uterine pouch (also known as the Pouch of Douglas) and rectum are seen deep to the cervix (Figure 8.1ii).

The probe is rotated 90 degrees counterclockwise for the transverse pelvic view with the probe marker pointed to the patient's right-hand side (Figure 8.2i). A transverse view of the uterus is seen with good delineation between the endometrium and myometrium (Figure 8.2ii). The fallopian tubes may be visible on either side of the uterus although can be obscured by bowel gas. The user should fan through the entire uterus in both the sagittal and transverse windows.

From the transverse view the tail of the probe is rocked to the patient's right side to visualise the left ovary (Figure 8.3i). This can be repeated in the

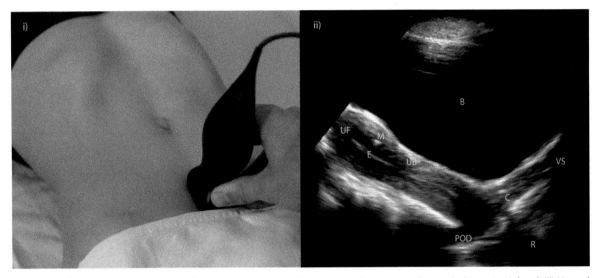

Figure 8.1 **(i) Probe position to acquire the sagittal pelvic view. The probe marker is pointed towards the patient's head. (ii) Normal anatomy of the pelvic organs.** B, bladder; UB, uterine body; UF, uterine fundus; E, endometrium; M, myometrium; POD, Pouch of Douglas; C, cervix; VS, vaginal stripe; R, rectum.

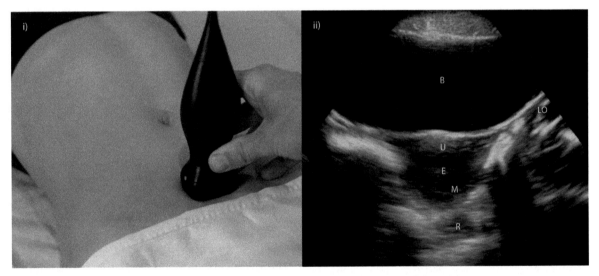

Figure 8.2 **(i) Probe position to acquire the transverse pelvic view. (ii) Normal anatomy of the pelvic organs.** B, bladder; U, uterus; E, endometrium; M, myocardium; LO, left ovary; R, rectum.

opposite direction for the right ovary. The ovaries lie lateral and/or posterior to the uterus and appear as hypoechoic follicular structures that typically measure 2–3 cm in diameter (Figure 8.3ii). They may be challenging to identify in a poorly opti-mised patient.

Free Fluid within the Pelvic Cavity

Free fluid accumulates in dependent regions within the abdomen. This has been previously discussed

within Chapter 4. In females, the Pouch of Douglas (POD), also known as the posterior cul de sac and recto-uterine pouch, is a dependent region that may contain small volumes of fluid in healthy individuals. This is particularly noted during ovula-tion and is usually around 10–20 ml in volume (Figure 8.4).

Larger volumes of fluid should be considered to be pathological and may represent a significant condition such as pelvic inflammatory disease,

181

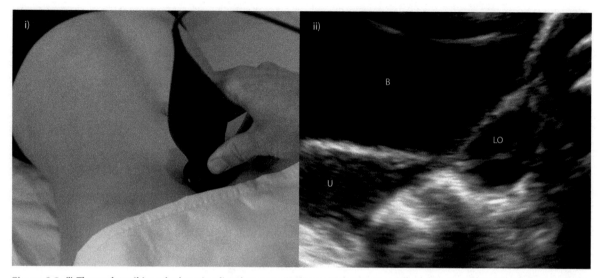

Figure 8.3 (i) The probe tail is rocked to visualise the ovary. (ii) Normal appearance of the left ovary. Note the anechoic follicular structure. B, bladder; U, uterus; LO, left ovary.

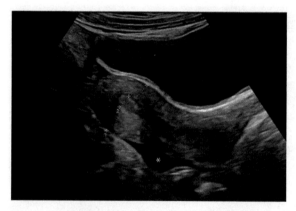

Figure 8.4 Free fluid within the Pouch of Douglas (*).

ectopic pregnancy, endometriosis, leiomyoma or malignancy.

If free fluid is seen within the pelvis it is useful to image the right upper quadrant (RUQ) and left upper quadrant (LUQ) to evaluate for more fluid. Figure 8.5 demonstrates fluid in Morison's Pouch and LUQ. The presence of fluid within these regions is more likely to indicate an acute surgical emergency and should be urgently correlated with other clinical features and referred for specialist opinion.

It is important to remember that any acute surgical emergency or chronic medical conditions, such as cardiac, renal or hepatic failure, may also lead to free abdominal fluid.

Confirmation of Intrauterine Pregnancy

Intrauterine pregnancy (IUP) is diagnosed by confirming the presence of a yolk sac or foetal pole located within a gestational sac inside the uterus. Transabdominal ultrasound is sufficiently sensitive to identify a gestational sac from approximately 6 weeks gestation. It may be identified from 3 to 5 weeks using TVUS.

Gestational Sac

The gestational sac appears as an anechoic circular structure surrounded by an echogenic ring of trophoblasts located eccentrically within the endometrium. The lining of this is called the decidua capsularis and is surrounded by a second hyperechoic ring which is the lining of the uterine cavity – the decidua parietalis. The presence of these two sacs is called the 'double decidual sac sign' and is a useful feature for confirming IUP if the yolk sac or foetal pole is not seen.

A pseudogestational sac describes the presence of intrauterine fluid with a positive pregnancy test that is mistakenly considered to be a true gestational sac. This potentially misses the presence of an ectopic pregnancy. Key sonographic findings of pseudogestational sacs include:

- Located within the endometrial cavity rather than gestational sacs which are eccentrically positioned within the endometrium.

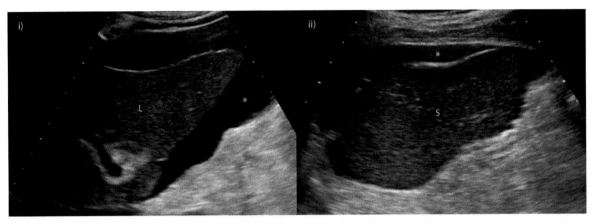

Figure 8.5 Free fluid (*) in (i) the right upper quadrant and (ii) the left upper quadrant. L, liver; S, spleen.

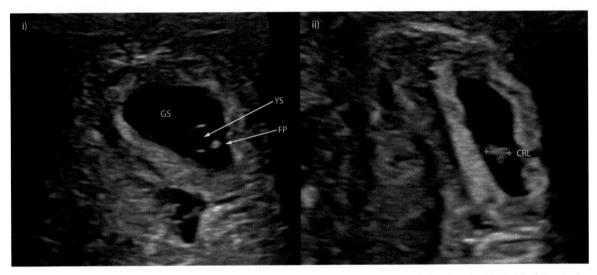

Figure 8.6 (i) Key findings with the gestational sac. Note the two echogenic outer lines which is the 'double decidual sac sign'. (ii) The crown-rump length has been measured. GS, gestational sac; YS, yolk sac; FP, foetal pole; CRL, crown-rump length.

- Fluid may appear to fill a more 'angular' cavity whereas gestational sacs are round and regular.
- The border is less echogenic than a gestational sac.
- Fluid may be hypoechoic and contain debris rather than anechoic.
- Does not contain a yolk sac or foetal pole.
- Absence of double decidual sac sign.

Intrauterine fluid collections are common and occur in up to 20% of ectopic pregnancies highlighting the importance of recognising these features.

Yolk Sac

The yolk sac is the first structure to be identified within the maturing gestational sac and provides nutrients to the embryo during the initial stages of development. It is visible on transabdominal US from approximately 7 weeks gestation. It appears as a circular anechoic structure with an echogenic wall located within the gestational sac (Figure 8.6i). A yolk sac is only present in an IUP and therefore is a key feature to differentiate IUP from ectopic pregnancy.

Foetal Pole

The foetal pole is the first finding of the developing embryo during pregnancy. It can normally be seen with transabdominal US from the seventh week although may appear later. The appearance is of an echogenic thickening on the border of the yolk sac.

The long axis of the foetal pole – the crown-rump length (CRL) – will eventually become visible as the distance between the top of the head from the bottom of the torso (Figure 8.6ii). This measurement is used to estimate gestational age and from a CRL of ≥7 mm the foetal heartbeat should be detected.

The absence of a foetal pole with a yolk sac diameter of >25mm on transabdominal US is suggestive of a failed pregnancy. In these cases, the patient should be considered for TVUS and the scan repeated after 7 days.

Foetal heart rate is measured when the CRL is ≥7 mm and is preferentially performed using M-mode US. M-mode is preferred to pulsed wave (PW) Doppler as it subjects the developing foetus to lower US energy levels. This is performed by placing the M-mode cursor through the foetal pole and ensuring an O&G preset is selected. The heart rate is seen as deflections in the M-mode trace and the machine will automatically calculate the heart rate.

Again, if no foetal heartbeat is detected then the patient should be urgently referred for specialist assessment and repeat transabdominal US or TVUS.

Ectopic Pregnancy

Ectopic pregnancy is a pregnancy occurring outside of the uterus and is the most common gynaecological emergency and the leading cause of maternal mortality in the first trimester. Incidence ranges from 0.5% to 1.5% of all pregnancies. The majority of ectopic pregnancies occur within the fallopian tubes but many other sites may be affected.

Patients will typically present with abdominal pain, pelvic pain or vaginal bleeding. The primary role of US should **not** be to definitively 'rule-in' an ectopic pregnancy but rather to **confirm the presence of an IUP** which makes an ectopic pregnancy less likely. This is particularly important within an emergency setting where rapid identification of an IUP may guide the clinician to consider alternative diagnoses.

Two key steps should be followed when considering ectopic pregnancy in a patient with abdominal pain and a positive beta human chorionic gonadotropin (beta-HCG):

Step 1 – The uterus should be scanned to identify a gestational sac with a yolk sac and foetal pole. If detected, the patient has an IUP and is unlikely to have a concurrent ectopic unless having in vitro fertilisation (IVF) therapy.

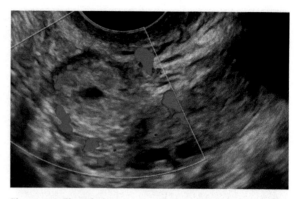

Figure 8.7 The tubal ring sign and ring of fire sign in a patient with ectopic pregnancy.

Step 2 – If no IUP is detected and the patient is haemodynamically stable then the adnexa may be assessed for direct signs of an ectopic pregnancy.

The most reliable finding of ectopic pregnancy is the presence of an extra-uterine gestational sac but this may not be present in up to one-third of patients. The **tubal ring sign** describes the presence of a hyperechoic ring of trophoblastic cells around an adnexal mass and is a common US finding in an ectopic pregnancy (Figure 8.7). The **ring of fire sign** is the presence of a hypervascular ring on the periphery of a tubal ectopic (Figure 8.7). Both the tubal ring sign and the ring of fire sign are also seen in a corpus luteum cyst and bimanual examination may be required to differentiate.

Any patient with a suspected ectopic pregnancy should be clinically optimised prior to any US assessment. A positive beta-HCG with the presence of free fluid in the POD ± the RUQ or LUQ should prompt urgent referral for surgical intervention.

Pregnancy of unknown location describes a positive pregnancy test with no evidence of an IUP or extrauterine pregnancy on TVUS. It is essential not to diagnose a complete miscarriage due to the absence of an intrauterine gestational sac unless the patient has previously been demonstrated to have an IUP.

Case – Emergency Department Diagnosis of Ruptured Ectopic Pregnancy using Ultrasound'

A 32-year-old female presented to the ED with acute lower abdominal pain and vomiting. She was hypotensive, tachycardic and tachypnoeic. On examination, her abdomen was peritonitic and bedside tests demonstrated a positive beta-HCG with no evidence of an intrauterine pregnancy on US. A significant

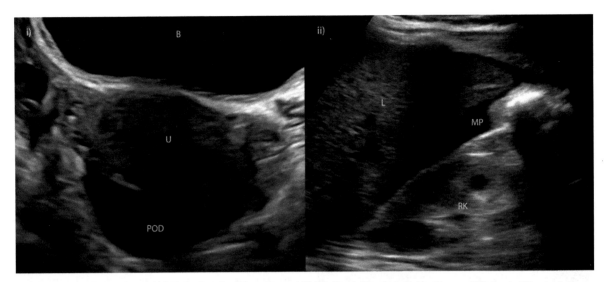

Figure 8.8 Free fluid seen within (i) the Pouch of Douglas and (ii) Morison's Pouch. B, bladder; U, uterus; POD, Pouch of Douglas; L, liver; MP, Morison's Pouch; RK, right kidney.

amount of free fluid was visualised within the POD and Morison's Pouch (Figure 8.8).

Urgent laparoscopic surgery was undertaken and demonstrated a ruptured tubal ectopic pregnancy requiring salpingectomy. She subsequently made a good recovery.

The presence of free intraperitoneal fluid in the context of a positive beta-HCG and an empty uterus is approximately 70% specific and 63% sensitive for an ectopic pregnancy.

Molar Pregnancy

Molar pregnancy is the most common form of gestational trophoblastic disease and occurs when a non-viable fertilised egg implants into the uterus. It commonly presents as painless vaginal bleeding, severe nausea and vomiting and excessive uterine enlargement. Histopathology of the products of conception still remains the gold standard for diagnosis of trophoblastic disease but the diagnosis may be readily made using US.

The US findings in complete molar pregnancy are described as having a **'snow storm'** appearance as they have a complex echogenic mass with cystic spaces (Figure 8.9).

Fibroids (Leiomyomas)

Fibroids are the most common type of benign neoplasm. They can arise in a variety of locations within

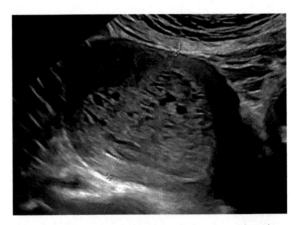

Figure 8.9 'Snow storm' appearance in keeping with molar pregnancy.

the smooth muscle layer of the uterus and can produce a spectrum of symptoms depending on the size and location of the mass.

Most patients are asymptomatic but can experience abnormal uterine bleeding or infertility.

On US, fibroids are detected by heterogeneous enlargement of the uterus due to the presence of well demarcated, hypoechoic masses within the myometrium. However, fibroids may also appear isoechoic or hyperechoic. Note fibroids can extend beyond the normal contours of the uterus and may only be found outside the myometrium.

Intrauterine Device Malposition or Displacement

An intrauterine device (IUD) on US appears as a hyperechoic structure exhibiting posterior shadowing and should be located within the endometrial cavity (Figure 8.10). US is a simple, quick method commonly used to confirm placement. US can also detect complications including migration, expulsion and uterine perforation. This would be an ideal modality for general practice where loss of strings or expulsion are common complaints and are reported in approximately 2–3% of women with an IUD.

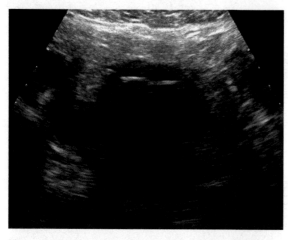

Figure 8.10 Appearance of a correctly sited intrauterine device. Note the hyperechoic device with post-acoustic shadowing.

Ovarian Masses

Ovarian masses are common incidental findings and can readily be interrogated by US. We will discuss the appearance of simple and corpus luteum cysts, ruptured/haemorrhagic cyst, ovarian torsion, tubo-ovarian abscess and ovarian tumours.

Ovarian Cysts

Ovarian cysts are extremely common and appear on US in a variety of ways depending on their subtype. Typically, they are characterised by anechoic fluid filling the cyst with thin walls.

Corpus Luteum Cysts

Corpus luteum cysts are a normal part of the menstrual cycle. They are usually <3 cm and appear as a fluid-filled mass with a thick wall. As previously mentioned, these may demonstrate the tubal ring sign and ring of fire sign and may be confused for ectopic pregnancy. Corpus luteum cysts tend to be less echogenic than ectopic pregnancy.

Simple Ovarian Cysts

Simple ovarian cysts are common and appear as smooth, thin-walled sacs containing anechoic fluid (Figure 8.11). The vast majority of cysts are benign and are related to ovulation. Most are asymptomatic but may cause pelvic or lower back pain. Above a certain size threshold, ≥5 cm for pre-menopausal and ≥3 cm for post-menopausal women, surveillance is recommended.

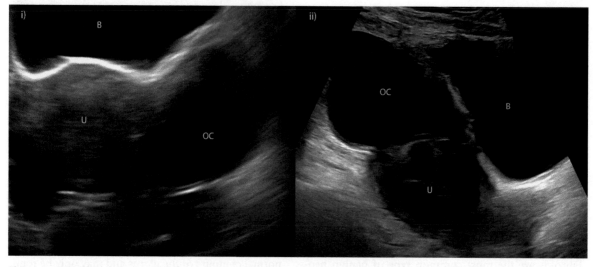

Figure 8.11 (i) Transverse view with an ovarian cyst adjacent to the uterus. Note the anechoic appearance. (ii) Sagittal view of a different patient demonstrating a very large ovarian cyst. B, bladder; U, uterus; OC, ovarian cyst.

Ruptured/Haemorrhagic Ovarian Cysts

Haemorrhagic cysts are usually seen in premenopausal women and are usually the result of bleeding into a simple cyst, follicle or corpus luteum cyst.

Patients present with acute pelvic or abdominal pain and may have a pelvic mass. They may, however, be completely asymptomatic and the cyst is an incidental finding.

Ultrasound demonstrates a 'cob web' appearance of internal echos due to fibrinous strands (Figure 8.12). A fluid level may be visible. The wall of the cyst remains thin and internal clot may be visible.

Rupture of a haemorrhagic cyst into the peritoneum is a serious condition presenting with pain, tenderness, nausea and vomiting and may progress to peritonitis. Free fluid will be identified in the pelvic and abdominal windows. Urgent surgical intervention may be required.

Ovarian Tumours

Ovarian tumours are notoriously challenging to diagnose from symptoms alone. On US their appearance is very variable from a cystic to solid structure with or without septae. In general, the more solid an ovarian mass is, the more likely it is to represent malignancy.

Case – Red Flag Symptoms

A 65-year-old lady presented with abdominal distension and pain combined with generally feeling unwell and a history of weight loss. On examination she had a distended lower abdomen and blood results revealed an acute kidney injury.

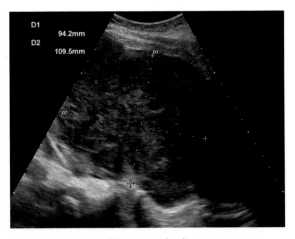

Figure 8.13 Large pelvic mass with a heterogeneous appearance. Note the solid regions interspersed with cystic regions.

A POCUS scan was undertaken within the ED which showed a large pelvic mass measuring 11 cm × 9.5 cm (Figure 8.13). Further abdominal US revealed mild bilateral hydronephrosis. She underwent an urgent CT scan which confirmed an ovarian tumour with hydroureter and mild bilateral hydronephrosis. She was referred swiftly to the gynaecology team.

Ovarian Torsion

Ovarian torsion is a gynaecological emergency where the ovary has twisted upon its ligaments and blood supply. It is often seen in patients with ovarian cysts. Rotation of the ovary leads to compression of the arteries, veins and lymphatics causing congestion, ovarian oedema and potentially infarction if left untreated.

Patients present with acute pelvic or lower abdominal pain with nausea and vomiting. Studies have shown the right ovary is more commonly affected due to the sigmoid colon conferring some protection to the left.

Ultrasound will demonstrate unilateral findings with an oedematous enlarged ovary of >4 cm with the **string of pearls sign** (Figure 8.14). The string of pearls sign describes peripheral anechoic follicles being visible due to central lymphatic congestion. In addition, the **whirlpool sign** may be seen which is the wrapping of vessels around the central axis of the pedicle shown with colour Doppler or power Doppler.

The string of pearls sign may also be present in polycystic ovary syndrome but the remainder of the ovary is normal in morphology.

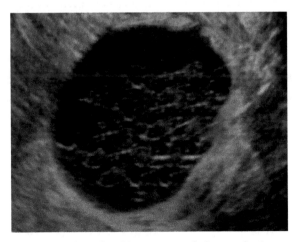

Figure 8.12 The 'cob web' appearance of a haemorrhagic cyst.

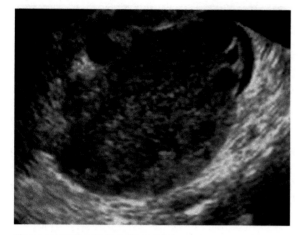

Figure 8.14 The 'string of pearls' sign.

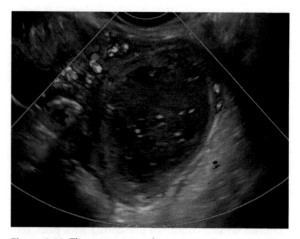

Figure 8.15 The appearance of an ovarian abscess. Note the thick and irregular walls with variable internal echogenicity.

Case – A String of Pearls in Ovarian Torsion

A 28-year-old woman presented to ED with sudden onset of right iliac fossa pain. It was constant, sharp in nature and associated with vomiting. She complained of similar episodes over the past few weeks but these had been shorter in duration and resolved spontaneously. She was haemodynamically stable with no fever but had guarding in the right iliac fossa. The team were concerned about appendicitis and POCUS was performed. The scan showed no features of appendicitis but a swollen, oedematous ovary in keeping with torsion.

She underwent emergency laparoscopic surgery which revealed a torted oedematous ovary with an underlying cyst. An ovarian cystectomy was performed and the ovary was uncoiled and viable.

Tubo-Ovarian Abscess

A tubo-ovarian abscess is a complex, infected, pus filled mass in the adnexa that is most commonly secondary to pelvic inflammatory disease (PID). Patients present with lower abdominal and pelvic pain, fevers and vaginal discharge. Although antibiotics may be effective, approximately 25% of patients require surgery.

Ultrasound will reveal an adnexal mass with septated, irregular/thick walls and variable internal echogenicity. Solid areas may be present. The ovary will have an irregular, thickened wall and hydrosalpinx may be present as shown in Figure 8.15.

Hydrosalpinx

Hydrosalpinx is the abnormal accumulation of fluid in the fallopian tubes causing tubal swelling. Causes

include PID, endometriosis, tubal obstruction or as a complication of hysterectomy. Patients may present with pelvic pain and infertility.

Fallopian tubes are not normally visible on US unless surrounded by intraperitoneal fluid. In hydrosalpinx, the fallopian tubes become dilated and may be seen with the following characteristics:

- A tubular-shaped cystic mass discontinuous with the ipsilateral ovary.
- Indentations on both sides of the tubular mass (waist sign).
- Appearance like 'beads on a string'.

Pelvic Inflammatory Disease

Pelvic inflammatory disease is a very common gynaecological condition which is increasing in frequency. It is the result of ascending spread of infection within the pelvis, most commonly due to Chlamydia trachomatis or Neisseria gonorrhoeae. Patients present with pelvic pain, vaginal discharge, fever and uterine/adnexal tenderness.

Although PID is a clinical diagnosis, US is the first-line imaging modality and may demonstrate:

- Adnexal mass.
- Free fluid in POD.
- Hydrosalpinx.
- Multiple cysts in the ovaries.
- Tubo-ovarian abscesses.

Case – Pelvic Free Fluid and Pelvic Inflammatory Disease

A 21-year-old woman presented to the ED with lower abdominal pain, dysuria, brown vaginal discharge

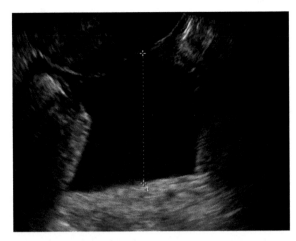

Figure 8.16 **Pelvic free fluid in a patient with pelvic inflammatory disease.**

and mild fever to the Gynaecology Ambulatory Clinic. She has a history of sexually transmitted infections. The clinician was concerned about PID but wanted to exclude an ectopic pregnancy or UTI. Her pregnancy and urine tests were negative. On clinical examination she had adnexal tenderness and high vaginal swabs were taken. A US was undertaken which revealed free fluid in the POD (Figure 8.16). There was no free fluid in Morison's pouch and no evidence of an intrauterine or ectopic pregnancy.

The patient was initiated on an appropriate antibiotic regimen for PID and discharged home with safety netting advice and follow-up planned after 7 days.

Summary

- Ultrasound plays a major role in women presenting as an emergency with abdominal pain. It can aid with diagnosing intrauterine pregnancy and fetal viability during a time which can be very anxious for patients and provides valuable bedside information in life-threatening gynaecological emergencies such as ectopic pregnancy, ruptured and torted ovarian cysts where time is of the essence.

- Outside the emergency care environment US is critical within general practice/family medicine empowering them to diagnose common obstetric and gynaecological conditions that can be managed safely in the community.

- The portability of US makes this modality ideal in remote, low-resource settings where poor access to healthcare leads to a high rate of preventable maternal morbidity. Numerous humanitarian and teleultrasound projects are focusing on delivering O&G US and training to communities who need it the most. This is discussed more in Chapter 11.

A full list of references and further reading is available at www.GeneralistUltrasound.com

Hospital at Home

Hospital at Home provides an alternative pathway of acute care that is traditionally delivered within hospital settings. This pioneering concept of care provides a potential solution to the increasing demand on acute hospital trusts and dwindling availability of hospital beds. The primary goal is to provide hospital admission avoidance whilst delivering high-quality acute care in a multi-disciplinary fashion. Senior decision-making and mobile diagnostics, such as point-of-care ultrasound (POCUS), are critical to this model.

Point-of-care ultrasound can empower clinicians to justify a patient's transfer to hospital whilst maintaining confidence in the decision to keep others at home. It is invaluable in the provision of acute care in the community and offers high quality diagnostic capability that has previously been reserved for hospital environments. The Hospital at Home model has been shown to be cost effective and reduces the harm associated with unnecessarily exposing vulnerable patients to the hospital environment.

We present a snapshot of cases showcasing the use of POCUS by the Hospital at Home team. These cases emphasise how swift intervention in a residential setting may safely avoid hospital admission and, if admission is required, how this may be performed swiftly and efficiently to streamline the patient journey.

Case – Ultrasound-Guided Acute Care at Home

A 94-year-old lady from a care home with a background of dementia, heart failure (ejection fraction of 25%) and previous aortic valve repair was reported by the nursing team to be increasingly drowsy. A COVID-19 swab had been performed several days earlier and was negative. The paramedics had assessed her and reported a BP of 77/42. The GP was contacted for advice as the patient's family had requested that she should not be transferred or admitted to hospital. The Hospital at Home team were called for input and

upon arrival they found her alert and sat upright but non-communicative and with poor oral intake. Her BP was 95/62 and remaining observations were within normal range.

Basic point-of-care blood tests were undertaken and they revealed acute on chronic kidney injury with a significantly elevated urea. A POCUS scan of her heart, inferior vena cava (IVC), lungs and kidneys were undertaken. Lung ultrasound (LUS) showed multiple B lines (Figure 9.1).

Focused echo demonstrated features of hypovolaemia with an acceptable left ventricular (LV) contractility given her known history of heart failure (Figure 9.2).

Renal ultrasound showed no evidence of hydronephrosis (Figure 9.3) and her IVC was small in calibre with >50% inspiratory collapse (Figure 9.3).

Her drug history was reviewed and it was noted she was prescribed multiple nephrotoxic agents. The patient's family insisted they did not want her to be admitted to hospital and for her care to remain within the care home.

Nephrotoxic agents were discontinued and intravenous (IV) fluids were administered daily for 48 hours with close monitoring. She made a significant improvement and on day three she was sat out of bed, eating and drinking and engaging with her carers. This case demonstrates the importance of POCUS in assessing volume status and excluding other significant pathology in a patient with undifferentiated symptoms. These findings enabled simple interventions to lead to an excellent clinical outcome without moving the patient out of her own environment.

Case – Another Hospital Admission Avoided

An 88-year-old man with cardiomyopathy, atrial fibrillation (AF), chronic kidney disease (CKD) and prostate cancer was referred to the Hospital at Home team with the possibility of needing IV fluids as he had been anuric for 10 hours. He was under the community heart failure team who were administering IV diuretics every morning and being closely monitored due to previous deterioration in renal function.

On examination he was agitated, in pain and dyspnoeic at rest.

Lung ultrasound (LUS) showed bilateral effusions with B lines consistent with heart failure (Figure 9.4i). Focused echo confirmed poor LV function (Figure 9.4ii).

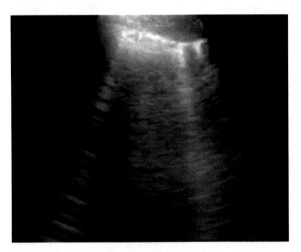

Figure 9.1 **B lines were present but these did not coalesce.** *A video is available to view in the online video library.*

Point-of-care ultrasound of his bladder demonstrated a distended bladder in keeping with urinary retention (Figure 9.5).

Renal ultrasound (US) showed no signs of hydronephrosis. The patient was catheterised and he immediately drained 500 ml of urine which relieved his symptoms. A simple scan identifying urinary retention relieved the patient's symptoms and prevented unnecessary transfer to hospital.

The main differential in this case would be urinary tract obstruction and hydronephrosis secondary to prostate cancer. If catheterisation was unsuccessful, bedside US-guided percutaneous nephrostomy or suprapubic catheter insertion could be performed in a patient's home to relieve this obstruction in a patient who is not appropriate for acute hospital transfer.

Case – It's not always about Dehydration and Heart Failure

A 90-year-old man, living with his wife, was escalated to the Hospital at Home team for IV fluids by the GP. His renal function had been deteriorating for the past 3 months and recent blood tests demonstrated a sharp decline in function. Past medical history included chronic kidney disease, type 2 diabetes mellitus (T2DM), ischaemic heart disease and diastolic dysfunction.

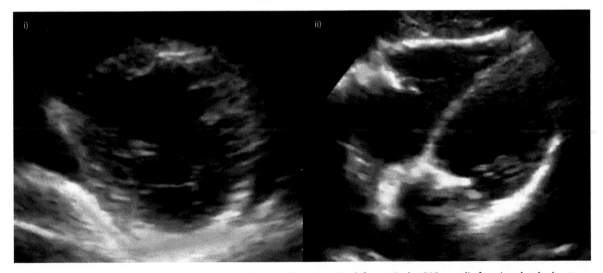

Figure 9.2 **(i) Parasternal short-axis and (ii) subcostal views demonstrating left ventricular (LV) systolic function that had not deteriorated from known levels. At the time of this study the LV systolic function appears to be more than the previously documented 25%.** *Videos are available to view in the online video library.*

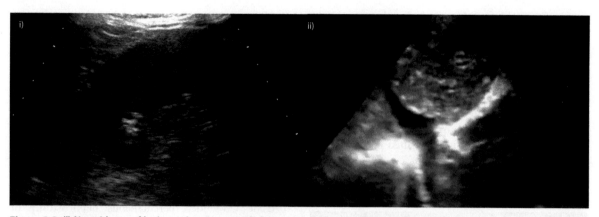

Figure 9.3 (i) No evidence of hydronephrosis on renal ultrasound. (ii) Small calibre IVC with >50% inspiratory collapse suggestive of hypovolaemia. *Videos are available to view in the online video library.*

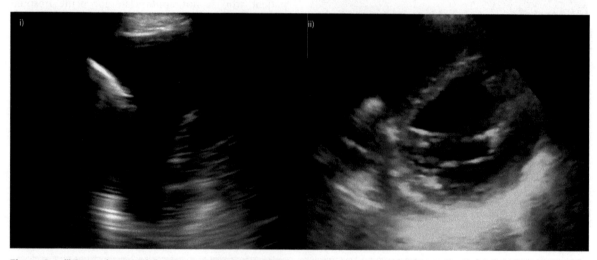

Figure 9.4 (i) Lung ultrasound showing a small pleural effusion in keeping with longstanding heart failure. (ii) Parasternal short-axisview at the mitral valve level demonstrating poor LV systolic function. *Videos are available to view in the online video library.*

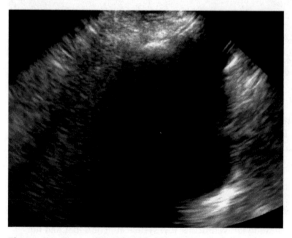

Figure 9.5 Large, distended bladder in keeping with urinary retention. *Note the artefact from bowel gas on the left of the screen.*

On examination the patient was frail, found to be hypoglycaemic and extremely short of breath. He was given IV 20% glucose to reverse his hypoglycaemia and a POCUS screen was undertaken.

The clinician was expecting to see features of heart failure in view of the acute kidney injury but instead identified an interstitial syndrome with a thickened pleural line and subpleural consolidation consistent with COVID-19 (Figure 9.6). Further questioning revealed clinical symptoms in keeping with this diagnosis.

At his own request, the patient was made comfortable in his own home with anticipatory medications tailored to his symptoms. He passed away a few days later but remained comfortable and distress free in his last days of life.

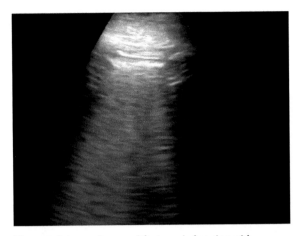

Figure 9.6 **Lung ultrasound features in keeping with COVID-19 pneumonitis.** *A video is available to view in the online video library.*

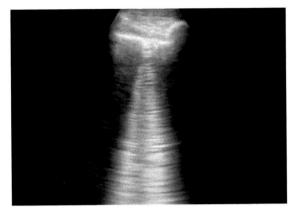

Figure 9.8 **Lung ultrasound demonstrating B lines secondary to heart failure.** *A video is available to view in the online video library.*

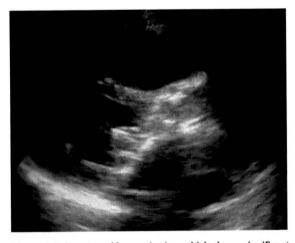

Figure 9.7 **Parasternal long-axis view which shows significant artefact from the aortic and mitral valve replacements, severe bradycardia and impaired LV systolic function.** *A video is available to view in the online video library.*

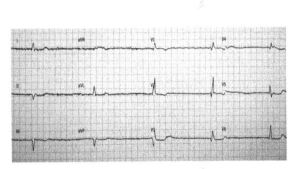

Figure 9.9 **Upon arrival to hospital his ECG demonstrated complete heart block.**

Case – Reversing the Reversible

An 89-year-old man was referred to the Hospital at Home team with a one-week history of fatigue, reduced appetite and had 'taken to his bed'. His background included atrial fibrillation (AF), ischaemic heart disease (IHD), mitral and aortic valve replacements.

On assessment he was lying flat in bed and complained of dyspnoea on exertion. He insisted he wanted to stay at home and had felt he had come to the end of his life. His point-of-care blood results showed significant acute kidney injury.

A POCUS scan was undertaken which revealed bradycardia and impaired LV systolic function on echo (Figure 9.7) with features of fluid overload on the lung scan (Figure 9.8).

A portable ECG showed complete heart block (Figure 9.9) which explained his decompensation.

Despite the patient wanting to stay at home it was explained that all his symptoms could be reversed with insertion of a pacemaker. He eventually agreed for admission and he was directly admitted to the cardiology unit and temporised on an isoprenaline infusion. A pacemaker was inserted the following morning and he made a full recovery with resolution of his renal failure.

This case highlights how POCUS identified a reversible cause and justified an urgent hospital transfer for definitive intervention.

Summary

- Hospital at Home provides an alternative pathway to hospital admission and delivers safe acute care within the patient's home environment.
- Point-of-care ultrasound can empower clinicians to justify patient transfers to hospital whilst maintaining confidence in the decision to keep other patients at home.
- The holistic approach of a generalist coupled with the diagnostic capability of POCUS provides clinicians and patients with confidence in this unique service.

A full list of references and further reading is available at www.GeneralistUltrasound.com

Palliative Care and End of Life Care

Palliative and end of life care is everybody's business. Generalists need to be competent in not only recognising the dying process and prescribing anticipatory medication, but also have the ability to correctly diagnose the pathology of a symptom that is causing distress. Although not in widespread use, POCUS is a skill that provides invaluable diagnostic and procedural capabilities to clinicians involved in palliative care.

Common examples of POCUS applications include drainage of pleural effusions and ascites, peripheral nerve blockade for refractory pain, identification of deep vein thromboses (DVTs) and challenging peripheral vascular access. All of these interventions may be delivered without moving the patient, allowing them to remain in their home environment which is of tremendous value at the end of life.

Additionally, POCUS may aid in the decision to de-escalate a patient's level of care and justify treatment limitations which may at times be challenging. This chapter presents several cases where POCUS can be applied by all generalists within palliative and end of life care settings.

Case – I Would Like to Die at Home

A 63-year-old male had been diagnosed with metastatic renal carcinoma 3 months earlier. The tumour was inoperable and the disease had progressed resulting in peritoneal, liver and pulmonary metastases. The patient was involved in a community-based palliative care programme and his wife was his informal carer.

The patient called the community palliative care team due to dyspnoea. He complained of some abdominal pressure and distension which was making him dyspnoeic. The pain was relatively well controlled with opiates and he was adamant he wanted to stay at home because he did not want to 'waste time' with people he did not know.

The GP palliative care physician performed a physical examination and found the patient to be tachypnoeic with abdominal distension. The clinician was not 100% confident this was ascites.

Differential diagnosis prior to POCUS included constipation, ileus, ascites, pleural effusion or pulmonary embolism. POCUS was undertaken examining the chest for effusions, heart for right ventricular dilatation and abdomen for ascites and bowel oedema.

Point-of-care ultrasound confirmed large quantities of ascites (Figure 10.1) causing dyspnoea, tachypnoea and discomfort.

Ultrasound (US) is not currently mandated for drainage of ascites but can be particularly useful to avoid inadvertent bowel wall or blood vessel puncture when inserting a drain. Gaseous or fluid distension of the bowel due to obstruction or ileus may simulate ascites clinically and POCUS can confirm the absence of ascites avoiding unnecessary blind taps.

Bedside US-guided abdominal paracentesis was performed within his own home. Long-term, indwelling peritoneal catheters, tunnelled or non-tunnelled, are good options to treat recurrent malignant ascites. It is beneficial symptomatically, avoids hazards of multiple repeated procedures and reduces treatment costs.

A differential here was acute or subacute bowel obstruction. Typically abdominal radiographs are the first-line diagnostic imaging modality. However US has a greater sensitivity and specificity for the diagnosis of small bowel obstruction. This has been described in detail in Chapter 4. Some of the features on US for small bowel obstruction are dilated fluid-filled bowel loops, a 'to-and-fro motion' known as pendulum peristalsis, the absence of peristalsis in paralytic ileus and prominent jejunal valvulae conniventes referred to as the 'keyboard sign' (Figure 10.2).

The patient required two further abdominal paracenteses over the course of the month and his dyspnoea was well managed. During his review, regular POCUS of his chest was undertaken where he was found to have developed clinically insignificant

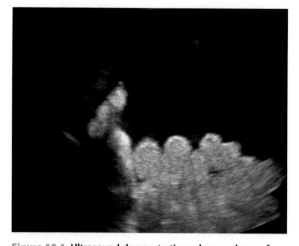

Figure 10.1 Ultrasound demonstrating a large volume of ascites with underlying bowel loops. *A video is available to view in the online video library.*

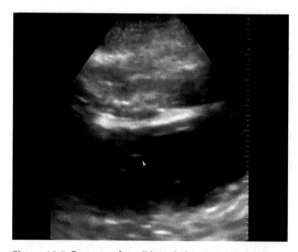

Figure 10.2 Features of small bowel obstruction include bowel dilatation (>2 cm), fluid-filled bowel with hyperechoic gas bubbles (arrow) and 'to-and-fro' or pendulum peristalsis. *A video is available to view in the online video library.*

pleural effusions. He died at home as he had wished, 5 months after his initial diagnosis, surrounded by his family.

Case – I Am Scared of Hospitals

A 37-year-old female was diagnosed two years previously with disseminated cervical carcinoma. The malignancy progressed rapidly despite treatment. She had developed metastases in her pelvic organs, peripheral lymph nodes and bones. She was under the care of the community-based palliative team and she had wished to spend as much time as possible with her husband and son. She had a fear of hospitals and refused to attend for any further tests.

She visited her GP complaining of unilateral lower limb swelling that had appeared 2 weeks previously. The pain in her leg was relatively well controlled, but she was complaining of fatigue and weight loss. In addition, she was dyspnoeic on minimal exertion. The GP performed a physical examination and noticed tachycardia, normal lung and heart examination but a significantly swollen left lower limb oedema from foot to thigh as well as bilateral indurated inguinal lymph nodes.

Differential diagnosis prior to POCUS was DVT causing a pulmonary embolism (PE) and possible peripheral lymphoedema. POCUS was undertaken examining the leg for a DVT or subcutaneous oedema and a focused echo to identify right heart dilatation.

A DVT was excluded (Figure 10.3) and her right heart size was normal. The US scan did confirm extensive subcutaneous oedema (Figure 10.4) of her left lower limb and the diagnosis of lymphoedema due to lymph node metastases was made. The GP commenced her on elastic compression for her lower limb.

Diffuse pain and unilateral limb swelling is a common occurrence in advanced malignancy. Causes include DVT, lymphoedema due to metastatic lymph nodes, cellulitis or generalised oedema due to poor nutrition or renal impairment.

In this patient a D-dimer would not be helpful in diagnosing DVT in view of her underlying cancer.

With elastic compression the lymphoedema became less pronounced and she had no related complications such as erysipelas and pain. The patient died two months later at home with her family. This case demonstrated how her symptoms were managed optimally and confidently whilst avoiding hospital visits.

Case – I Am not Ready until I See my Great-Granddaughter

A 91-year-old female who lived in a nursing home became gradually dyspnoeic and refused to engage with her fellow residents. She had a background of heart failure with severe inoperable aortic stenosis. She was mobile using a walker and was cognitively intact.

The nursing home GP reviewed her after concerns were raised about her respiratory deterioration. The patient stated 'I know my heart is very weak and this cannot be changed, but I have a granddaughter who is pregnant with a girl. I have four great-grandsons,

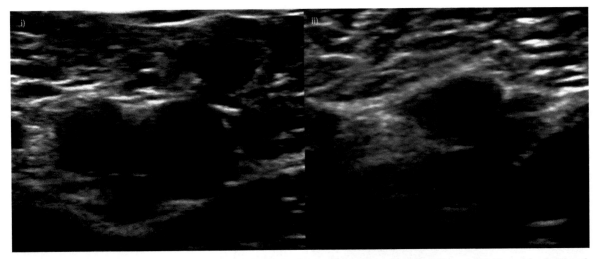

Figure 10.3 Compression ultrasound performed at the levels of the saphenofemoral junction (i), superficial femoral vein (ii) and popliteal vein (not displayed here).

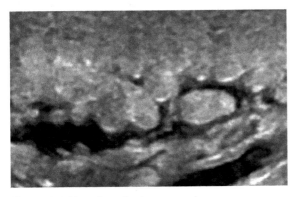

Figure 10.4 Extensive subcutaneous oedema.

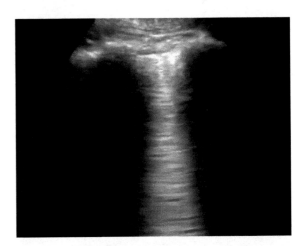

Figure 10.5 B line lung profile is consistent with the suspected diagnosis of pulmonary oedema secondary to heart failure.

but I would like to live long enough to see a great-granddaughter'.

The GP carried out POCUS focusing on the suspicion of decompensated congestive heart failure and a possible pleural effusion.

Point-of-care ultrasound did demonstrate features of heart failure with the lung scan showing B lines (Figure 10.5) and bilateral pleural effusions.

The focused echo showed severe systolic dysfunction with a dilated left ventricle (LV) with a heavily calcified aortic valve (Figure 10.6).

The patient's diuretic therapy was increased and she received close monitoring of fluid intake/output and weight. The GP attempted to identify different precipitants for decompensation including infection, exertion and diuretic non-compliance but no

additional cause was found. Following the up-titration of diuretics and regular review her symptoms improved and she managed to see her great-granddaughter before she passed away.

This case illustrates how palliation should not just be focused around cancer patients but all chronic conditions including end stage heart failure, chronic obstructive pulmonary disease (COPD), liver and renal failure.

Case – Withdrawing Medical Care

A 78-year-old female smoker with hypertension, diabetes and COPD presented to the ED with features of septic shock. Baseline exercise tolerance was 50 metres and she used a mobility scooter daily. She had been unwell for several weeks with fevers, dyspnoea and a cough productive of green sputum. Her GP had prescribed a course of antibiotics and prednisolone with little improvement. On arrival to ED she was hypotensive, tachycardic, tachypnoeic and required 15 litres of oxygen to maintain saturations of 92%. Her level of consciousness was scored as 14 on the Glasgow Coma Scale (GCS).

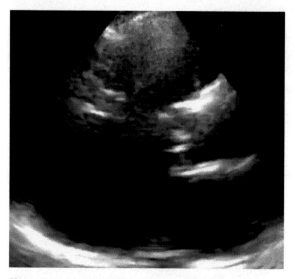

Figure 10.6 Limited quality parasternal long-axis view showing calcified aortic valve and severely impaired left ventricular systolic function. *A video is available to view in the online video library.*

Her chest X-ray confirmed extensive right-sided consolidation and blood results revealed an acute kidney injury (AKI), a C-reactive protein (CRP) of 350 mg/L, a white cell count (WCC) of 28×10^9/L and a lactate of 9mmol/L with a significant metabolic acidosis. The patient was diagnosed with septic shock and treated with fluid resuscitation and IV antibiotics. After 2 hours of aggressive treatment she was reviewed and had unfortunately deteriorated further. Her GCS was now 11 and she was becoming fluid overloaded. She was peripherally shut down with mottled skin and remained anuric with a lactate that had risen to 11 mmol/L.

A focused echo was undertaken which demonstrated a dilated LV with severe global LV dysfunction (Figure 10.7).

The patient had multi-organ failure and despite aggressive treatment there was no improvement. Her poor LV function made her a poor candidate for escalation of treatment including cardiovascular or renal support. The decision was made to switch to a symptomatic, comfort-focused approach as she was dying. The family were informed and involved in the decision-making process.

Assessment of cardiac function provided the clinician with valuable information and confidence in deciding the trajectory of care. The prognosis of multi-organ failure with poor cardiac reserve is grave. Making such decisions may be challenging and POCUS is an indispensable tool to guide front-line clinicians.

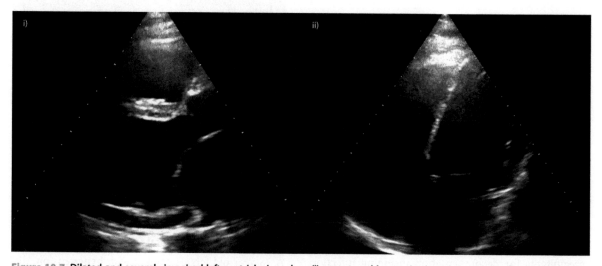

Figure 10.7 Dilated and severely impaired left ventricleviewed on (i) parasternal long-axis view view and (ii) off-axis apical four-chamber view. *Videos are available to view in the online video library.*

Summary

- Point-of-care ultrasound provides diagnostic confidence for all practitioners who care for palliative and end of life patients.
- It is critical in provision of distress relieving interventions including drains, nerve blocks and vascular access.
- Safe delivery of interventions within the patient's home negates the need for hospital transfer.
- Point-of-care ultrasound provides generalist clinicians with valuable information to guide escalation of care decisions.

A full list of references and further reading is available at www.GeneralistUltrasound.com

Ultrasound in Prehospital, Remote and Austere Environments

Introduction

The portability and versatility of ultrasound (US) makes it ideally suited to diagnostic imaging in remote settings. The falling prices and diminishing size of high-quality devices are increasing the availability of US to clinicians working outside of hospital environments. Generalist healthcare professionals with US experience now have advanced diagnostic capabilities in settings where they would previously be reliant upon clinical examination alone.

Ultrasound for the Generalist is designed to provide clinicians with the building blocks to use US in whatever healthcare setting, environment or level of acuity from the ED or ICU to a GP practice. US will never replace high resolution imaging modalities, such as CT and MRI, but their deployment is limited by the prohibitive initial expense and the advanced technical expertise required for use and maintenance. The portability, low power consumption and low cost of US makes it uniquely suited to remote, low resource and austere environments and will elevate the diagnostic capability of the individual clinicians (Figure 11.1).

This chapter will aim to provide the reader with examples of how the techniques described in previous chapters may be applied to these low-resource settings. The key areas considered include:

- Prehospital Emergency Medicine and Transfer Medicine
- Remote, Wilderness and Austere Medicine
- Military Medicine
- Humanitarian and Post Disaster Medicine

Prehospital Emergency Medicine and Transfer Medicine

Prehospital ultrasound (PHUS) is becoming increasingly used to provide advanced clinical assessment within prehospital teams. The potential benefit is amplified in remote regions where long travel times may mandate therapeutic interventions prior to departure or arrival at regional centres. It has been successfully deployed within helicopters and fixed-wing aircraft where conventional examination techniques, such as auscultation, are technically challenging.

Early adopters focused on the use of PHUS within trauma by performing serial focused assessment with sonography in trauma (FAST) scans during transportation of patients to trauma centres. The identification of abdominal free fluid could alert the receiving team of probable significant intra-abdominal pathology to facilitate early mobilisation of operative teams. Modern Prehospital Emergency Medicine (PHEM) teams are delivering increasingly complex clinical interventions at the roadside, such as extracorporeal membrane oxygenation (ECMO) and resuscitative endovascular balloon occlusion of the aorta (REBOA), where the use of US can vastly improve the speed and accuracy of vascular access.

Potential applications for PHUS will be discussed here. The technique for performing each individual assessment is considered in the relevant chapters.

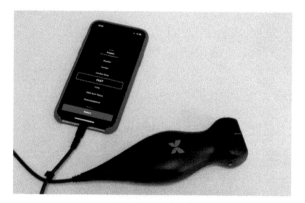

Figure 11.1 The Butterfly iQ is an example of an 'all-in-one' ultrasound probe. Other examples of portable US probes include: Philips Lumify, EchoNous Kosmos, GE Vscan, Sonosite iViz, Clarius C3 and the Healcerion Sonon.

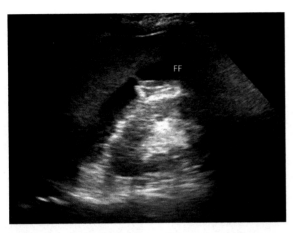

Figure 11.2 Focused assessment with sonography in trauma scan with free fluid (FF) seen in Morison's Pouch.

Trauma

Although the role of FAST has largely been superseded by CT within trauma centres, when performed by PHEM practitioners it may provide valuable information to guide triage, patient management and destination hospital.

Performing extended FAST (e-FAST) has been demonstrated to be feasible during rotary and fixed-wing transport without extending the transport time in even the shortest of journeys. It has been suggested to change the prehospital management of patients in 30%, and hospital management in 22% of cases and therefore may prove to be of value in the triage of major trauma patients. Furthermore, identification of multisystem injury may provide justification for the PHEM team to redirect to a major trauma centre. Figure 11.2 shows a positive FAST scan with free fluid in Morison's Pouch.

The real value of prehospital e-FAST is in delivery of *serial imaging* during prolonged transportation. All imaging modalities provide a snapshot at the time of assessment and, through repetition, the sensitivity of the study will increase. As time elapses the likelihood of blood being visualised increases and a negative initial study does not necessarily exclude major visceral injury.

Key regions that should be assessed during an e-FAST include:

- Abdomen – this should be assessed in the right upper quadrant (RUQ), left upper quadrant (LUQ) and pelvic views.

- Pericardium – the subcostal view is commonly used to achieve this although the parasternal or apical views are also suitable. Haemopericardium is a potentially reversible cause of traumatic cardiac arrest and early identification is essential.
- Lung bases – by sliding the probe superiorly from the RUQ and LUQ views the diaphragm and lung bases may be visualised. In the setting of trauma, any fluid in this region should be considered to be a haemothorax.
- Anterior lung fields – in the supine patient any traumatic pneumothorax will be visible in the upper anterior lung zones. The absence of pleural sliding is suggestive of a pneumothorax.

Any key finding during transportation can be alerted to the receiving team to allow planning of urgent interventions or mobilisation of the operative teams if the patient is clinically unstable. A trauma CT should still be performed upon arrival if patient stability allows due to the complex nature of polytrauma and the need to accurately characterise injuries.

Thoracic Ultrasound

We have already considered the possibility of pneumothorax and haemothorax in patients who have sustained major trauma. These are key findings that can transform patient management. In unpressurised aeromedical transportation the risk of a pneumothorax expanding and causing tension physiology is increased due to falling pressure causing gas volume to expand (Boyle's Law). Identifying pneumothoraces early, prior to patient deterioration, is extremely valuable and can guide the PHEM practitioners to perform needle decompression or thoracostomy. Additionally, the *presence* of pleural sliding can reduce the need for unnecessary decompression in patients without pneumothoraces (Figure 11.3).

Other causes of acute dyspnoea may be identified using lung ultrasound (LUS) including pneumonia or pulmonary oedema. Although these have been described in the prehospital setting, they are less likely to require urgent intervention and have not been frequently reported within the literature.

Many prehospital services deployed LUS during the COVID-19 pandemic to triage patients who may require hospital transfer and admission. It is not clear whether this affected overall outcome but acted as an additional tool to guide patient management during a time when services were stretched.

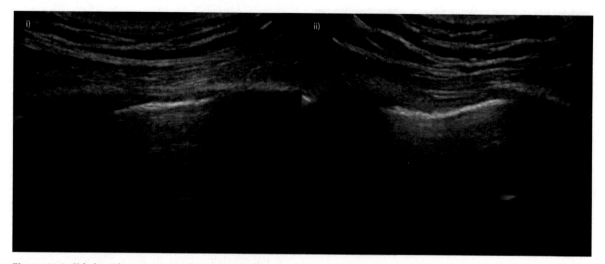

Figure 11.3 **Side-by-side comparison of (i) pleural sliding versus (ii) absence of pleural sliding.** This can only be visualised if viewing the online material. *Videos are available to view in the online video library.*

Confirming Endotracheal Intubation

The gold standard for confirming endotracheal tube (ETT) placement is with end tidal capnography (EtCO2) to detect expiratory CO_2. This is achievable in most modern PHEM services. However, the presence of EtCO2 does not distinguish between endotracheal and endobronchial intubation and auscultation to confirm bilateral air entry is often challenging within prehospital settings due to excessive ambient noise. This may lead to significant hypoxia and diagnostic uncertainty. Confirming bilateral pleural sliding will reassure the clinician that the ETT is sited in an acceptable location to ventilate both lungs.

Using pleural sliding for two separate applications, diagnosing pneumothoraces and confirming ETT position, may cause confusion and uncertainty. As with any examination or investigation the sensitivity and specificity are guided by the pre-test probability. Many major trauma services will perform bilateral finger thoracostomies as a routine intervention at the roadside and therefore, unless they lose patency and require re-fingering, a significant sized or tension pneumothorax is improbable. Furthermore, the transportation of unwell patients is not isolated to trauma and the displacement of ETTs or spontaneous pneumothoraces are possible during any high-risk transfer.

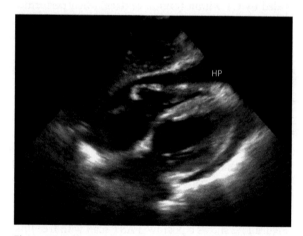

Figure 11.4 **Haemopericardium (HP) visualised on the subcostal view in a patient following major trauma.**

Cardiac Arrest

The use of prehospital echocardiography in cardiac arrest is essential to identify cardiac tamponade (Figure 11.4) and can reliably distinguish between cardiac activity and standstill which can be used as a marker of prognosis. This is described in more detail in the Chapter 2.

Vascular and Procedural Ultrasound

Intraosseous access has become commonplace within prehospital teams to deliver parenteral medication. In more controlled environments, US may be used to aid successful intravenous cannulation but this is less likely to be required in the acute setting.

A new area of work by prehospital services is the introduction of extracorporeal life support in the form of percutaneous venoarterial extracorporal membrane oxygenation (VA-ECMO). Furthermore, prehospital REBOA has been described in patients with severe pelvic trauma to reduce the risk of haemorrhagic shock. These are extremely specialised services and interventions that rely on highly trained staff to perform vascular access using ultrasound at the roadside.

Early Pregnancy Complications

In patients with suspected early pregnancy complications, such as ruptured ectopic pregnancy, the identification of free abdominal fluid highlights patients who are at risk of deterioration. A similar technique to 'FAST' may be used to identify the regions where fluid is most likely to accumulate. This is described in more detail in Chapters 4 and 8.

Remote, Wilderness and Austere Medicine

Since the 1980s, the demographic of visitors travelling to remote environments has changed from predominantly young, fit and healthy individuals to an increasing number of older visitors with medical comorbidities reflective of their age.

Medics in remote and austere environments are faced with significant clinical, logistical and resource challenges. They must diagnose and manage patients within potentially extreme environments with long and complex evacuation processes. The available resources are a fraction of what is found in most hospitals and many rely on basic history and examination for diagnosis whilst subjected to adverse conditions. These challenges are more manageable with the use of US for advanced diagnostics, severity assessment and to provide therapeutic management of pain. This can focus the initial management, guide appropriate logistical decision-making and justify a potentially high-cost evacuation to a destination suited to the patient's needs.

Wilderness medical providers must carry much of the equipment required to deliver medical care for their team. The development of cheaper, smaller, lighter and more portable devices with image quality capable of advanced diagnostics has made US a uniquely useful tool for experienced practitioners.

Ultrasound has been adopted in expedition and wilderness medicine for many applications. Musculoskeletal injuries form a large proportion of the healthcare needs on expeditions and US can diagnose pathology such as long bone fractures, joint dislocations, joint effusions and tendon ruptures. It is used for triage and destination planning for trauma patients using e-FAST, differentiating between causes of dyspnoea using LUS and echo and for identification of ophthalmic pathology including retinal detachment, globe rupture and vitreal haemorrhage.

Although all techniques described in this book may be applied within remote settings, there are some additional findings that may be unique to particular environments. These will be discussed below.

Respiratory

Acute dyspnoea is a presentation with a vast differential diagnosis. LUS can quickly and accurately identify pathology and, when combined with history, examination and multisystem POCUS, the diagnosis is often clear.

In high altitude settings dyspnoea is a common symptom due to a reduced partial pressure of oxygen leading to hypoxia. This causes the release of *hypoxia-inducible factor* to promote many physiological adaptations known as *acclimatisation* including:

- Hyperventilation – to increase alveolar oxygen partial pressure.
- Renal adaptation – hyperventilation is limited by the development of alkalaemia due to reduction in the arterial partial pressure of carbon dioxide. Renal excretion of bicarbonate normalises the pH and allows further hyperventilation.
- Tachycardia – to increase cardiac output and therefore tissue perfusion and oxygen delivery.
- Erythropoeisis – increasing the number of red blood cells and haemoglobin concentration to optimise tissue delivery of oxygen.

Altitude-related illnesses are a consequence of these adaptations and include high altitude headache, acute mountain sickness (AMS), high altitude cerebral oedema (HACE) and high altitude pulmonary oedema (HAPE).

High Altitude Pulmonary Oedema

High altitude pulmonary oedema is an uncommon but serious complication of altitude. It is characterised by tachycardia, dyspnoea, crackles/wheeze, cough, reduced exercise tolerance and fatigue. Risk factors include rapid ascent of altitude, pulmonary hypertension, congestive cardiac failure, COPD, exaggerated hypoxic pulmonary vasoconstrictor response, excessive physical exercise, cold weather and respiratory tract infection.

Lung ultrasound findings in HAPE are consistent with other types of pulmonary oedema causing B lines or comet tails. As severity of HAPE increases, LUS demonstrates an increased number of B lines with coalescing (Figure 11.5).

Recent evidence suggests that even subclinical pulmonary oedema may be recognised in asymptomatic patients by the identification of a B-type lung pattern. This may be used to identify individuals at risk of developing worsening HAPE with increasing altitude although more research is required to confirm this.

Lung ultrasound is a key tool to diagnose HAPE in individuals at altitude in whom dyspnoea is a common and expected symptom. Furthermore, it can aid in the differentiation between HAPE and other respiratory illnesses such as pneumonia, pneumothorax and pulmonary embolism.

Pulmonary Hypertension

Altitude is associated with exaggerated hypoxic pulmonary vasoconstriction leading to raised pulmonary vascular resistance and pulmonary artery pressure.

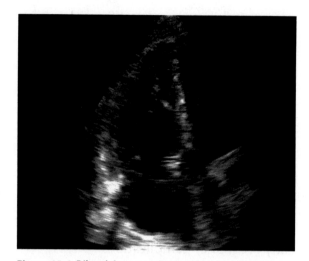

Figure 11.6 Dilated, hypertrophied and impaired RV in a patient with longstanding pulmonary hypertension and cor pulmonale. *A video is available to view in the online video library.*

High altitude pulmonary hypertension (HAPH) is a specific condition seen in high-altitude dwellers and can lead to reduced exercise capacity and eventual morbidity and mortality from right-sided heart failure.

Echocardiography may be used to assess the severity of pulmonary hypertension and identify remodelling of the right heart. Furthermore, acute right heart failure may be seen in patients with pre-existing pulmonary hypertension who ascend to altitude. Figure 11.6 shows a four-chamber view with a dilated, hypertrophied and impaired right ventricle (RV) in a patient with pulmonary hypertension and cor pulmonale.

Neurology

Research into the pathophysiology of AMS and HACE has focused on the use of optic nerve sheath diameter (ONSD) as a surrogate of intracranial pressure. This method is described in more detail in Chapter 7.

Acute Mountain Sickness and High Altitude Cerebral Oedema

Acute mountain sickness (AMS) is the most common altitude-related illness and is characterised by headache, poor appetite, fatigue and dizziness. It usually occurs in unacclimatised individuals ascending beyond 2500 m although has been reported in susceptible people at much lower altitudes. Risk factors include rate of ascent, altitude reached and pre-existing risk

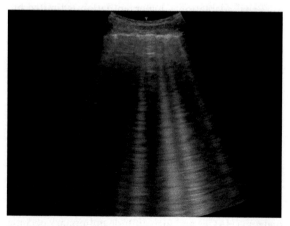

Figure 11.5 B line pattern in high altitude pulmonary oedema. *A video is available to view in the online video library.*

factors. Severity is measured using a recognised scoring tool known as the 'Lake Louise Score'.

In contrast, HACE is a medical emergency presenting with a change in mental status, hallucinations, headache, papilloedema, tachycardia, tachypnoea and can lead to seizures, coma and death. It is most common in individuals with pre-existing AMS or HAPE. It is thought to be a consequence of the autoregulatory processes to maintain cerebral perfusion and oxygenation during acclimatisation.

Optic nerve sheath diameter (ONSD) has been shown to correlate accurately with the severity of AMS as measured by the Lake Louise Score (Figure 11.7). One study demonstrated a mean ONSD of 5.34 mm in individuals with AMS compared with 4.46 mm in those without. Raised ONSD is also seen in people with evidence of HAPE on LUS demonstrating how the spectrum of altitude illnesses are intrinsically linked. ONSD has not been extensively studied for the diagnosis of HACE and, although theoretically useful, should not replace clinical history and examination.

Optic nerve sheath diameter may be used to recognise alternative causes of raised intracranial pressure such as traumatic brain injury or intracranial haemorrhage. In settings with limited resources, where the differential diagnosis for reduced level of consciousness is vast, US may be of value in cases of diagnostic uncertainty.

Transcranial Doppler (TCD) is a tool that has been used extensively in hospital settings. This technique is described in Chapter 7. TCD of the middle cerebral artery (MCA) has been deployed as part of research expeditions to measure the effect of altitude on intracranial blood flow. It has also been proposed to be a useful tool for the identification of MCA ischaemic stroke in the prehospital setting and may recognise absence of flow prior to any ischaemic features being present on CT imaging.

Transcranial Doppler was successfully used to diagnose a left MCA infarct at 5900 m on Cho Oyu in Tibet. The medical team were contacted due to a previously fit and healthy 49-year-old collapsing whilst at rest. The predominant concern was of HACE due to reduced level of consciousness. He was noted to have reduced airway protective reflexes, dysphasia, a dense right hemiparesis and right-sided neglect. Bilateral TCD was performed showing good flow in the right MCA but absent flow in the left suggestive of an ischaemic stroke. He was treated with aspirin and continuous TCD was maintained prior to evacuation due to the theoretical benefit of improved thrombolysis.

In this case, US enabled rapid identification of the causative pathology in an environment where diagnosis is challenging.

Vascular

The risk of venous thrombosis is increased in remote environments due to numerous risk factors such as cold weather, dehydration, prolonged immobility in tents owing to adverse weather conditions and long transportation times. DVT scanning is quick, simple and feasible in remote environments and is described in detail in Chapter 5 (Figure 11.8).

Venous thromboembolism is a potentially life-threatening cause of acute dyspnoea. The use of focused

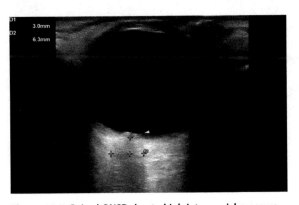

Figure 11.7 Raised ONSD due to high intracranial pressure and papilloedema. Note the bulging optic disc (arrow) which is another feature of papilloedema.

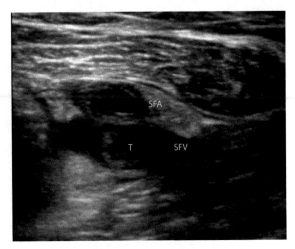

Figure 11.8 Thrombus (T) in the superficial femoral vein. SFV, superficial femoral vein; SFA, superficial femoral artery.

echo in patients with suspected pulmonary embolism may identify right heart dilatation and failure. This technique is described in Chapter 2.

Venous US and echocardiography have been used to detect venous gas emboli (VGE) in divers to assess post-dive decompression stress. With ascent from depth, a reduction in pressure causes dissolved nitrogen particles to be released as gas bubbles in blood vessels and tissues which can cause flow occlusion in tissues. This causes 'decompression sickness' (DCS) or 'the bends'. The symptoms of decompression sickness are extremely varied and range from mild joint discomfort and fatigue to severe neurological and respiratory injury.

Echocardiography has been used following ascent from depth to quantify the decompression VGE by acquiring a modified A4C view of the right heart. The number of bubbles visible in the right ventricle and right atrium in a single frame in mid-diastole may be counted and correlates with the risk of DCS (Figure 11.9)

Musculoskeletal Injury and Peripheral Nerve Blockade

Musculoskeletal injury is the most common cause of patients requiring medical assistance in remote settings. Conventional methods of confirming diagnosis, such as X-ray and CT, are frequently unavailable and portable US may be a suitable alternative for medical providers. Diagnosis of basic injuries is described in more detail in Chapter 6 which discusses musculoskeletal ultrasound.

Peripheral nerve blockade is a highly valuable tool to provide long-lasting, opiate-sparing analgesia to patients who have sustained significant injuries. US-guided regional anaesthesia (UGRA) is becoming widely accepted as the safest method for delivering peripheral nerve blockade and increases likelihood of successful pain relief. Femoral and fascia iliaca nerve blocks are excellent for femoral shaft and neck of femur fractures, median nerve blocks for hand and finger injuries and transversus abdominis plane (TAP) blocks provide good pain relief for the abdominal wall.

Ultrasound-guided regional anaesthesia is a dedicated skill that requires knowledge and expertise. We recommend only appropriately trained practitioners who use UGRA as part of their daily practice should use it in remote settings.

Foreign Body

Foreign bodies are readily visible with US which can directly localise the region to attempt removal. This is discussed in Chapter 6.

Tropical Diseases

In tropical remote settings US may often be the only diagnostic tool available to clinicians. Common US techniques may reveal findings that, in the correct

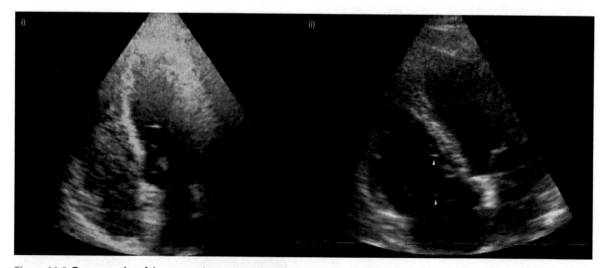

Figure 11.9 Two examples of decompression venous gas emboli (VGE) seen in the right heart following ascent from dive. (i) Large number of VGE that fill the RA and RV. The chroma setting on (ii) is used to aid identification of bubbles when few are present (arrows). Images kindly provided by Prof. Costantino Balestra, Prof. Murat Egi and Dr. Burak Parlak.

environment, may be interpreted as specific tropical diseases. US has been reported to be useful in the diagnosis of many infections including, but not limited to, amoebic liver abscesses, echinococcosis, ascariasis, schistosomiasis and dengue fever.

Furthermore, in sub-Saharan Africa, a resurgence of extra-pulmonary tuberculosis (TB) due to HIV co-infection has led to the development of a dedicated US protocol named the focused assessment with sonography for HIV-associated tuberculosis (FASH). This protocol aims to identify extra-pulmonary features such as pericardial or pleural effusion and signs of abdominal TB including retroperitoneal and mesenteric lymphadenopathy, hypoechoic splenic nodules and ascites.

These are non-specific clinical findings that will require accurate clinical correlation and experience to gauge significance.

Case – A Diagnostic Dilemma at the South Pole

During mid-summer at the South Pole there are 24 hours of sunshine with a temperature of −40 degrees Celsius and extremely high winds. The medical provider was accompanying an overnight expedition group to a South Pole camp where a couple were planning to get married (Figure 11.10).

During wedding preparation, the team were informed of a medical evacuation (medevac) for clients undertaking a *last degree*. A South Pole last degree is an expedition where participants are flown from base camp at Union Glacier which is 660 m above sea level to a latitude of 89 degrees south and 2800 m altitude. They then ski from 89 degrees to 90 degrees south which is an equivalent of 60 nautical miles or 110 km. Due to the low barometric pressure of the Antarctic Plateau, an altitude of 2800 m equates to a physiological altitude of 3400 m. This increases the risk of developing symptoms of AMS and cases of HAPE have been reported.

In response to the medevac call the medical team boarded the DC3 aircraft and flew out over the wind swept, sastrugi-filled ice cap of Antarctica (Figure 11.11). The expeditioners were found and taken back to the base camp. Initial assessment revealed that the patient was acutely unwell with severe dysnpoea and only able to speak in single

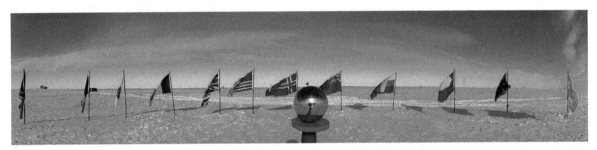

Figure 11.10 **The ceremonial South Pole.**

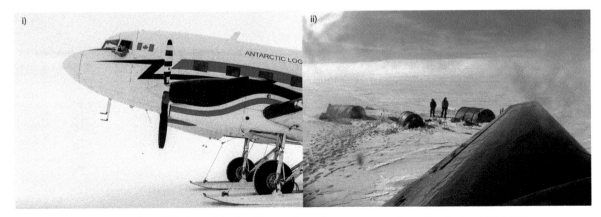

Figure 11.11 **(i) DC3 aircraft and (ii) view of the Last Degree Group temporary camp from the window of the DC3.**

words. Observations demonstrated a temperature of 37.8°C, heart rate 104, respiratory rate 32 and oxygen saturations of only 79%. After initial assessment, the working diagnosis was pneumonia with a differential diagnosis including HAPE and PE. His oxygen saturation improved to 96% on 3 L oxygen via nasal cannulae with an improvement in dyspnoea. The major challenge in this case was differentiating between causes of dyspnoea and logistical planning. If a diagnosis of HAPE was suspected, he would require emergent evacuation to a lower altitude.

The altitude at the South Pole is due to a giant ice cap covering the continent which is around 2.5 km thick at 90 degrees south. Unlike descent in an alpine environment, descending to a lower altitude from the South Pole requires hundreds of kilometres to be travelled and therefore a flight is required. The next scheduled flight out was the following day for the wedding party. There was not an option of two flights and they were keen to stay to celebrate at 90 degrees south. If medevac was required then the entire wedding party would need to be on the plane. The key question was whether the patient had HAPE and whether the medical practitioner had the resources to manage him at the South Pole (Figure 11.12 and Figure 11.13).

Ultrasound was used to evaluate the patient's lungs, heart and vasculature to look for DVT. LUS revealed no evidence of B lines that would indicate the presence of HAPE (Figure 11.14i). Furthermore, pleural sliding was present excluding a pneumothorax. Echocardiography demonstrated no features of raised right ventricular pressure and, although this does not exclude a PE, it reduced the likelihood of a large clot (Figure 11.14ii).

There was also no evidence of a DVT (Figure 11.15).

The patient was medically managed overnight at the South Pole with a working diagnosis of a lower respiratory tract infection. The following day the wedding party and medevac expeditioners were flown back to base camp.

Case – Diagnostic and Therapeutic Advantage of Ultrasound in Remote Locations

A 64-year-old female slipped whilst skiing on an icy slope 4 km from base camp on Union Glacier in Antarctica. She had severe hip pain and was unable to mobilise. The medic and field guides packaged and then transported her to the medical unit in camp. Clinically she had an isolated left neck of femur fracture with a shortened, externally rotated leg (Figure 11.16).

A medevac was initiated immediately but would be delayed due to mandatory crew stand-down time.

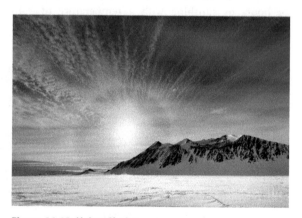

Figure 11.13 **Union Glacier.**

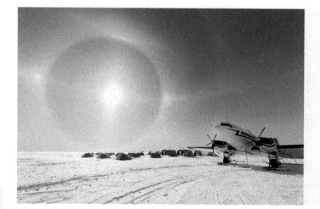

Figure 11.12 **The South Pole camp.**

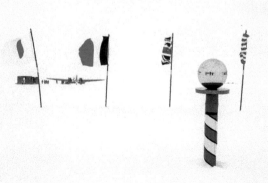

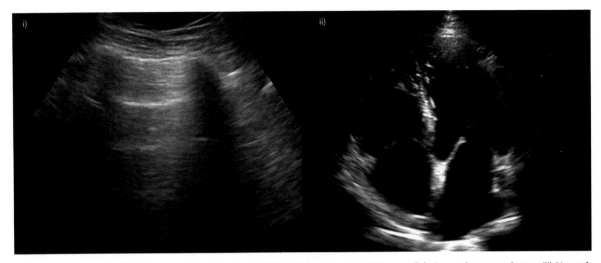

Figure 11.14 (i) Normal lung appearance with pleural sliding. This excludes HAPE, consolidation and pneumothorax. (ii) Normal A4C view of the heart with no RV dilatation. This makes a significant sized pulmonary embolism very unlikely.

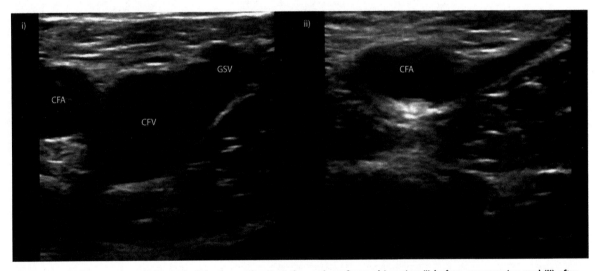

Figure 11.15 Compression ultrasound of the femoral vein at the saphenofemoral junction (i) before compression and (ii) after compression revealing no evidence of DVT. CFV, common femoral vein; CFA, common femoral artery; GSV, great saphenous vein.

US of her left hip confirmed the diagnosis of a fractured neck of femur (Figure 11.17).

An US-guided femoral nerve block was performed and provided excellent pain control which improved the patient's ability to tolerate the evacuation from Union Glacier to Punta Arenas, Chile (Figure 11.18).

Case – A Needle in a Hay Stack in the Jungle

Expeditions in the Amazon jungle are remote, hot and sweaty and retrieval is challenging (Figure 11.19). The role of the medical provider is to keep the team safe and attempt to manage medical issues in the field whilst keeping the team members mobile.

One team member stepped onto a thorny branch and it penetrated his foot through a hole in his shoe into the plantar aspect of his foot. He attempted to remove the thorn but only the superficial segment was retrieved. A 3 cm foreign body was confirmed to be in situ via US (Figure 11.20) and a posterior tibial nerve block was applied to allow exploration of the area.

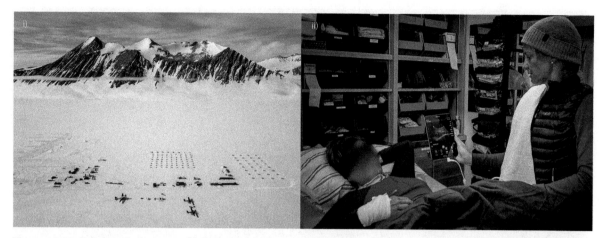

Figure 11.16 (i) Union Glacier camp with heated medical unit. (ii) Diagnosing neck of femur fracture using the Philips Lumify.

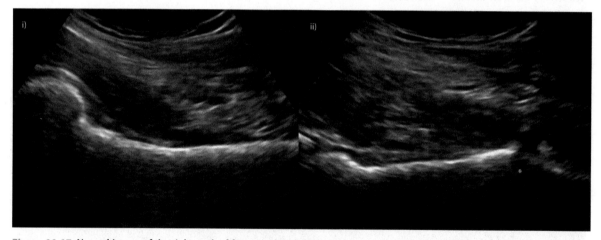

Figure 11.17 Normal image of the right neck of femur and (ii) left neck of femur with cortical discontinuity indicating a fracture.

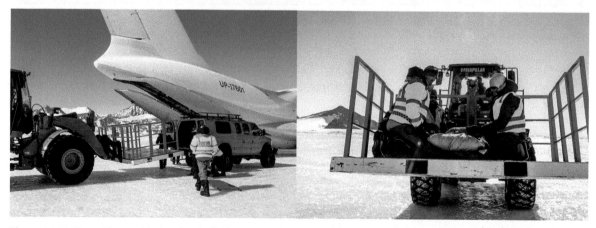

Figure 11.18 Femoral nerve block provided sufficient analgesia for transfer of the patient to the Ilyushin aircraft for evacuation.

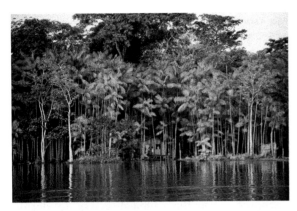

Figure 11.19 **The Amazon river.**

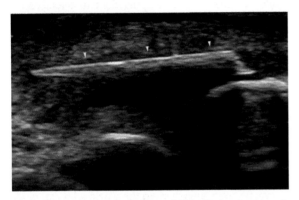

Figure 11.20 **Foreign body (arrows) identified and retrieved using US guidance.**

Using US-guidance and a needle location technique the foreign body was removed with minimal tissue damage. The team member was able to continue with minimal disruption to the expedition.

Equipment Maintenance and General Considerations

The use of unproven electronic equipment within austere, harsh environments will have inevitable difficulties. As with any medical expedition planning, thorough preparation is required to ensure these difficulties have been anticipated. Although not a comprehensive list of potential problems, the following text will provide an example of encountered issues within remote environments.

Cold Temperature

Any battery-operated equipment will face reduced performance in significantly cold temperatures. At the South Pole, where temperatures are on average −30 to −50 degrees Celsius, this reduction in battery life is significant. A potential solution for this environment is to keep the tablet, which for many portable US devices such as the Philips Lumify is the battery source, underneath the middle layers of clothing. If the US probe also contains a battery source, for example the Butterfly iQ, this should also be kept in a warm place. Hand warmers can be kept within carry cases as a contingency plan if this is not possible.

On any expedition a system of charging necessary items needs to be developed. This is determined by the length of the expedition, type of expedition and the equipment required. In certain environments, such as Antarctica in the summer, 24 hours of sunshine allow solar charging almost all the time. Backup generators are also available if this system should fail. Solar panels are increasingly reliable and affordable and are becoming essential carry items on most expeditions.

Extreme cold weather can freeze the piezoelectric crystal elements of the probe. Although this does not appear to affect the integrity of the crystals, they require rewarming (e.g. in warm water) prior to use. Some modern probes use solid-state technology rather than individual crystals that are less susceptible to freezing.

The probe cords have a tendency to become extremely stiff and brittle in cold weather. This may increase the risk of cords breaking. Basic battery saving measures, such as keeping the probe in a heated tent or medical unit, inside sleeping bags with a hot water bottle or within inner layers of clothes, will also reduce the risk of crystals freezing or cords breaking.

Ultrasound necessitates the use of gel to allow transmission of sound waves into the body. As this gel is water-based the freezing point is at 0 degrees Celsius. Strategies to prevent the gel from freezing are essential to allow the device to function when required.

Exposing patients to the extreme cold to assess with US has the potential to cause or worsen hypothermia. Robust planning is required to develop a process for performing US in the field. In Antarctica, all patients were retrieved from the field and assessed in a heated medical unit (insulated, heated wooden construction or heated tent). Medical and research teams at altitude tend to perform US within heated tents at set camp locations. Whatever the process, careful planning prior to departure is essential to ensure the safety of the team.

Ambient Light

Excessive ambient lighting may impact the user's ability to optimise and interpret the US images. Inevitably, the situations where US is required are unlikely to have optimal lighting. Certain environments, such as alpine or polar regions, will have extremely high ambient lighting and strategies for optimising imaging conditions should be developed. In the case of US being performed on the summit of Denali, the users were required to cover themselves with multiple layers of sleeping bags in order to permit visualisation of the US screen.

Hot, Wet, and Humid Weather

Moisture within any humid conditions, such as the jungle, is extremely problematic for all equipment. Using waterproof covers for tablets and for probe storage is essential. The probe itself tends not to be affected by moisture but should be used under a shelter and out of direct rain.

Training and Quality Assurance

Delivery of medical care within remote environments must be performed by individuals with appropriate clinical experience and not beyond their regular scope of practice. US is no different and requires a period of training, adequate supervision and accreditation prior to integration into patient care. At present, there is no accreditation pathway aimed at US in prehospital or remote settings and clinicians must extrapolate knowledge from their base specialty. Users must not use US to infer diagnoses beyond their level of expertise.

Reporting scans, reliable anonymised storage and quality assurance are essential for applications of US in any environment.

Research

Ultrasound is proven to be a reliable and uniquely useful tool for researching the response of human physiology to extreme environments. This has been most notable within the field of altitude research where many techniques have been used including TCD, ONSD, B lines in pulmonary oedema, echocardiography, venous compression US and IVC calibre for fluid status. The limitations of training requirements and potential inter-user variability are frequently considered but have not been a barrier to the completion of research projects.

Furthermore, US has been deployed on the International Space Station where a non-physician was reported to have achieved normal FAST views in 5.5 minutes. These images were interpreted by an expert on Earth in real time with only a 2 second latency period.

With devices reducing in size and potential US applications developing this is a field that is likely to increase in popularity in the coming years.

Telemedicine

The delivery of healthcare in remote, rural environments is limited by the availability of resources, diagnostic capabilities, limited access to doctors and the lack of specialised medical professionals. Teleultrasound is a developing field in telemedicine aimed at providing diagnostic imaging services to regions lacking this expertise. As internet connection increases in speed and becomes more widespread, the potential benefit of real-time telemedicine is enormous for diagnosis, guiding procedures, remote expert opinion and healthcare education.

Online cloud-based storage networks for US images have been developed by multiple companies that have now been adapted to facilitate telemedicine. An example of this is the Butterfly iQ Teleguidance platform. This allows clinicians to remotely connect to practitioners anywhere in the world who can guide on how to scan and optimise images. This has the potential to be an excellent educational tool for resource-limited regions and offers a safety net for second opinions from expert clinicians.

To date, most teleultrasound research has focused on obstetric health and foetal medicine due to the immense global burden of preventable maternal death. US can aid in confirmation of pregnancy, monitor foetal growth and identify pregnancy-related complications such as ectopic pregnancy and placenta praevia.

The potential for teleultrasound in the management of acutely unwell patients, trauma, procedural guidance and diagnosis and monitoring in outpatient settings is enormous and will continue to develop with continuing technological advancements.

Military Medicine

Advances in healthcare are frequently associated with military operations. The recent war in Afghanistan provided the British Military with a wealth of clinical knowledge and experience in the management of major trauma casualties. Although formal training is in its infancy, POCUS within military medicine is an emerging field that can provide improved examination and diagnostics to clinicians throughout the Operational Patient Care Pathway.

In Camp Bastion, basic haemodynamic transthoracic echocardiography (TTE) for volume assessment following damage control resuscitation and surgery was performed upon arrival to critical care due to the absence of any deployed cardiac output monitoring. These patients were young and physically fit and therefore frequently maintained normal physiological parameters despite hypovolaemia. Many had already received high volume blood transfusions pre- and intraoperatively. Basic TTE, focusing on chamber size, stroke distance measurements and IVC calibre, revealed marked variation in the filling status and enabled targeted resuscitation to avoid subsequent haemodynamic instability and the deleterious effects of over resuscitation (Figure 11.21). TTE had the additional benefit of identifying potential complications of major blunt trauma or blast injuries including myocardial contusion and cardiac tamponade.

The British Military have identified US as a potentially invaluable tool for clinicians in a forward deployed setting leading to significant investment in portable devices. A pilot project has been developed, named Project Morpho, aimed at providing POCUS capabilities to General Practitioners and Special Forces personnel and is due to be implemented into formal training.

Historically, US has been reserved for use in Role 2 or Role 3 medical treatment facilities. Role 1 describes the delivery of primary care within a small unit. Role 2 facilities deliver triage, resuscitation, and basic treatment of patients in a larger unit level. US is available for use in these settings although there is no radiologist present and therefore any provision of US must be extrapolated from a clinician's regular practice. Role 3 describes the 'field hospital' level of facility and is capable of delivering advanced diagnostics with surgical and medical interventions prior to evacuation. A radiologist with US capability is based within Role 3 treatment facilities and was utilised to perform eFAST during the initial resuscitation phase. US was available for use within the Medical Emergency Response Team (MERT) helicopters although did not form part of any standard operating procedure.

The aim of Project Morpho is to extend the diagnostic potential of US to general medical providers within Role 1 medical treatment facilities. Rather than focus on specific organ systems, the aim of the curriculum is to answer specific questions:

- Is there raised intra-cranial pressure (ONSD)?
- Is there a pneumothorax?
- Is there free fluid in the pleural space?
- Is there free fluid in the peritoneal space?
- Is there critical hypovolaemia?

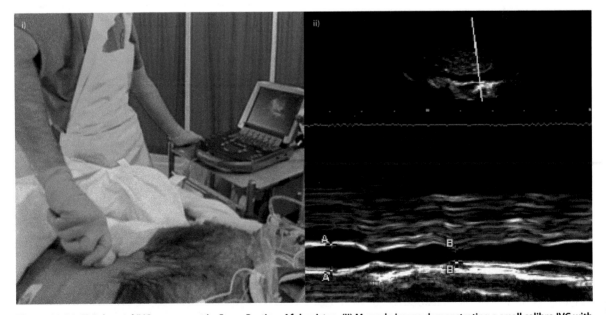

Figure 11.21 (i) Subcostal IVC assessment in Camp Bastion, Afghanistan. (ii) M-mode image demonstrating a small calibre IVC with respiratory variability in keeping with hypvolaemia. The British Military have identified US as a potentially invaluable tool for clinicians in a forward deployed setting leading to significant investment in portable devices. A pilot project has been developed, named Project Morpho, aimed at providing POCUS capabilities to general practitioners and Special Forces personnel and is due to be implemented into formal training.

- Is there pericardial fluid?
- Is there a rib/long bone/sternal fracture?
- Is there a foreign body/fluid collection?
- Is there a DVT?
- Can I cannulate a peripheral vein guided by ultrasound?

These questions have been specifically tailored to the scenarios the clinicians are exposed to. Special Forces personnel carry a limited supply of resuscitation fluid (including packed red cells and plasma) and hypertonic saline and therefore prioritising administration to patients with objective evidence of hypovolaemia or raised intracranial pressure allows for an efficient use of resources.

Clinicians are required to perform a minimum number of scans as part of the training pathway. Training US-naïve clinicians to perform diagnostic imaging of course leads to questions regarding quality assurance. The military have utilised the Butterfly iQ all-in-one device with the integrated cloud-based storage to allow remote supervision and imaging review.

If this pilot continues to be successful then the aim is to deploy a portable device to all Role 1 medical treatment facilities.

Humanitarian and Disaster Relief Medicine

One of the biggest challenges for all healthcare systems is the provision of equal access to advanced healthcare resources for all populations and communities. Many countries have a vast geographical landscape which isolates patients and limits access to healthcare services. This is particularly prevalent in patients from disadvantaged communities which further exacerbates the increased rates of morbidity and mortality. US can provide a solution to this with portable equipment enabling clinicians to aid these communities to provide critical diagnostics to the patient. This is a potentially cost-effective strategy for screening in resource-limited settings.

Education and training in these environments, either through humanitarian aid or teleultrasound, will help to develop the expertise within resource-poor settings which is an essential step in improving global health.

Natural or man-made disasters have the potential to render even the most developed of communities as resource poor. In 2011 the Japanese Great Northeast Earthquake and tsunami destroyed the local infrastructure, electrical grid and hospitals leaving portable

US devices as the only diagnostic imaging tools available. In Haiti, following the earthquake disaster of January 2010, a portable US device was deployed as part of the New Mexico Disaster Medical Assistance Team. This was used to aid in the assessment of hypotension, trauma, abdominal pain, dyspnoea, DVT and PE, fractures, abscess, foreign bodies and parasitic infections. It also became essential in the confirmation of pregnancy after pregnancy tests became unavailable. US was reported to have influenced management decisions in up to 70% of cases which highlights its value in these settings.

Numerous global humanitarian projects are using US to screen populations in low resource settings.

Cape Town in South Africa is an example of a community with enormous inequality of healthcare provision. Exclusive hotels, restaurants and shopping centres within the private Victoria and Albert Marina are only a few miles away from townships where poverty and illness is rife.

One project we have had the privilege to be involved in is with the British Society of Echocardiography (BSE) 'Echo in Africa' project (Figure 11.22). Since 2014 the BSE has partnered with SunHeart in Cape Town to deliver an echo programme within resource-poor settings in South Africa.

During that time over 200 volunteers have travelled to South Africa to offer vital skills to an underprivileged population (Figure 11.23). To date, almost 7500 children have been scanned and enabled detection of over 200 cases of previously unrecognised

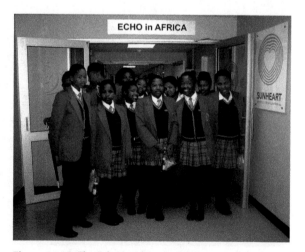

Figure 11.22 The Echo in Africa project is a partnership between SUNHeart in Cape Town, South Africa and the British Society of Echocardiography.

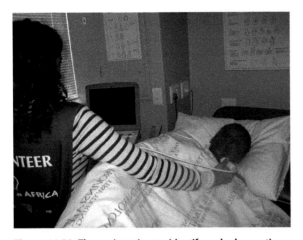

Figure 11.23 The project aims to identify early rheumatic heart disease. This project has also involved an education programme for the children which focuses upon public health awareness and how to access healthcare.

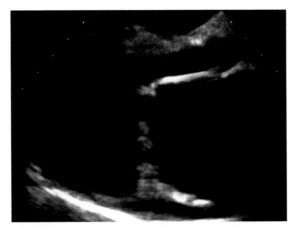

Figure 11.24 Typical features of rheumatic mitral valve disease including leaflet thickening, diastolic 'hockey stick' doming of the anterior mitral valve leaflet and left atrial dilatation. He was asymptomatic and had a further detailed scan which confirmed the diagnosis of early RHD. He was managed with antibiotic prophylaxis and had regular follow-up at the tertiary centre.

rheumatic heart disease (RHD) and a further 55 cases of congenital abnormalities. Handheld scanners were used within the townships and those with abnormal scans were brought to the tertiary hospital for detailed assessment.

Case – Echo Screening Saves Lives

A 13-year old boy was screened using a portable echo which revealed early changes of RHD. This included anterior and posterior MV leaflet thickening, excessive leaflet tip motion, diastolic doming known as a 'hockey stick appearance' and mild MV regurgitation. The AV was also involved showing focal thickening and anterior regurgitation (Figure 11.24).

Rheumatic heart disease is estimated to affect over 20 million people worldwide with the vast majority being in developing countries. Screening for RHD has been recommended by the World Health Organization (WHO) since 2004. A three- to ten-fold increase in prevalence of RHD has been detected by using portable echo when compared with the conventional method of auscultation.

Case – Incidental Important Findings on Ultrasound

A 14-year-old girl was scanned as part of the RHD screening project and had an incidental diagnosis of a bicuspid aortic valve (Figure 11.25).

Bicuspid aortic valves are the most common cause of congenital heart disease with a prevalence of one to two in 100 people. Over time, bicuspid AVs lead to aortic stenosis, aortic regurgitation and are associated with a higher incidence of aortic dissection. It is the

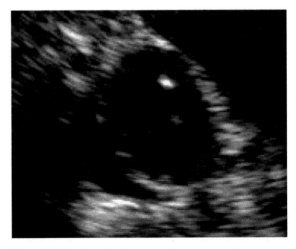

Figure 11.25 Bicuspid aortic valve seen in the parasternal short-axis view.

most common reason for patients under 60 years old to require an aortic valve replacement. Bicuspid AV should alert the clinician to consider other associated conditions including subacute bacterial endocarditis and coarctation of the aorta. As this is a congenital condition, close family members should also receive screening.

This humanitarian work is simply one example of how US has and will transform the lives of some of the least fortunate people by giving them access to prophylactic treatment, long-term management plans and the best chance of a good quality of life.

Summary

- Modern portable US machines can offer advanced diagnostic capabilities to people in low-resource settings.
- Ultrasound is increasingly being utilised in prehospital, transfer, remote and austere environments.

- Robust quality assurance measures are essential and clinicians should only perform US if part of their regular clinical practice.

A full list of references and further reading is available at www.GeneralistUltrasound.com

COVID-19 – A World Stage

During the writing of this book we were hit hard by the Coronavirus disease 2019 (COVID-19) pandemic and it is only appropriate to include a chapter describing how point-of-care ultrasound (POCUS) played a critical role in triage, diagnosis, management and prognostication. COVID-19 is a disease caused by the virus Severe Acute Respiratory Syndrome Coronavirus 2 (SARS-CoV-2) and has stretched healthcare systems beyond anything seen in our lifetimes. Interest and utilisation of POCUS has soared during the pandemic as increasing numbers of clinicians identified the role of lung ultrasound (LUS) in the diagnosis of COVID-19 within minutes without the need for further imaging. Increased accessibility to portable scanners led to the education and rapid upskilling of many clinicians.

Originating in Wuhan, China, the first cluster of cases were reported in December 2019. Cases exponentially increased and spread throughout the world to Europe, UK, USA and beyond (see Figure 12.1). The virulence of this disease led to lockdown in many countries, severely impacted economies and caused a high degree of morbidity and mortality. It is phenomenal news that we have several vaccines that have been developed and sanctioned by regulatory bodies across the world. These are currently being deployed and provide hope for many, however the impact of this deadly virus will stay with us for the rest of our careers.

COVID-19 is primarily a disease of the respiratory system presenting with symptoms of fever, dry cough and shortness of breath. Other recognised symptoms include anosmia, myalgia, diarrhoea and anorexia. However, what made this virus very challenging were the atypical presentations, particularly within the elderly population, with symptoms including confusion, being generally unwell and falls. Diabetes, hypertension, cardiovascular disease, older age and multisystem comorbidity are associated with a higher mortality rate. In addition, social deprivation and ethnic minorities were disproportionately affected as they were unable to social distance and continued to work in public-facing roles. Many healthcare workers have been affected, with at least 7000 global deaths directly attributed to COVID-19.

Blood results typically demonstrated a normal white cell count with lymphopenia and a high C-reactive protein (CRP). The higher CRP has been found to be associated with increased mortality. Chest X-ray (CXR) findings demonstrate bilateral infiltrates similar to that seen with historical acute respiratory distress syndrome (ARDS) (Figure 12.2). CT thorax commonly demonstrates ground glass opacities which can be bilateral, subpleural and peripheral. Other features include interlobar septal thickening, air space consolidation and traction bronchiectasis (Figure 12.2).

Frontline departments, particularly acute/general medicine and critical care were overwhelmed with attendances outstripping the hospital resources. Colleagues throughout the world applied POCUS as a tool for triage, diagnosis and to assess response to treatment.

We have already discussed in Chapter 3 that LUS is superior to CXR and studies suggest diagnostic accuracy may be comparable to CT imaging. With such a virulent disease, POCUS was exceptionally useful to avoid the unnecessary transfer of patients to radiology for X-ray and CT. Stethoscopes were of minimal use in COVID-19 and many departments advocated against auscultation for the protection of clinicians. For trained clinicians POCUS became the natural successor to auscultation – a step that many enthusiasts have recommended for years.

Key findings and progression of disease are easy to identify and prognostically important. They are summarised in Figure 12.3 (this poster is freely available on our website at *www.GeneralistUltrasound.com*).

We recommend a focused LUS and echo in all patients with suspected and confirmed COVID-19.

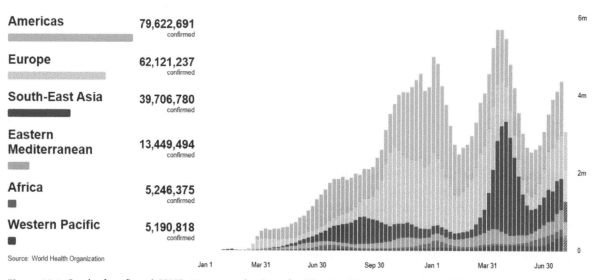

Americas 79,622,691
       confirmed

Europe   62,121,237
       confirmed

South-East Asia 39,706,780
       confirmed

Eastern
Mediterranean 13,449,494
       confirmed

Africa   5,246,375
       confirmed

Western Pacific 5,190,818
       confirmed

Source: World Health Organization

Figure 12.1 Graph of confirmed COVID-19 cases at the time of publication. Up-to-date graph available on the World Health Organization website. https://covid19.who.int/

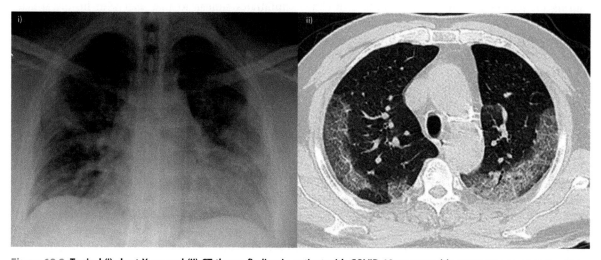

Figure 12.2 Typical (i) chest X-ray and (ii) CT thorax finding in patient with COVID-19 pneumonitis. COVID-19 causes bilateral multilobar ground glass opacification which tends to be peripheral and basal.

Method

Please refer to Chapters 3 and 4 for introduction to these techniques.

In supine patients, the technique for LUS is the same as that described in Chapter 4, by scanning the 'BLUE protocol' regions. It is important to note that COVID-19 results in patchy changes interspersed with normal lung and therefore a more comprehensive assessment for diagnosis may be required.

Due to the propensity for COVID-19 to affect the posterior lung regions, proning was incorporated into the management of both self-ventilating and intubated patients. Dependent regions of the lung receive a higher proportion of pulmonary blood flow due to the effect of gravity. Normal physiological adaptation is to preferentially ventilate dependent lung regions to optimise matching of ventilation and perfusion (V/Q). If pathology is affecting the function of dependent lung regions, then gas exchange is limited whilst still receiving a greater degree of blood

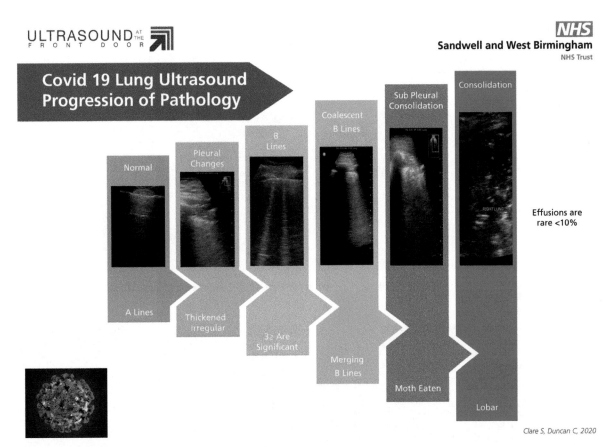

Figure 12.3 Progression of disease on lung ultrasound.

flow – leading to significant VQ mismatch. Proning enables the less diseased areas of the lungs to become the 'dependent' lung, therefore receiving more ventilation and perfusion and reducing the mismatch leading to improved oxygenation. This may have the added benefit of posterior lung recruitment, reduced atelectasis and aiding drainage of secretions.

Lung ultrasound can help to identify patients with posterior atelectasis and consolidation and therefore this patient cohort is most likely to benefit from proning.

It is key to understand that the LUS features in COVID-19 are not unique to this disease. Indeed, they appear very similar to other causes of viral pneumonitis or ARDS. This further highlights the need to incorporate LUS into history and examination to avoid error.

Scanning in the proned position is simple and straightforward. The technique is demonstrated in Figure 12.4.

Progression of COVID-19 on Lung Ultrasound

Normal Lung

A lines are demonstrated in all lung fields. There will be normal lung sliding and the pleural line will be thin (Figure 12.5). Note patients may have COVID-19 infection and have a normal LUS.

Thickened and/or Irregular Pleural Line

The first change on LUS is a thickened and/or irregular pleural line (Figure 12.6). Changing to a higher frequency probe may aid in imaging the pleural line in detail.

B Lines

B lines (comet tails) are vertical lines that arise from the pleural line and can be seen to extend to the

219

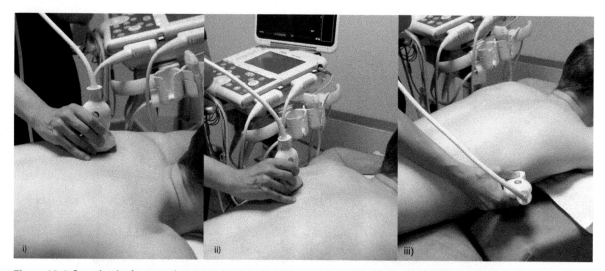

Figure 12.4 Scanning in the proned position: (i) posterior left upper zone; (ii) posterior left mid zone; (iii) right lower zone.

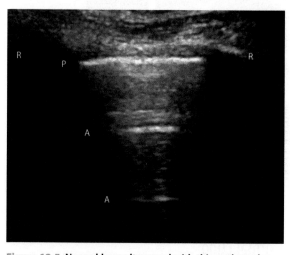

Figure 12.5 Normal lung ultrasound with thin and regular pleural line, pleural sliding and A lines. P, pleural line; R, rib; A, A lines. *A video is available to view in the online video library.*

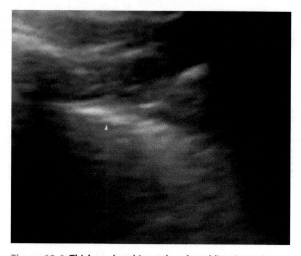

Figure 12.6 Thickened and irregular pleural line (arrow). *A video is available to view in the online video library.*

bottom of the lung window. This is caused by a 'ring down artefact' that is described in more detail in Chapter 1. More than or equal to three B Lines are pathological and result from the combination of air in the alveoli and thickening of the interlobular septa due to fluid or fibrosis (Figure 12.7).

Coalesced B Lines

This appearance is when multiple B lines converge and merge to create a white lung. This is often described as a waterfall appearance (Figure 12.8).

The lung becomes less aerated and oxygenation requirements increase.

Subpleural Consolidation

This is where consolidation occurs just beneath the pleurae. Note the irregular pleural line (Figure 12.9).

Consolidation

Consolidation is easily identifiable on LUS. Consolidated lung has high fluid content and can appear similar to the liver/spleen. It may contain

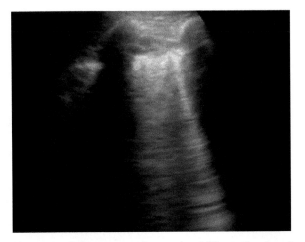

Figure 12.7 B lines can now be seen in addition to the pleural line thickening and irregularity. *A video is available to view in the online video library.*

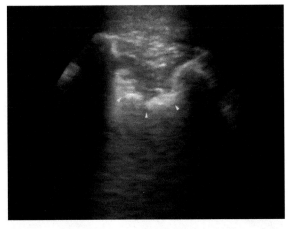

Figure 12.9 Subpleural consolidation (arrows). Not the absence of the regular pleural line. *A video is available to view in the online video library.*

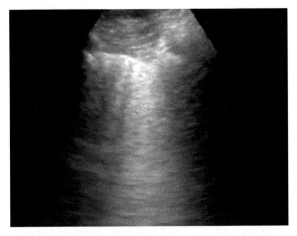

Figure 12.8 B lines increase in severity and begin to coalesce. *A video is available to view in the online video library.*

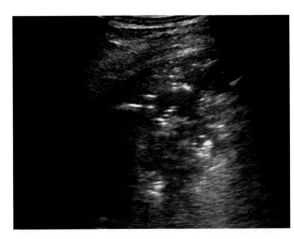

Figure 12.10 Lung consolidation in patient with COVID-19 pneumonitis. *A video is available to view in the online video library.*

air and fluid bronchograms (Figure 12.10). This is described in more detail in Chapter 3.

Consolidation is a much less common feature within COVID-19. Its identification should prompt consideration of superadded bacterial infection.

Pleural Effusions

Pleural effusions are rare in COVID-19 affecting <10% of cases. They are typically seen in more severe cases and, much like consolidation, should be considered a potential feature of superadded infection (Figure 12.11). Development of bilateral transudative pleural effusions may be a feature of long-term critical illness.

Our Experience in a Busy District General Hospital with the Use of Lung Ultrasound in COVID-19

Many hospitals experienced a significantly inflated workload which outstripped available resources. Already stretched staffing levels were required to manage a larger number of patients as wards dramatically expanded. Symptomatic but stable patients had a tendency to deteriorate rapidly due to profound hypoxia without overt features of respiratory distress – often described as 'happy hypoxia'.

Novel approaches were required to rapidly risk assess patients to identify those requiring admission

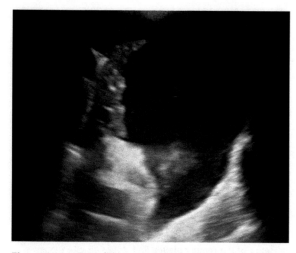

Figure 12.11 Consolidation with parapneumonic effusion.
A video is available to view in the online video library.

to the increasingly scarce hospital beds. Our experience suggested that LUS was essential in this rapid triage process. In some regions this approach was also taken into the prehospital setting with paramedics performing focused LUS to identify those potentially needing transfer to hospital for further assessment. Categorisation of patients was as follows:

Asymptomatic and Normal Scan

With large volumes of patients presenting to the ED, LUS was a quick tool to use to reassure patients at the front door. The visualisation of A lines and a thin, sliding pleural line led to patients being discharged promptly without the need for CXR and a clinical workup.

Symptomatic and Normal Scan

Many COVID-19 patients presented with respiratory symptoms with normal observations including oxygen saturations. Demonstrating A lines and a thin, sliding, pleural line reassured both clinicians and patients. These patients were discharged and advised to self-isolate in line with national guidance. Many were given access to saturation probes and advised to monitor at home.

Asymptomatic and Abnormal Scan

This group of patients were worrying as they were asymptomatic but displayed typical LUS COVID-19 findings at the peak of the pandemic. This group of patients were the asymptomatic carriers which studies worldwide estimated to be between 5–80%. Signs

tended to be confined to a thickened pleural line, subpleural consolidation and B lines. These patients were able to be discharged but with clear advice to urgently return if they became short of breath.

Symptomatic and Abnormal Scan

Patients that needed admission were those that required oxygenation and these patients had the typical CXR findings of bilateral infiltrates. LUS changes varied in severity as described earlier. See Figure 12.3. Clearly these patients should not be discharged from hospital and vigilance for deterioration was essential.

Important Additional Findings

Lobar Pneumonia

Patients that were COVID-19 positive who had lobar pneumonia on CXR did not have typical consolidation on LUS but in fact multiple B lines and coalescing B lines. This is a key feature to delineate an atypical radiographic presentation of COVID-19 from bacterial pneumonia. Furthermore, hospital patients remained at high risk of hospital-acquired infections, such as hospital-acquired pneumonia, particularly after the introduction of routine dexamethasone therapy resulting in a degree of immunosuppression. LUS features of classical consolidation, rather than a B line profile, should prompt the consideration of superadded bacterial infection.

Case – Ultrasound Opens a New Chapter in Learning

A 76-year-old male presented with shortness of breath, fever and cough for 2 weeks. CXR showed left basal and mid-zone consolidation (Figure 12.12i). LUS showed multiple B lines which coalesced (Figure 12.12ii). He was COVID-19 swab positive and his oxygen requirement increased during his admission.

This is an example of a patient presenting with radiographic features suggesting lobar bacterial consolidation but with LUS features of COVID-19 pneumonitis. He demonstrated no other features suggestive of bacterial infection and therefore continued to be managed without antibacterial cover.

Progression of Disease and Management Pathways

Lung ultrasound was key in assessing and managing deterioration of patients. When patients deteriorated,

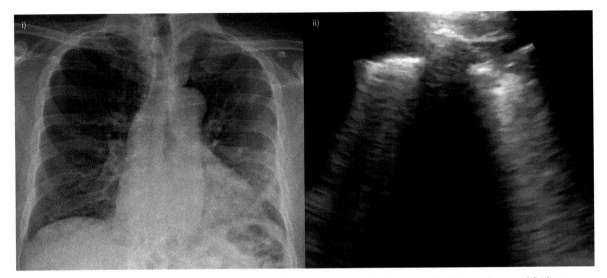

Figure 12.12 (i) Chest X-ray demonstrating left middle and lower zone consolidation but with (ii) lung ultrasound findings of COVID-19.

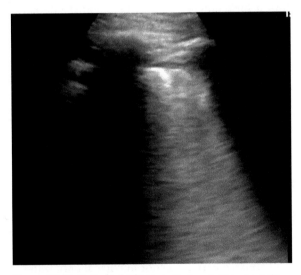

Figure 12.13 **Coalesced B lines.** *A video is available to view in the online video library.*

requiring increasing amounts of oxygenation, the LUS findings appeared to correlate with progression of disease. This appeared as increased B lines throughout the lung with extension up into the upper zones and increasing subpleural and lobar consolidation (Figure 12.13). Rather than exposing patients to repeat CXR and CT scanning, LUS played a key role which aided escalation to CPAP, high flow nasal oxygenation or invasive ventilation.

Case – Silent Hypoxia

A 34-year-old Indian male was admitted with dyspnoea and a small oxygen requirement (initially only 28% oxygen). He was COVID-19 swab positive and CXR confirmed classical bilateral infiltrates – particularly in the basal regions (Figure 12.14i). The following day he deteriorated requiring 40% oxygen to maintain saturations and was increasingly tachypnoeic. LUS demonstrated widespread coalescent B lines which had progressed to both upper zones (Figure 12.14ii). Despite self-proning, his symptoms and oxygenation did not improve, and he was taken to the intensive care unit where he was intubated to facilitate invasive mechanical ventilation. LUS demonstrated extensive disease in all zones without need for CT scanning.

Case – Lung Disease Progression

An 84-year-old male with COPD presented with COVID-19 symptoms and classic radiographic features (Figure 12.15). He was initially requiring 24% oxygen but rapidly deteriorated overnight requiring 15 L of oxygen via a non-rebreathe mask. His LUS demonstrated extensive B lines, coalescing with subpleural consolidation. The patient was too unwell to transfer for CT imaging and the LUS progression empowered the clinicians to escalate to ward-based continuous positive airway pressure (CPAP) therapy. A sub-massive/massive pulmonary embolism was also deemed unlikely based upon focused echo due

223

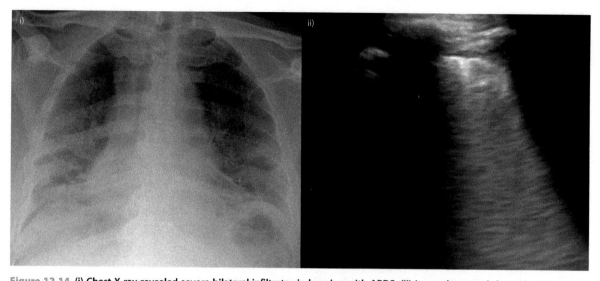

Figure 12.14 (i) Chest X-ray revealed severe bilateral infiltrates in keeping with ARDS. (ii) Lung ultrasound showed widespread features of COVID-19 pneumonitis. Although the findings of pneumonitis are similar to previously discussed cases, here they were widespread with no patches of normal lung suggesting a more significant disease severity.

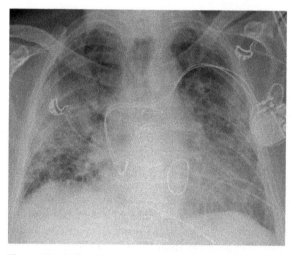

Figure 12.15 Chest X-ray in severe ARDS due to COVID-19 pneumonitis.

to the absence of RV dilatation and strain. He was managed with CPAP for several days but unfortunately deteriorated further and sadly passed away. Although a negative outcome, POCUS provided the clinicians with an extra diagnostic tool in an unwell patient and empowered them to escalate therapy when time and resources were at a premium.

Critical Care

The COVID-19 pandemic saw critical-care-level interventions being delivered in remote settings. Despite

this, a high number of patients required intubation and mechanical ventilation for prolonged periods of time. Although initially labelled as 'ARDS', it quickly became clear that COVID-19 pneumonitis behaved in a unique manner unlike anything we had managed previously.

The role of POCUS within a critical care setting was different to the risk stratification being used in the front-line specialties such as the ambulance service and emergency/acute medicine. Diagnosis for critical care patients had (usually) already been made and POCUS was targeted at titration of ventilatory strategies or for identification of complications associated with long-term critical care and mechanical ventilation.

Two key patterns on LUS were identified for mechanically ventilated patients:

1. Diffuse, bilateral, anterior multiple B lines with pleural abnormalities (Figure 12.16). These patients were more likely to respond to increased positive end-expiratory pressure and careful titration based upon conventional techniques may be employed.
2. Features of posterior consolidation/atelectasis (Figure 12.17). These were the key patients to identify as basal atelectasis suggested the patient was far more likely to respond to proned ventilation.

Although these factors were a useful additional tool it was not employed in many critical care settings due to high workload and limited time. Early reports

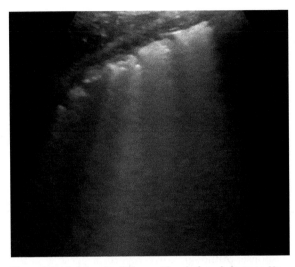

Figure 12.16 Extensive B lines with subpleural changes. No evidence of lobar consolidation. *A video is available to view in the online video library.*

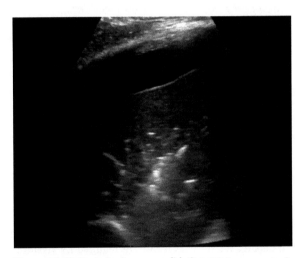

Figure 12.17 Posterior lung consolidation. This is an example of the tissue sign of hepatisation. Note the parapneumonic effusion. *A video is available to view in the online video library.*

suggested that LUS could be used to guide weaning of ventilation and when A lines began to develop this represented an improvement in lung function and facilitated weaning of mechanical ventilation. In reality, clinicians relied on conventional measures of lung function, spontaneous breathing trials, clinical experience and tracheostomies to wean due to the long duration of critical illness.

The main utility of skilled POCUS users was in identification of complications and for efficient, precise clinical interventions:

1. Ultrasound-guided vascular access is an essential element to critical care and limiting complications, such as pneumothoraces, in a cohort with high FiO_2 requirements is crucial. Rapid vascular access performed with a single needle puncture limited the duration of time these patients had to undergo positional changes and reduced the risk of line-related infections.

2. Myocarditis was a recognised complication of COVID-19. The majority of critical care patients did not demonstrate a significant degree of cardiovascular instability and the requirement for high doses of vasoconstrictors necessitated focused echocardiography to identify complications.

3. Following ~Day 10 of the illness it was noted that the lung compliance for mechanically ventilated patients deteriorated and represented a more 'classical ARDS picture'. Higher inspiratory ventilation pressures were required which increased the risk of iatrogenic complications – notably pneumothoraces. LUS in acutely deteriorating patients was exceptionally useful to identify and manage these complications – particularly given the delay in conventional portable X-ray imaging.

4. Other mechanical ventilation-related complications that are detected by POCUS include ventilator-associated pneumonia, diaphragmatic dysfunction and acute cor pulmonale.

Other areas within critical care where POCUS played a role was the management of fluid administration and haemodynamic monitoring, in particular assessing cardiac output and pulmonary artery pressures.

Recovery

As patients recovered, they reported improved shortness of breath and a reduction in oxygen requirement. This correlated with a reduction in pathological LUS signs and the reappearance of A lines (Figure 12.18). The reappearance of A lines was a reassuring sign of clinical improvement, not only for clinicians, but also patients who were able to view the results at the bedside.

The overall frequency and severity of B lines, pleural line thickening and subpleural consolidation appeared to decrease although residual changes persisted. At time of publication, it is unclear how long

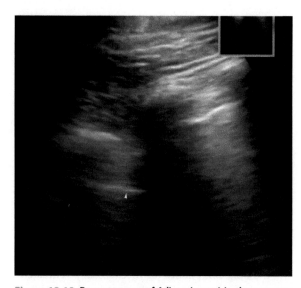

Figure 12.18 Reappearance of A lines (arrow) in the recovery phase of COVID-19 pneumonitis. *A video is available to view in the online video library.*

these findings will persist during the recovery phase. Similar findings are seen in patients with classical ARDS and may persist for months or years due to fibrotic response to lung injury.

British Thoracic Society guidance suggests patients receive a CXR 12 weeks following discharge from hospital wards or 6 weeks after discharge from critical care. If CXR findings persist then pulmonary function tests, high-resolution computed tomography (exclude pulmonary fibrosis) and CT pulmonary angiogram (exclude pulmonary emboli) are required. In addition, an echocardiogram is advised to identify features of heart failure as a cause.

We do not truly know the long-term sequelae of this illness. 'Long COVID' is a diagnosis given to individuals with residual symptoms more than 1 month after COVID-19 and is reported to affect as many as 20% of patients. Fatigue, dyspnoea, muscle aches, chest pain, anxiety and inability to concentrate are just a few symptoms that have been reported.

Do All Viruses Cause Lung Ultrasound Changes that We See in COVID-19?

All patients presenting to the acute medical department were routinely having LUS as part of the standard initial assessment. This resulted in identifying patients with typical COVID-19 symptoms and LUS changes secondary to alternative viral infections such as influenza and Epstein Barr Virus (EBV). This is a reminder that the LUS changes seen are not specific to COVID-19 and to be vigilant when entering the winter months when influenza and COVID-19 will both be presenting as emergencies.

Echocardiography

For a detailed description on performing bedside echocardiography please see Chapter 2.

COVID-19 Myocarditis

COVID-19 is a recognised cause of myocarditis and is thought to be due to a combination of direct viral injury and secondary to host-mediated immune response. Although early reports suggest a 7–10% incidence of *clinically significant* cardiac injury, this is likely to be an overestimate. Magnetic resonance imaging has revealed a much greater frequency of *subclinical* cardiac involvement (~60–70%).

COVID-19 myocarditis should be suspected in patients with tachyarrhythmias, ECG changes and cardiovascular instability. Some patients may rapidly progress to develop acute onset heart failure and cardiogenic shock. Right heart dilatation is common in COVID-19 due to a combination of impaired hypoxic pulmonary vasoconstriction, raised pulmonary artery pressure and pulmonary vascular resistance and the impact of positive pressure ventilation. Right ventricular failure is a recognised complication in severe cases but is likely to be overestimated due to the difficulty of imaging the right heart in acutely unwell patients.

Echocardiographic features of COVID-19 myocarditis are extremely variable and remain subject to debate. We have seen cases of regional LV dysfunction in patients with no coronary artery disease, right ventricular failure independent of ventilation and classically presenting fulminant myocarditis 2–3 weeks following exposure.

Fulminant myocarditis may present as a nonspecific illness with low grade fevers, tachycardia with hypotension and cold, mottled peripheries suggesting cardiogenic shock. Echocardiography will reveal a globally impaired left ventricle with or without dilatation (Figure 12.19). LV walls may appear thinned, normal or thickened depending on the acuity of the disease. Mitral and tricuspid regurgitation are a common feature.

COVID-19 myocarditis remains an unclear disease that is under investigation. Management is supportive and should be discussed with local cardiology teams for consideration of further investigation and follow-up.

Post COVID-19 Pericardial Effusion

Several weeks following COVID-19 exposure a cohort of patients began re-presenting with progressive shortness of breath. This is the perfect environment for rapid assessment using POCUS. Many clinicians were concerned about venous thromboembolism due to the

higher incidence in COVID-19 and recent hospital admission. The differential diagnosis in these patients is vast and rapid differentiation between a cardiac and respiratory cause can transform the patient journey – particularly in the setting where resources are limited and CT pulmonary angiography may be delayed.

Pericardial effusion is a recognised sequela of viral illness and frontline clinicians using POCUS enabled swift diagnosis at the bedside (Figure 12.20). Blindly anticoagulating these patients may be disastrous and increases the risk of intervention in tamponade or potentially leads to haemorrhagic transformation precipitating tamponade. The majority of viral pericardial effusions will self-resolve with little or no intervention.

Pulmonary Embolism and COVID-19

Venous thromboembolism (VTE) causes significant morbidity and mortality among hospitalised patients. It is estimated that 1–2 per 1000 population develop VTE each year and 7–8 per 10,000 individuals develop PE. COVID-19 infection is associated with a significantly increased risk of VTE due to a number of reasons. Firstly, COVID-19 is recognised to be an intrinsically thrombogenic condition. Risk is further increased with dehydration, reduced mobility and the weight gain that was observed during lockdown. Lastly, COVID-19 led to prolonged periods of convalescence with reports of extreme fatigue even in the fittest of individuals.

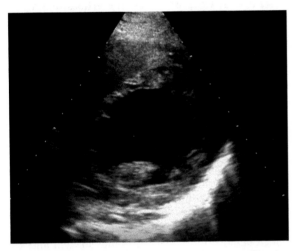

Figure 12.19 Parasternal short-axis view showing a dilated, poorly contracting left ventricle in a patient with suspected COVID-19 myocarditis. *A video is available to view in the online video library.*

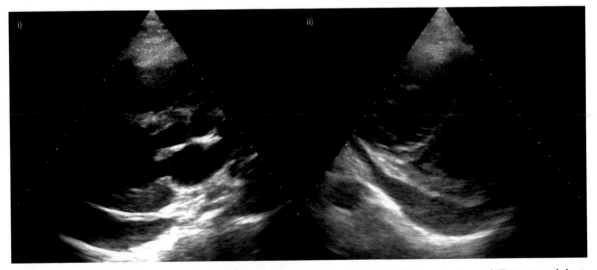

Figure 12.20 Global pericardial effusion in a COVID-19 patient seen in the (i) parasternal long-axis view and (ii) parasternal short-axis view. *Videos are available to view in the online video library.*

Though we do not have accurate figures, one study in Amsterdam reported that 20% of patients with COVID-19 developed symptomatic VTE. There is also concern that patients develop VTE despite receiving standard thromboprophylaxis with numerous reports of fatal massive/submassive PE. This has led many organisations amending their prophylaxis guidance to higher doses and weight-based dosing.

Point-of-care ultrasound is key when COVID-19 patients deteriorate and oxygen requirement increases. Bedside TTE and LUS will help you differentiate between progression of pneumonitis or an alternative diagnosis such as PE.

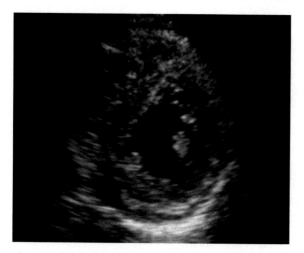

Figure 12.21 Septal flattening is consistent with RV overload.

Think about VTE in:

– Patients who have recently had COVID-19.

– Patients who have an increasing oxygen requirement.

– Patients who develop cardiovascular instability. This is not a typical feature of COVID-19 infection without additional complications.

– Patients who are not following a typical pattern of clinical and symptomatic improvement.

The vascular ultrasound features of DVT are described in Chapter 5, and the echocardiographic features of massive/submassive PE are described in Chapter 2.

Case – Consequences of COVID-19

A 56-year-old lady presented with acute shortness of breath and chest pain. She had been admitted 2 weeks previously with COVID-19 viral pneumonitis, confirmed by swab. On this acute admission she was hypoxic, hypotensive, and peri-arrest. Bedside TTE demonstrated right heart strain with septal flattening suggesting RV overload (Figure 12.21).

Lung ultrasound demonstrated consolidation and B Lines right and middle zone. She was intubated and underwent a CT pulmonary angiogram (Figure 12.22) which demonstrated large thrombus in right and left pulmonary artery as well as segmental branches in both right and left lungs. There were ground glass changes bilaterally in keeping with COVID-19 pneumonitis as well as features of a right lower zone

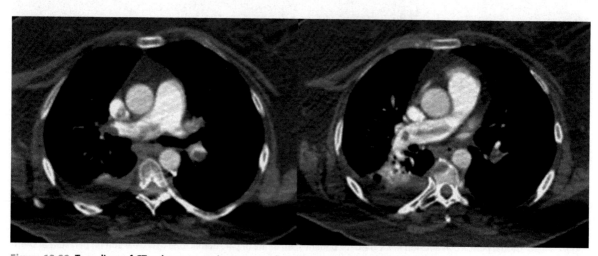

Figure 12.22 Two slices of CT pulmonary angiogram revealing large bilateral pulmonary emboli.

pulmonary infarction and consolidation with evidence of right heart strain.

Paediatric Multisystem Inflammatory Syndrome Temporarily Associated with COVID-19

Several weeks after the pandemic peak a new illness within children was described called 'Paediatric Multisystem Inflammatory Syndrome Temporarily Associated with COVID-19' (PIMS-TS). Children presented with symptoms similar to those seen in toxic shock syndrome and Kawasaki disease and exhibited multisystem involvement. Patients have been treated with immunoglobulins with good effect and it is still an area of evolving research.

Point-of-care ultrasound plays a critical role here where patients can present with features of cardiogenic shock and bedside echocardiography is a key diagnostic tool. In our hospital our handful of cases were identified with focused echocardiography which revealed reduced LV function. LUS in all cases was normal.

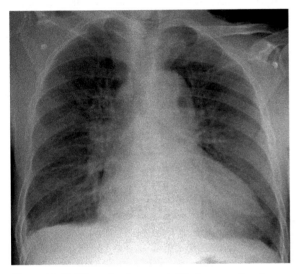

Figure 12.23 Bilateral pulmonary infiltrates secondary to heart failure.

Differentiating from Pulmonary Oedema

Our personal experience has demonstrated the utility of LUS in differentiating between a COVID-19 pneumonitis and pulmonary oedema secondary to heart failure. This was critical due to the increased incidence of patients with late presentations of acute myocardial infarctions and heart failure. Many had been assumed to have COVID-19 upon initial assessment. The CXR for both COVID-19 pneumonitis and pulmonary oedema are similar, demonstrating bilateral infiltrates (Figure 12.23). This may lead to diagnostic challenges particularly when the patient presents in extremis.

Lung ultrasound in pulmonary oedema is distinctly different to pneumonitis. They both form part of the differential of an 'interstitial syndrome' – the presence of a B line profile on LUS (Figure 12.24).

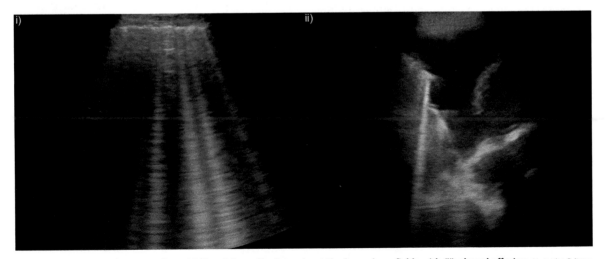

Figure 12.24 (i) Significant number of B lines bilaterally throughout the lower lung fields with (ii) pleural effusion. Note the B lines within the lung base adjacent to the pleural effusion. *Videos are available to view in the online video library.*

Table 12.1 Differences between acute respiratory distress syndrome/COVID-19 and pulmonary oedema on lung ultrasound

	ARDS/COVID-19	Pulmonary oedema
Pleural line	Irregular and thickened	Thin
B lines	Multiple throughout lung B lines do not improve with diuresis	Predominate at bases Number of B lines decreases with diuresis
Lung parenchyma	Subpleural and lobar consolidation	No consolidation
Effusions	Rarely seen <10%	Common at bases

Pulmonary oedema tends to present with a widespread B line profile which is increasingly severe at the lung bases due to the effect of gravity. As you ascend the thorax the B lines become less frequent except for in very severe cases. The pleural line is thin and there are commonly bilateral pleural effusions present (Figure 12.24).

In COVID-19 pneumonitis there are widespread B lines throughout the lung fields which may be patchy and interspersed with normal lung tissue. The pleural line is characteristically irregular and thickened with subpleural consolidation. Pleural effusions are rare.

Diuresis will lead to a rapid improvement in B line profile in pulmonary oedema whereas, as previously mentioned, lung changes appear to remain for weeks or months following COVID-19 pneumonitis.

The comparison in features between pulmonary oedema and COVID-19 pneumonitis or other forms of ARDS are summarised in Table 12.1.

The key benefit of POCUS is to apply the skill to the overall clinical picture and combine multiple systems within your assessment. In the case of pulmonary oedema, detailed history and examination should reveal atypical features for a COVID-19 infection and, in the case of cardiogenic pulmonary oedema, combined focused echocardiography should reveal features of LV systolic or diastolic dysfunction.

Summary

- Point-of-care ultrasound has been critical in triage, diagnosis, medical management and prognostication of COVID-19.
- Applying diagnostic imaging to the bedside is essential to reducing the transportation of acutely unwell patients around the hospital as well as reducing nosocomial infection.
- Other features of COVID-19 may be identified with POCUS including myocarditis, pericardial effusion and pulmonary embolism.
- The COVID-19 pandemic has exemplified and accelerated the argument that POCUS should be a mandatory skill for all generalist clinicians.

A full list of references and further reading is available at www.GeneralistUltrasound.com

Governance and Quality Assurance

Comprehensive point-of-care ultrasound (POCUS) frameworks are essential to ensure we are providing safe and consistent high-quality care to our patients. Currently, within POCUS programmes, emphasis is biased towards education and accreditation without adequate governance, infrastructure, administration and quality assurance processes. The factors discussed in this chapter are essential to consider when setting up your POCUS service.

Quality Assurance (QA) within POCUS is an important tool to allow continuous assessment of the focused studies performed by all clinicians. Due to the infancy of POCUS the structures for governance and QA are frequently non-existent. Urgent ultrasound (US) is often performed by non-accredited clinicians without the saving of images and formal reporting which precludes robust QA processes. All departments, whether community- or hospital-based, should have a clear governance and QA structure which includes a POCUS lead who is accredited to govern and oversee the work that is occurring.

Within our own department we have a dedicated named POCUS lead who is an accredited US clinician. In addition, we have a clear governance policy which is documented in Table 13.1.

We have regular meetings with cardiology, respiratory and radiology colleagues offering shared learning and presentation of cases that we have scanned on the unit.

We recommend the following structures as in Figure 13.1 are in place and overseen by a lead POCUS clinician to provide QA within a department.

Equipment

Technological advances have allowed US equipment to become smaller, lighter, cheaper and intuitively designed. POCUS equipment should be appropriate for the clinical context and examination types being performed. When purchasing equipment, one must consider diagnostic capability, image quality, transducers, screen size, infection control, battery life, Wi-Fi/network and budget constraints. In some countries such as Australia there is clear Government guidance on imaging equipment standards.

We would recommend a minimum five-year warranty as part of the purchase contract to include annual service and software upgrades.

All machines must be cleaned after use for infection control purposes and to ensure probes do not become damaged from gel accumulation.

Equipment must be respected and any damage reported promptly to the POCUS lead.

Archive

Information technology is vital for any successful POCUS programme. Digital Imaging and Communications in Medicine (DICOM) compatibility and Wi-Fi connectivity are the most ideal modalities for image transfer to Picture Archive and Communication Systems (PACS). It is paramount that studies are archived for a complete patient imaging record for medico-legal and clinical QA purposes. Other archival options such as web- or cloud-based servers may be considered provided there is adequate security to maintain patient confidentiality. It is also important to ensure that all necessary views and measurements, including on-screen labelling, are recorded to answer the clinical question and justify the management plan.

In the acute scenario, e.g. cardiac arrest, there may be insufficient time for patient details to be recorded. In these circumstances we recommend recording the images and editing patient details post-scan. Regardless of clinical outcome clinicians should ensure a report is documented and archived for QA.

It is vital that storage of POCUS images is standardised throughout any organisation. This process has been dominated in recent years by DICOM which

Table 13.1

Point-of-care ultrasound governance and quality assurance policy
Education and training requirements for independent scanning to those in training
Standardised reporting form
How to look after the machine including storage and cleaning
How to record images (anonymise to export and how to use for learning and education)
Regular 3-monthly audit of POCUS scans (includes type, number, quality, scanner grade and outcome of patients)
Regular independent review of images and feedback to sonographers with particular focus on quality of scan images and report

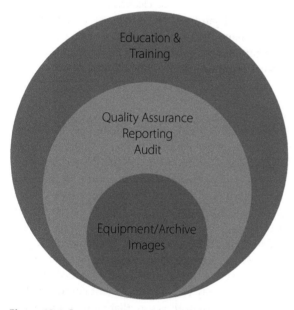

Figure 13.1 Structures required for robust quality assurance and governance.

allows all images to be stored on a central server, thus increasing the accessibility of images throughout the organisation. Additionally, this allows for easy comparison of images to previous studies enabling quick identification of new diagnoses and implementation of timely management plans. DICOM may be integrated with patient electronic medical records to streamline documentation and accessibility for clinical teams.

Quality Assurance

It is vital that images are reviewed regularly to ensure that all relevant guidance, views and protocols have been adhered to. All scans must be of sufficient quality with accurate and relevant measurements performed where required. QA provides evidence of consistent and reproducible reporting of focused studies and can highlight common errors made by clinicians. Strengths and weaknesses within the department may be identified and guide future training for both novice and experienced sonographers. Feedback and peer review ensure that all patients receive the highest achievable standard of care regardless of clinical setting.

Audit and quality improvement projects are essential within all aspects of modern clinical care for governance and education. A continuous audit evaluating image acquisition, optimisation, appropriate measurements and accurate reporting provides a high-quality training environment for novice sonographers and maintains high standards for the department. This, in turn, is likely to translate to better care and treatment for patients over a period of time.

Skill maintenance is an important aspect of quality and there is no clear consensus amongst POCUS accreditation pathways as to the number of scans required per annum to maintain competency. At present, clinicians must have insight into their own level of competence and seek out opportunities to maintain their skill set. More established accreditation pathways, e.g. British Society of Echocardiography Level 2 transthoracic echocardiography accreditation, have rigid re-accreditation requirements mandating a minimum number of studies and continuing professional development points in order to demonstrate a maintained level of competency.

If you work in remote environments or as a lone clinician, it is important to connect with colleagues who can offer external review of images for QA and professional development. The Internet has provided a key platform for remote QA and discussion of difficult cases even across international borders. Examples of these include platforms such as *www .SonoClipShare.com* and the *Butterfly iQ cloud*.

Image Optimisation

Image optimisation is discussed in Chapter 1 and therefore is not described at length here. This inclusion is to serve as a reminder for clinicians that simple adjustments may significantly alter the quality of a study.

For high quality images with greater resolution, one must optimise gain, sector width and depth. Figure 13.2 demonstrates the differences in gain and focus and how they can be optimised to prevent distortion of the image.

Figure 13.2i displays no ECG recording. The ECG is a vital part of any focused echo study as it allows accurate assessment of structural heart disease in relation to the stage of the cardiac cycle, fundamental in the assessment and identification of clinical conditions such as cardiac tamponade. It is vital the machine purchased for focused echo has the ability to monitor ECG.

A traffic light system (Table 13.2) is a simple system used by various bodies in ultrasonography to assess the quality of the scan. This system can also be applied to audit the quality of the final report.

Reporting

Obtaining high quality images will not necessarily improve patient care if the report produced is not of the same high quality. The main aim of the report is to describe key findings, answer the clinical question and to present the conclusions in a clear, concise and accurate manner to guide patient management. Departmental studies frequently include the phrase 'clinical correlation required' to allow the parent team to highlight the key relevant pathology and act accordingly. For POCUS, the clinician should have formulated a clinical question *before* performing the scan and the report should reflect any findings within the overall clinical context.

An example clinical question with example report conclusion is shown below:

Clinical question: *?Pericardial effusion.*

Report conclusion: *Global pericardial effusion identified with a maximal diameter of 1 cm around the RV free wall in diastole. There is no chamber collapse suggesting there is no evidence of pericardial tamponade. This correlates well with the haemodynamic status of the patient.*

It is imperative to understand that there may be a wide range of clinicians with different levels of experience reading and acting upon your report. Reports therefore need to be standardised, consistent, relevant, precise and easy to understand.

Furthermore, it is important to only report findings that are within your level of accreditation. For example,

Table 13.2 Traffic light system assessing image quality

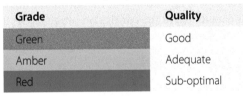

Grade	Quality
Green	Good
Amber	Adequate
Red	Sub-optimal

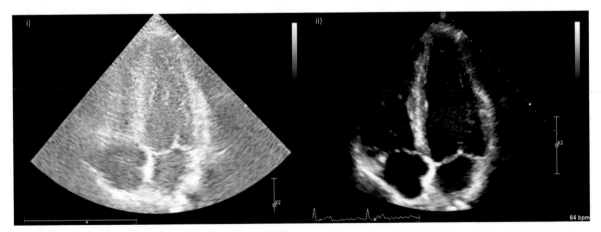

Figure 13.2 The above images have been taken on the same individual. (i) has no ECG, gain settings are too high and focus is incorrectly placed. (ii) has a clear ECG, appropriate gain and optimised focus allowing clear identification of cardiac cycle, endocardial border and valvular structure.

if the clinician was accredited in basic echocardiography (e.g. focused ultrasound in intensive care (FUSIC) heart or British Society of Echocardiography (BSE) Level 1) then attempting to sonographically differentiate between a pericardial effusion and cardiac tamponade is not appropriate. The report may therefore read as such:

Clinical question: *?Pericardial effusion.*

Report conclusion: *Global pericardial effusion identified with a maximal diameter of 1 cm around the RV free wall in diastole. There are no clinical features of tamponade upon patient examination. Cardiology Specialist Registrar contacted who will kindly attend to perform a formal study and advise upon further management.*

This report answers the question in a clear and concise manner within the limitations of the expertise of the performing clinician. Furthermore, it documents a snapshot of the patient's clinical condition at the time of the study and outlines the steps taken to

ensure definitive imaging has been arranged in the presence of a positive finding.

Physicians involved in POCUS need a mechanism to document scan findings and archive these alongside the images for medicolegal purposes. Electronic medical records may act as an alternative solution in certain centres. Our centre requests users to document a written report within the patient notes, within the US machine and complete a dedicated reporting sheet which is kept on the US machine for audit purposes. These reports must include the following details.

– Patient details

– Operator

– Date

– Scan type

– Indication and clinical details

– Quality of scan

– Report of scan

See Figure 13.3 for a sample report template that our unit uses for audit purposes.

Reporting audits are part of QA and should be conducted to ensure that the final report answers the clinical question. If the clinical question cannot be answered, it is important that the reason for this is clearly documented in the conclusion of the report to reduce unnecessary repeat scans being requested.

Education, Training and Continuing Professional Development

Ultrasound is a complex motor skill and POCUS education involves skill acquisition, accreditation, continuing professional development and maintenance of competency.

Point-of-care ultrasound education and training can be achieved in many ways and there are numerous international training programmes and accreditation pathways as described in further detail in Chapter 14. The ideal model for an accreditation pathway is to have dedicated widely available POCUS-qualified trainers, protected teaching time, adequate resources and an appropriate QA structure.

Sharing good practice is imperative to improve the development of novice or junior team members. Interesting and informative cases should be regularly discussed in review meetings in addition to dedicated teaching programmes. This is beneficial for all POCUS users regardless of level of experience. We

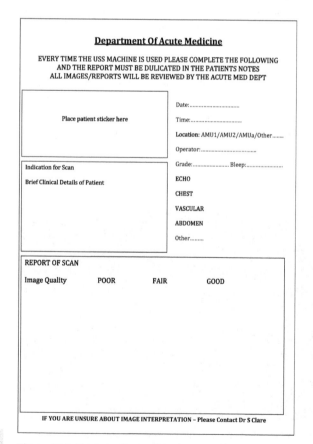

Figure 13.3 **Example of reporting sheet used in our department.**

have regular shared meetings with specialists, including radiologists, cardiologists and respiratory physicians, which has been a powerful collaborative process to guarantee QA, improve scanning ability and nurture relations between speciality teams.

After accreditation it is vital that clinicians maintain their skills within US. Extended hiatuses without performing any scans (often immediately following completion of accreditation!) may lead to the clinician becoming deskilled. As adult learners it is vital that we continue to learn from each other, feedback and continue a logbook for professional development and evidence of regular scanning. There are many websites and social media platforms that share both commonly faced and interesting cases amongst POCUS communities which is another novel form of learning and sharing. Continual professional development (CPD) is an essential element to the appraisal and revalidation process and evidence of scanning is likely to become mandatory to retain accreditation.

Summary

- Governance and Quality Assurance is a fundamental element of POCUS.
- Equipment purchasing, maintenance, imaging archives and reporting processes are a mandatory initial investment for any POCUS lead.
- Education, training, accreditation, peer review and CPD creates a robust and safe POCUS service.

A full list of references and further reading is available at www.GeneralistUltrasound.com

Training and Accreditation

Training and accreditation in POCUS varies widely in the expected standards and level of expertise. In some countries there is increasing exposure for undergraduates whereas others it is solely a postgraduate discipline. The momentum and interest in POCUS is increasing around the world and many colleges, societies and academies are implementing new and novel pathways to suit their discipline.

Ultrasound (US) requires continued exposure, practice, and continuing professional development (CPD) to maintain skill. Feedback and quality assurance processes need to be robust and clinicians should only use US within their skillset.

It is impossible to discuss every accreditation pathway in the world and this would not be relevant for most readers. The following table will provide a brief summary of the most commonly completed accreditation pathways for our readers and provide links to further information. This list only contains accreditation pathways/curricula described in the English language.

Ultrasound fellowships are becoming increasingly popular around the world and are key in raising the profile of POCUS and maintaining a high quality of imaging. This is embedded within North America where a dedicated society, The Society of Clinical Ultrasound Fellowships (SCUF), lists over 70 fellowships on their website (https://eusfellowships.com/). In the UK and Australasia, US fellowships in emergency medicine, critical care and acute medicine are increasing in frequency and popularity.

Undergraduate level – Only several medical schools include US training within mandatory curriculum. This focuses on US-guided vascular access.
Postgraduate level – Well established within the UK with numerous accreditation pathways for various acute specialities. Emergency medicine (EM), respiratory and cardiology mandate the completion of US training prior to completion of training. Key pathways for general clinicians will be described below.
General practice/family medicine – At present there is no formal accreditation pathway for general practitioners or family medics. A dedicated GP POCUS committee is currently working on this.
Musculoskeletal ultrasound – There is no singular organisation overseeing the training in MSK US but rather many university-based postgraduate certificates in MSK US.

Organisation	Accreditation	Speciality	Systems (total number of scans if applicable)	Requirements and assessment	Further information
Royal College of Emergency Medicine	Core (Level 1) US	EM (mandatory for EM trainees.)	FAST AAA Echo in life support Vascular access	Logbook – must complete all disciplines, e-learning and triggered assessment.	www.rcem.ac.uk
Intensive Care Society and British Society of Echocardiography	Focused intensive care ultrasound (FUSIC)	ICM	Basic TTE (50) Thoracic (30) Abdominal (25) Vascular access (10) DVT (5)	Course, logbook for each discipline, e-learning and triggered assessment.	www.ics.ac.uk
Society of Acute Medicine	Focused acute medicine ultrasound (FAMUS)	AM	Thoracic (40) Abdominal (40) Vascular access (5) DVT (10)	Course, logbook for each discipline, e-learning and triggered assessment.	www.acutemedicine.org.uk/famus
British Thoracic Society	Thoracic ultrasound	Respiratory (mandatory for Respiratory trainees.)	Thoracic	Emergency, primary, advanced and expert pathways with individualised requirements.	www.brit-thoracic.org.uk/
Royal College of Radiology	RCR ultrasound training recommendations	Any non-radiology	Urology, gynaecology, GI, vascular, breast, thoracic, cranial, 'emergency US', head and neck, MSK	Individualised requirements to achieve level 1, 2 and 3 competencies in each discipline	www.rcr.ac.uk

Organisation	Accreditation	Speciality	Systems (total number of scans if applicable)	Requirements and assessment	Further information
British Society of Echocardiography (BSE)	BSE level 1	Emergency TTE (mandatory for first year cardiology trainees)	TTE (75)	Logbook of 75 cases. Practical assessment.	https://bsecho.org
BSE	BSE level 2	Formal TTE (mandatory for cardiology trainees/ or equivalent)	TTE (250)	Written examination, logbook of 250 cases, five video cases, practical assessment	https://bsecho.org
BSE	Adult critical care echo (level 2)	Formal TTE in ICM	TTE (250)	Written examination, logbook of 250 cases, five video cases, practical assessment	https://bsecho.org

United States of America

Undergraduate level – The Society of Radiologists of Ultrasound and the Alliance of Medical School Educators in Radiology have collaborated and created an US curriculum for medical students. Although not mandated, over half of medical schools report having formal US curriculum covering anatomy, physiology and pathology courses. US enhanced examination is taught as an adjunct to traditional physical examination. Some medical schools are loaning incoming medical students a hand-held US device.

Family medicine – POCUS training has expanded substantially within the family medicine speciality with two-thirds of residencies having core curricula or elective opportunities within POCUS. The remaining programmes without established POCUS training are reported to be in the process of incorporating it into the curriculum.

Organisation	Accreditation	Speciality	Systems (total number of scans if applicable)	Requirements and assessment	Further information
American Academy of Family Physicians (AAFP)	AAFP family medicine resident curriculum	Family medicine	O&G, cardiac, trauma, aorta, biliary, urinary tract, DVT, soft tissue/ MSK, thoracic, ocular, procedural	Logbook and competency assessment during residency. Absolute requirements vary	www.aafp.org/home.html
American College of Emergency Physicans (ACEP)	Clinical ultrasound accreditation program	EM	Trauma, pregnancy, cardiac/haemodynamic, AAA, airway/thoracic, biliary, urinary tract, DVT, soft tissue/MSK, ocular, bowel, procedural	EM residency 'emergency ultrasound' education program. Standardised checklists and 150 examinations	www.acep.org/by-medical-focus/ultrasound/cuap/cuap-home/
Society of Critical Care Medicine	SCCM programme	ICM	Focused TTE (30), Lung/pleural (20), Abdominal (30), Vascular access (20)	Logbook, variable assessment requirements determined by external bodies.	https://sccm.org/

Organization	Certification	Target	Requirements	Assessment	Website
American College of Chest Physicians (ACCP)	Certification in critical care ultrasound	Respiratory and ICM	Cardiac (10 studies, 50 images), lung/pleural (4 studies, 12 images), abdominal (4 studies, 16 images), vascular access (not specified)	Online learning module, course, online logbook of 102 video clips reviewed by faculty, practical assessment	www.chestnet.org/
American Society of Echocardiography (ASE)	Level 1 competency	Physicians	TTE (75, 150 interpreted)	Assessment of competencies within fellowship programme	www.asecho.org/
ASE	Level 2 competency	Physicians	TTE (150, 300 interpreted)	Assessment of competencies within fellowship programme.	www.asecho.org/
ASE	Level 3 competency	Physicians	TTE (300, 750 interpreted)	Assessment of competencies within fellowship programme	www.asecho.org/
National Board of Echocardiography (NBE)	Examination of special competence in adult echo	Physicians, sonographers, cardiac technicians	TTE (150, 300 interpreted)	Fellowship programme, written examination, logbook submission	https://echoboards.org/
NBE	Critical care echocardiography	ICM	TTE (150)	CCEeXAM or ASCeXAM (until 2022) written examination, logbook, board approval	https://echoboards.org/
POCUS Certification Academy	POCUS generalist certification	General clinicians	AAA (15), cardiac (30) lung (20), MSK (20), biliary (25), OB first trimester (25), DVT (20), renal (20)	POCUS fundamentals certificate (e-learning), case-based assessments, peer evaluations, video cases	www.pocus.org/
POCUS Certification Academy	POCUS EM certification	EM	AAA (15), DVT (20), abdominal trauma (20), lung (20), cardiac (30), OB first trimester (25), biliary (25).	POCUS fundamentals certificate (e-learning), case-based assessments, peer evaluations, video cases	www.pocus.org/

Organization	Certification	Specialty	Content	Assessment	Website
POCUS Certification Academy	POCUS MSK certification	Family and sports medicine, orthopaedics, internal medicine, PT	Upper extremity MSK (20), lower extremity MSK (20), soft tissue (20).	POCUS fundamentals certificate (e-learning), case-based assessments, peer evaluations, video cases	www.pocus.org/

Canada 🇨🇦

Undergraduate Level – A significant proportion of medical schools incorporate focused ultrasound into the undergraduate curriculum. The Canadian Ultrasound Consensus for undergraduate medical education has recommended 85 curricular elements for inclusion in the Canadian Medical School focused ultrasound curriculum.

General practice and family medicine – There is a strong consensus that focused ultrasound should be incorporated into family medicine. There are currently only a few family medicine residency programmes with established US curriculum but this trend is growing in momentum.

Organization	Certification	Specialty	Content	Assessment	Website
Royal College of Physicians and Surgeons of Canada	Emergency ultrasound	EM	Confirming IUP, echo in life support, abdominal, vascular access, AAA.	Individual residency programmes	www.royalcollege.ca/rcsite/home-e
Canadian Critical Care Society	Critical care ultrasound	ICM	Basic TTE (30), lung (20), vascular access (10), abdominal free fluid (10)	Individual residency programmes	https://canadiancriticalcare.org/
Canadian Society of Internal Medicine	Canadian internal medicine ultrasound	Internal medicine	Basic TTE and haemodynamic assessment, lung, abdominal free fluid, venous and arterial access, knee effusion + aspiration	Individual residency programmes	https://csim.ca/
Canadian POCUS Society	Acute care core independent practitioner (IP) certification	EM, family medicine, internal medicine, ICM, surgery	Subxiphoid TTE, AAA, abdominal free fluid, first trimester OB, lung	Written, visual and practical examinations, logbook	www.cpocus.ca/
Canadian POCUS Society	Family medicine core IP certification	Family medicine	Subxiphoid TTE, AAA, abdominal free fluid, first Trimester OB, lung	Written, visual and practical examinations, logbook	www.cpocus.ca/
Canadian POCUS Society	Resuscitation expanded IP certification	EM, internal medicine, ICM	TTE (PLAX/PSAX/A4C), expanded lung, IVC.	Written, visual and practical examinations, logbook	www.cpocus.ca/

Organisation	Level/Certification	Target group	Scope/numbers	Assessment	Website
Canadian POCUS Society	Diagnostic expanded IP certification	General physicians	Gallbladder, renal, bladder, DVT, ocular.	Written, visual and practical examinations, logbook	www.cpocus.ca/
Canadian POCUS Society	Musculoskeletal expanded IP certification	General physicians	Dislocation, effusion, tendon, fracture, soft tissue.	Written, visual and practical examinations, logbook	www.cpocus.ca/
Canadian Society of Echocardiography	Level 1	Cardiology, radiology, IM, EM, ICM, anaesthesia	Focused TTE (40)	Discretion of individual residency/fellowship programmes	http://csecho.ca/
Canadian Society of Echocardiography	Level 2	Cardiology, radiology, IM, EM, ICM, anaesthesia	Formal TTE (150, 450 interpreted)	Discretion of individual residency/fellowship programmes	http://csecho.ca/
Canadian Society of Echocardiography	Level 3	Cardiology, select others	Formal TTE (300, 550 interpreted)	Discretion of individual residency/fellowship programmes	http://csecho.ca/

Europe

Undergraduate Level – Many countries within Europe have well established US training as part of the undergraduate curriculum.

Postgraduate Level – POCUS in Europe is difficult to summarise as there is no central authority that determines the scope of practice or training. Most countries have individualised curricula and an exhaustive list is not appropriate for inclusion within this text. Various European societies are attempting to develop formalised education pathways including ESICM, EACVI, EUSEM and ESM but many remain under development.

General practice and family medicine – POCUS is commonly utilised within general practice and is regulated by national societies. The Austrian Society for US in Medicine, German Society of US and Denmark College of General Practitioners are just several examples.

Organisation	Level/Certification	Target group	Scope/numbers	Assessment	Website
European Society of Intensive Care Medicine (ESICM)	Core critical care US	ICM	TTE (30), lung/pleural, abdominal, vascular access. Only TTE number specified	10 hours echo and 10 hours CCUS theoretical content, logbook	www.esicm.org/
ESICM	European Diploma of Echo	ICM	Formal TTE (100) TOE (35)	Course, theoretical content (e-learning), logbook, written and practical assessment	www.esicm.org/
European Association of Cardiovascular Imaging	Adult TTE	Physician, sonographer	Formal TTE (250)	Written examination, logbook submission.	www.escardio.org/

European Society for Emergency Medicine	EUSEM US curriculum	EM	Focused TTE, lung, FAST, abdominal, soft tissue, DVT, procedural, MSK, ocular	Course, departmental training, accreditation pathway under development	https://eusem.org/

Australia and New Zealand

Undergraduate Level – Of the 22 medical schools within Australia and New Zealand, POCUS training is scarce, ranging from using US during anatomy lessons to several practical sessions scanning classmates. The Australasian Society of Ultrasound in Medicine (ASUM) advocates that POCUS be incorporated into medical undergraduate curriculum starting from Year 1.

Postgraduate Level – Australasian accreditation in general ultrasound is predominantly delivered by the Australasian Society for Ultrasound in Medicine (ASUM). They have varying levels of accreditation pathways and are aimed at all clinical practitioners.

General practice and family medicine – The Royal Australian College of General Practitioners (RACGP) and Australian College of Rural and Remote Medicine (ACRR) provide POCUS courses focusing on general practitioners working within remote environments. They do not directly accredit but their courses are endorsed by ASUM.

ASUM	Certificate in allied health performed ultrasound	AHPs	Basic early pregnancy (25) advanced early pregnancy (50) soft tissue (20) follicle tracing (50) vascular access (3) fetal monitoring (25) e-FAST (25) lung/diaphragm (40)	Each topic is an individual module. Each requires logbook, formative and summative assessments	www.asum.com.au/
ASUM	Certificate in clinician performed ultrasound	Non-imaging specialists	AAA, advanced neonatal, early pregnancy, O&G, soft tissue, breast, e-FAST, lung/pleural, basic TTE, rheum., acute scrotum, biliary, endocrine, neonatal, DVT, renal, vascular access	Each topic is an individual module. Each requires logbook, formative and summative assessments	www.asum.com.au/

ASUM	Diploma of diagnostic ultrasound (DDU) – critical care	EM, ICM, anaesthesia, retrieval	Formal TTE (300), TOE (25), lung (50), abdominal (50), vascular (50), procedures (50 lines, 25 other).	Formative and summative case studies and assessments. Two year minimum duration. Extensive logbook	www.asum.com.au/
ASUM	DDU – Emergency	EM	Abdominal (400), G&B obs (100), small parts (25), MSK (50), peripheral vascular (25), lung (50), basic echo (50), procedures (50).	Formative and summative case studies amd assessments. Two year minimum duration. Extensive logbook	www.asum.com.au/
ASUM	DDU – O&G	O&G, women's health	first trimester (100), second trimester (100), third trimester (200), early pregnancy (200), gynae (300)	Formative and summative case studies and assessments. Two year minimum duration. Extensive logbook	www.asum.com.au/
College of Intensive Care Medicine of Australia and New Zealand (CICM)	Focused cardiac ultrasound	ICM	Basic TTE (30)	Course, online examination, triggered assessment	www.cicm.org.au/
CICM	Advanced critical care echo (CCE)	ICM	Formal TTE (300) separate TOE (50) pathway available	Accredited course with exit exam and CPD	www.cicm.org.au/

Malaysia

Ultrasound education has been developing in Malaysia and the Society of Critical and Emergency Sonography (SUCCES) has been developed to govern US within critical and emergency care.

ASUM also offer a Postgraduate Diploma of Medical Ultrasonography through Vision College, Malaysia.

SUCCES	Ultrasound life support basic level 1	ICM EM	Focused TTE (80) lung (40), abdominal (50), head and neck (10), vessels (20)	Course, logbook, theoretical and practical examinations	www .criticalultrasoundmalaysia .org/

| Vision College and ASUM | Graduate diploma in diagnostic medical ultrasound | Any qualified healthcare provider | Logbook (500), written and practical examinations, full-time course | https://vision.edu.my/ |

South Africa

Ultrasound is widely performed in SA and is part of the curriculum for many acute specialties. Furthermore, US within rural medicine is increasing in popularity and a specific protocol, Focused Assessment with Sonography for HIV-Associated Tuberculosis (FASH), has been developed for use in rural Southern African settings. Multiple organisations have advocated for accreditation pathways to become mandated but this remains under development. The Emergency Medicine Society of South Africa (EMSSA) provide basic POCUS accreditation pathways for all acute care physicians.

| EMSSA | Basic emergency US | EM, ICM, AM | eFAST (20), AAA (15) focused echo evaluation in resuscitation (FEER, 15), DVT (10), CVC (5). | Course, logbook, triggered assessment | https://emssa.org.za/ |

India

In India there are an increasing number of US courses with POCUS particularly applied within EM. There remain no formal training accreditations pathways and clear discrepancies of US exposure throughout the country. New Delhi All India Institute of Medical Sciences (AIMMS) delivers several courses throughout the country including Ultrasound Trauma Life Support Course, Obstetric and Gynaecology Sonography and Keep It Simple Sonography for Neurosurgeons.

Singapore

Despite no formal curriculum or training, clinicians have reported a high exposure to POCUS particularly within EM and critical care settings. Knowledge and skills have been obtained as part of training programmes and incorporated into daily practice. POCUS courses are increasing in number but there is no formal accreditation to date.

A full list of references and further reading is available at www.GeneralistUltrasound.com

Meet the Authors

Dr Sarb Clare MBE
MBChB, FRCP, MSc Med Ed
BSE TTE Level 2 Proficiency Accreditation
RCR Level 2, FUSIC, FAMUS Mentor and Supervisor
FAMUS Committee Member
@AcuteMedSarbC

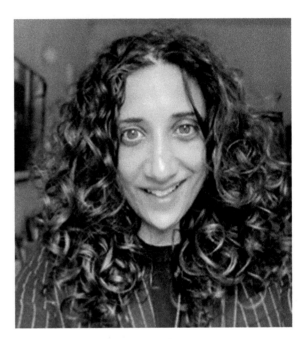

Dr Sarb Clare is a Consultant in Acute Medicine and Deputy Medical Director at Sandwell and West Birmingham NHS Trust, UK. She graduated from the University of Manchester in 1999 and embarked on her career within the field of medicine. As one of the first UK trained Acute Physicians she has over 17 years' experience in the field of point-of-care ultrasound (POCUS) and was the first Acute Medicine Consultant to acquire BSE TTE Accreditation within the UK. In 2010 she went on to set up an Echo Admission Avoidance Clinic to facilitate rapid discharge from the Acute Medicine Department and developed her yearly ultrasound course 'Ultrasound At the Front Door'. She has an extensive portfolio in ultrasound and is a pioneer, national speaker, and teacher in POCUS and has mentored and trained hundreds of trainees, colleagues and allied health professionals to achieve accreditation. Her mission is to get all clinicians to realise the power of POCUS.

She was awarded an MBE in the 2020 Queen's Birthday Honours for her services to the NHS and her leadership during the pandemic. She is passionate about healthcare leadership, widening participation and leads a movement entitled 'Women Empowering Women'. Outside medicine she is a flamenco dancer, runs marathons and she quotes her most important job is 'being mummy to her two young boys'.

Dr Chris Duncan
BMBS, BMedSci, MRCP, PGCert
BSE TTE Level 2 (Critical Care) Proficiency
Accreditation
FUSIC, FAMUS, RCR Level 1 and RCEM Core US
Mentor and Supervisor
@chrisfduncan

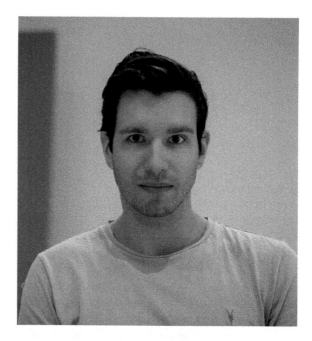

Dr Chris Duncan is a Specialist Registrar in Intensive Care Medicine in London, UK. He graduated from the University of Nottingham in 2014 and completed his early medical training in the Midlands before moving to the south of England. Early exposure to point-of-care ultrasound (POCUS) in Emergency and Acute Medicine highlighted the immense potential for patient care and he rapidly gained accreditation in the available specialty pathways. Since then, he has completed a Critical Care Echocardiography Fellowship at Queen Elizabeth Hospital Birmingham, specialising in echo within cardiothoracic critical care, transplantation and mechanical circulatory support.

Chris has experience in mentoring and has aided medical colleagues and allied health professionals to achieve proficiency accreditation in various ultrasound (US) disciplines. He has organised and taught on nationally approved US courses and given talks at regional and international conferences advocating for POCUS education. With an interest in IT, he has created the free open access medical education website www.GeneralistUltrasound.com and completed all the graphic design for this textbook.

Outside of medicine, Chris is an avid cyclist and has competed in multiple charity events. He has always had a passion for music and spent much of his school and university life playing the saxophone at restaurants, bars and weddings. He has written orchestral and hybrid music for television and film that has been aired on international TV channels and streaming platforms. Whenever not at work he is always looking for the next destination to travel!

For more information please contact
Website: www.GeneralistUltrasound.com
Twitter: @GeneralistUS

Index

A lines, 18, 74–5, 219–20, 225–6
A mode, 13
A2C view. *See* apical 2 chamber view
A3C view. *See* apical 3 chamber view
A4C view. *See* apical 4 chamber view
A5C view. *See* apical 5 chamber view
AAA. *See* abdominal aortic aneurysm
abdominal aorta
   abdominal US of, 99–103
   anatomy of, 99
abdominal aortic aneurysm (AAA),
   99–103
abdominal paracentesis, US guided,
   110–11, 195–6
abdominal ultrasound, 97, 126. *See also*
   focused assessment with
   sonography in trauma
   abdominal aorta on, 99–103
   appendicitis on, 121–2
   free fluid identification on, 105–12,
     201
   general principles of, 97–8
   hepatobiliary system on, 117–21
   IVC on, 103–5
   liver on, 117–18, 122–6
   probe selection for, 97–8
   renal tract on, 112–17
   scanning methods for, 97–8,
     100–5, 113, 117–18, 121–2
   small bowel obstruction on, 121,
     195–6
abscess
   liver, 123
   soft tissue US of, 143–5
   tubo-ovarian, 188
absorption, 7
ACA. *See* anterior cerebral artery
accreditation. *See* training and
   accreditation
acetabulum, 159
Achilles tendon, 162–4
acoustic enhancement, 17–18
acoustic impedance, 5–7
acoustic shadowing, 6, 18
acromioclavicular joint, 153–4
acute mountain sickness (AMS), 204–5
acute respiratory distress syndrome
   (ARDS)

COVID-19 with, 223–5
   LUS of, 84–5
air
   acoustic impedance of, 7
   on LUS, 74–5
   propagation velocity through, 4–5
air bronchograms, 76–7, 85–7
all-in-one probes, 2, 11, 200
altitude related illnesses, 203–5
alveolar syndrome, 85–8
Amazon jungle, foreign body removal
   in, 209–11
ambient light, US considerations in,
   212
amplitude, sound, 4–5, 12–13
AMS. *See* acute mountain sickness
anechoic structures, 5–6
aneurysm. *See* abdominal aortic
   aneurysm
angle of incidence, 7
ankle, MSKUS of, 162–7
anterior cerebral artery (ACA), 176–7
anterior consolidation, lung, 76–7, 95
anterior talofibular ligament, 164–5
aorta, 35–6. *See also* abdominal aorta
aortic aneurysm. *See* abdominal aortic
   aneurysm
aortic dissection
   abdominal US of, 99–100
   echo of, 65–7
aortic regurgitation (AR), 50, 65–7
aortic stenosis (AS), 49–50
aortic valve (AV)
   A3C view, 34
   A5C view of, 33–4
   bicuspid, 215
   PLAX view of, 29–30
   PSAX view, 30–2
apical 2 chamber (A2C) view, 34
apical 3 chamber (A3C) view, 34
apical 4 chamber (A4C) view, 32–3,
   52–3
apical 5 chamber (A5C) view, 33–4
appendicitis, 121–2
AR. *See* aortic regurgitation
archive, image, 231–2
ARDS. *See* acute respiratory distress
   syndrome

arm. *See* upper limb
arrhythmogenic right ventricular
   cardiomyopathy (ARVC), 49
artefacts, 17–21. *See also specific*
   artefacts and lung signs
   lung signs, 68–9
arterial access, US guided, 136–9, 225
arteries, 127–8. *See also* vascular
   ultrasound
ARVC. *See* arrhythmogenic right
   ventricular cardiomyopathy
AS. *See* aortic stenosis
ascites
   FAST of, 110–11
   US guided paracentesis of, 195–6
asthma, 95
atelectasis, lung, 85, 87, 224–5
attenuation, 7
augmentation technique, 131
austere medicine. *See* remote,
   wilderness and austere medicine
Australia, training and accreditation
   pathways in, 237–44
AV. *See* aortic valve
axial resolution, 5
axillary vein, 133–6

B lines
   COVID-19 with, 219–25, 229–30
   HAPE with, 204
   interstitial syndrome with, 82–5,
     229–30
   as lung sign, 76
   as ring down artefact, 18–19
   subpleural consolidation with, 86
B mode, 13
backscatter, 7
Baker's cyst, 148–9, 162
bar code sign, 75
basilic vein, 133–6
bat wing sign, 72–3
beam width artefact, 20
biceps muscle, 154–5
bicuspid aortic valve, 215
biliary tree. *See* hepatobiliary system
bladder
   abdominal US of, 114, 116–17
   FAST of, 107–9

bladder (cont.)
  Hospital at Home care for, 190–2
  transabdominal pelvic US of, 180–1
bladder cancer, 117
bladder residual volume, 116, 190–2
blood vessels, 141–3. *See also* vascular ultrasound
BLUE Protocol, 1–2, 69, 71–3
bone
  acoustic impedance of, 6–7
  fractures on, 147
  propagation velocity through, 4–5
  US characteristics of, 141–3
bowel ischaemia, 125–6
brachial veins, 133–6
brachiocephalic vein, 133–5
brightness, image optimisation with, 21–3
Butterfly IQ, 2, 11, 200

calcaneofibular ligament, 164
calculi, renal, 114–15
calf complex, 162–3
callipers, 24
Canada, training and accreditation pathways in, 237–44
capture, image, 24
cardiac arrest
  focused echo in, 36–8
  prehospital echo in, 202
cardiac masses, 63–5
cardiac output (CO), 60–1
cardiac tamponade, 50–5, 202
cardiogenic pulmonary oedema, 82–4
cardiopulmonary resuscitation (CPR), echo in, 36–8
carotid artery, 134–5
carpal tunnel syndrome, 156
cartilage, US characteristics of, 141–3
CBD. *See* common bile duct
cellulitis, 143–4
central venous access, US guided, 136–9
cerebral oedema, high altitude, 204–5
cervix, 180–1
CFM. *See* colour Doppler
chest anatomy, 69–70
chest X-ray (CXR), COVID-19 appearance on, 217–18, 222–4, 226, 229
cholecystitis, 117–19
choledocholithiasis, 119–20
cholelithiasis, 118–19
chronic kidney disease (CKD), 116
chronic pulmonary obstructive disease (COPD), 95
cirrhosis, 123
CKD. *See* chronic kidney disease
CO. *See* cardiac output

cobblestone appearance, cellulitis, 143–4
cold temperatures, equipment maintenance and considerations in, 211
collapsibility, IVC, 104–5
Colles' fractures, 147
colour Doppler (CFM), 15
  blood flow on, 127–8
  soft tissue and musculoskeletal US using, 140–1
comet tail artefact, 18–19, 76, 82–5, 219–21
common bile duct (CBD), 117–20
common extensor tendon, 154–6
common flexor origin, 156
complex effusions, 90–3
compound imaging, 24, 140–1
compression, probe, 14
compression, sound, 4–5
computed tomography (CT), COVID-19, 217–18, 226–8
congenital heart disease, 214–15
consolidation, lung, 76–8, 84–8, 91–2, 95, 220–1, 224–5
continual professional development (CPD), 234–5
continuous wave (CW) Doppler, 17
control panel, US machine, 8–9
COPD. *See* chronic pulmonary obstructive disease
Coronavirus disease 2019 (COVID-19), 218–19, 230
  B lines in, 219–25, 229–30
  case spread of, 217–18
  clinical presentations of, 217
  consolidation in, 220–1, 224–5
  critical care for, 224–5
  CT of, 217–18, 226–8
  CXR of, 217–18, 222–4, 226, 229
  disease progression and management pathways in, 222–4
  echo of, 226–8
  general hospital experience with LUS use in, 221–2
  Hospital at Home care for, 191–3
  lobar pneumonia in, 222–3
  LUS progression of, 84–5, 217, 219–26
  LUS scanning method for, 218–20
  myocarditis, 225–7
  patient categorisation by LUS scan in, 222
  pericardial effusion after, 227
  PIMS-TS, 229
  pleural effusions in, 221–2
  pleural line thickening in, 219–20
  POCUS role in, 201, 217, 221–5
  prehospital US of, 201

pulmonary embolism and, 227–8
pulmonary oedema differentiation from, 229–30
recovery from, 225–6
virus LUS changes compared to LUS changes of, 226
corpus luteum cysts, 186
COVID-19. *See* Coronavirus disease 2019
CPD. *See* continual professional development
CPR. *See* cardiopulmonary resuscitation
crown-rump length (CRL), 183–4
CT. *See* computed tomography
curtain sign, 80
curvilinear probe, 9–10
  abdominal US using, 97–8
  LUS using, 68
CW Doppler. *See* continuous wave Doppler
CXR. *See* chest X-ray
cysts
  Baker's, 148–9, 162
  ganglion, 146, 157
  labral, 152–3
  liver, 123–4
  ovarian, 186–7
  renal, 115–16
  sebaceous, 146

DCM. *See* dilated cardiomyopathy
decompression sickness, 206
deep vein thrombosis (DVT), 127, 139
  lower limb assessment for, 128–33
  lymphoedema differentiation from, 196–7
  remote, wilderness and austere medicine assessment of, 205–6
  upper limb assessment for, 133–6
depth, image optimisation with, 21
diaphragm
  FAST of, 105–7
  LUS of, 79–81
diastolic dysfunction, 39
Digital Imaging and Communications in Medicine (DICOM), 231–2
dilated cardiomyopathy (DCM), 42–5
disaster relief medicine. *See* humanitarian and disaster relief medicine
display marker, 11–12
distal biceps tendon, 154–5
Doppler effect, 14–15
double barrel shotgun, 120
double decidual sac sign, 182–3
DVT. *See* deep vein thrombosis
dyspnoea
  BLUE Protocol for, 1–2, 69, 71–3

remote, wilderness and austere
   medicine assessment of, 203–4

early pregnancy ultrasound. *See*
   obstetric and gynaecological
   ultrasound
ECG. *See* electrocardiogram
Echo in Africa project, 214–15
echocardiography (echo), 67
   A2C view, 34
   A3C view, 34
   A4C view, 32–3, 52–3
   A5C view, 33–4
   of acute MR, 41–2
   of aortic dissection, 65–7
   of ARVC, 49
   during cardiac arrest, 36–8
   of cardiac masses, 63–5
   of cardiac tamponade, 50–5
   clinical questions answered by, 26
   congenital heart disease detection
      on, 214–15
   COVID-19 on, 226–8
   of global LV dysfunction, 42–6
   of HCM, 33–4, 46–8
   heart block on, 193
   of hypertension, 45–7
   indications for, 26–7
   of ischaemic LV dysfunction, 39–42
   IVC view, 35–6
   LV function assessment with, 38–9
   of LV thrombus, 42–3
   of LVH, 33–4, 45–8
   of LVNCC, 48–9
   modified parasternal windows, 30–1
   normal useful reference ranges for,
      67
   of pericardial effusion, 50–5, 227
   PLAX view, 29–30, 52–3, 56–7, 78
   pleural and pericardial fluid on,
      29–30, 52–3, 78
   in post ROSC care, 37–8
   post-MI assessment with, 39–43
   prehospital, 202
   of proximal septal hypertrophy, 46–7
   PSAX view, 30–2, 52–3, 57–8
   of pulmonary embolism, 56–9,
      205–6
   remote, wilderness and austere
      medicine use of, 204–6
   rheumatic heart disease detection
      using, 214–15
   of RV dilatation, 56–7, 59
   RV function assessment with, 55–6
   SC view, 34–5, 52, 54
   scanning method for, 27–8
   shock, hypovolaemia, fluid
      responsiveness and fluid overload
      assessment with, 59–63

SSN view, 35–6
   of valvular heart disease, 49–51
   of ventricular septal rupture, 41–3
   windows used for, 28–9
echogenicity, 5–7
ectopic pregnancy, 110, 184–5
edge shadowing, 20
education. *See* training and
   accreditation
EF. *See* ejection fraction
e-FAST. *See* extended FAST
ejection fraction (EF), 38–9, 46–7, 55–6
elbow, MSKUS of, 154–6
electrical alternans, 51–2
electrocardiogram (ECG)
   in cardiac tamponade, 51–2
   echo with, 27
   heart block on, 193
   in massive PE, 56–7
emergency medicine, prehospital. *See*
   prehospital ultrasound
empyema, 90–3
end of life care. *See* palliative and end
   of life care
endocarditis, 64–5
endometrium, 180–1
endotracheal intubation, 202
epidermis, 141–3
Europe, training and accreditation
   pathways in, 237–44
extended FAST (e-FAST), 201
extensor tendons, 157–8

FAC. *See* fractional area change
fallopian tubes, 188
fascia, 141–3
FASH. *See* focused assessment with
   sonography for HIV-associated
   tuberculosis
FAST. *See* focused assessment with
   sonography in trauma
fat
   acoustic impedance of, 7
   propagation velocity through, 4–5
fatty liver, 123
FBs. *See* foreign bodies
femoral acetabular impingement,
   159
femoral artery, DVT assessment in,
   129–30
femoral head, 159
femoral nerve block, 208–10
femoral vein, DVT assessment in,
   129–33
FH. *See* frank hypovolaemia
fibroids, uterine, 185
field of view, probe, 9
flexor hallucis longus tendon, 166–7
flexor tendons, 158

fluid bronchograms, 76–7, 85–7
fluid overload
   echo assessment of, 59–63
   TTE assessment of, 213
fluid responsiveness, echo assessment
   of, 59–63
fluid tolerance, 60–1
focus, image optimisation with, 23–4
focused assessment with sonography
   for HIV-associated tuberculosis
   (FASH), 207
focused assessment with sonography in
   trauma (FAST)
   abdominal free fluid identification
      on, 105–12, 201
   ascites on, 110–11
   extended, 201
   general principles and scanning
      methods for, 105–9
   protocol of, 109–10
   rupture on, 110
foetal pole, 183–4
foot, MSKUS of, 162–7
footprint, probe, 9
foreign bodies (FBs)
   remote, wilderness and austere
      medicine, 206, 209–11
   soft tissue US of, 148–9
fractional area change (FAC), 55–6
fractures
   soft tissue US of, 147
   South Pole diagnosis and
      management of, 208–10
frame rate, 13
frank hypovolaemia (FH), 59–60
free fluid
   abdominal, 105–12, 201
   pelvic cavity, 181–5, 188–9
freeze, image, 24
frequency, 4–5, 7
fundoscopy, 168–70

gain, image optimisation with, 21–3
gallbladder. *See* hepatobiliary system
gallstones
   abdominal US of, 118–20
   acoustic shadowing by, 6
ganglion cysts
   dorsal wrist, 157
   soft tissue US of, 146
gastric perforation, 112
GCA. *See* giant cell arteritis
gel, US, 12, 70–1, 141, 169,
   211
gestational sac, 182–3
gestational trophoblastic disease, 185
giant cell arteritis (GCA), 174–6
glenohumeral joint, 152–3
gluteal medius tendinopathy, 159–60

governance, 231–2, 235. *See also* quality assurance
  education, training and continual professional development, 234–5
  equipment, 231
  image archive, 231–2
  image optimisation, 232–3
  reports, 233–4
great saphenous vein, 129–32
greater trochanteric pain syndrome, 159–60
gynaecological ultrasound. *See* obstetric and gynaecological ultrasound

HACE. *See* high altitude cerebral oedema
haematocrit sign, 93–4
haematoma, soft tissue US of, 147–8
haemodynamics
  echo assessment of, 60–1
  TTE assessment of, 213
haemopericardium, 201–2
haemorrhage, FAST protocol for, 109–10
haemorrhagic ovarian cysts, 187
haemothorax
  e-FAST of, 201
  LUS of, 93–4
halo sign, 174–5
hamstring tendinopathy, 160
hand, MSKUS of, 156–8
hand-held probes, 2, 11, 200
handlebar palsy, 157
HAPE. *See* high altitude pulmonary oedema
HAPH. *See* high altitude pulmonary hypertension
happy hypoxia, 221–2
HCM. *See* hypertrophic cardiomyopathy
headache, 169–71, 173–6
heart block, 193
heart failure
  COVID-19, 225–7
  at high altitude, 204
  palliative and end of life care for, 196–8
heart failure with preserved ejection fraction (HFpEF), 39
hepatic artery, 117–18, 120
hepatic veins
  abdominal US of, 123–5
  echo assessment of, 62–3
  flow within, 124–5
hepatisised lung, 77–8, 87
hepatitis, 123
hepatobiliary (HPB) system
  abdominal US of, 117–21

cholecystitis of, 117–19
choledocholithiasis of, 119–20
cholelithiasis of, 118–19
scanning method for, 117–18
HFpEF. *See* heart failure with preserved ejection fraction
high altitude cerebral oedema (HACE), 204–5
high altitude pulmonary hypertension (HAPH), 204
high altitude pulmonary oedema (HAPE), 204
hip
  fracture diagnosis and management, 208–10
  MSKUS of, 159–61
Hospital at Home, 190, 194
  COVID-19 case, 191–3
  heart block case, 193
  nephrotoxicity case, 190–2
  urinary retention case, 190–2
hot temperatures, equipment maintenance and considerations in, 212
HPB system. *See* hepatobiliary system
humanitarian and disaster relief medicine, 200, 214–16
humidity, equipment maintenance and considerations in, 212
hydronephrosis, 112–15
hydropneumothorax, 94
hydrosalpinx, 188
hyperechoic structures, 6
hypertension, 45–7
hypertrophic cardiomyopathy (HCM), 33–4, 46–8
hypervolaemia, 61–3
hypodermis, 141–3
hypoechoic structures, 6
hypovolaemia
  echo assessment of, 59–63
  TTE assessment of, 213

ICP. *See* intracranial pressure
idiopathic intracranial hypertension (IIH), 171, 173–4
iliopsoas, 159
iliotibial band, 161–3
image
  acquisition of, 12–21
  generation of, 12–13
  optimisation of, 21–4, 232–3
  saving of, 24, 231–2
imaging modes, 12–17
imaging planes, 12
India, training and accreditation pathways in, 237–44
inferior vena cava (IVC)

abdominal US of, 103–5
anatomy of, 103–4
in cardiac tamponade, 54
echo view of, 35–6
in frank hypovolaemia, 59–60
in pulmonary embolism, 58–9
right atrial pressure and, 62
internal jugular vein, 133–5
intersection syndrome, 157
interstitial syndrome
  COVID-19, 191–3, 229–30
  LUS of, 76, 82–5, 191–3, 229–30
intracranial pressure (ICP)
  papilloedema with raised, 168–71
  TCD estimation of, 178
intracranial vasospasm, TCD of, 177–8
intrauterine device (IUD), malposition or displacement of, 186
intrauterine pregnancy (IUP), 182–4
ischaemic LV dysfunction, 39–42
ischaemic stroke, 177, 205
ischial bursitis, 160–1
isoechoic structures, 6
IUD. *See* intrauterine device
IUP. *See* intrauterine pregnancy
IVC. *See* inferior vena cava

jellyfish sign, 83–4, 88–9
joints, US characteristics of, 141–3

keyboard sign, 121, 195–6
kidney
  abdominal US of, 112–17
  acoustic impedance of, 6–7
  anatomy of, 112–13
  cancer of, 116
  CKD of, 116
  cysts of, 115–16
  FAST of, 105–6
  Hospital at Home care for, 190–2
  hydronephrosis of, 112–15
  propagation velocity through, 4–5
  pyelonephritis of, 116
  renal calculi of, 114–15
  scanning methods for, 113
knee, MSKUS of, 160–3
knobology, 8–9

LA. *See* left atrium
labrum, 152–3
lateral collateral ligament, 161–2
lateral femoral cutaneous nerve, 159
lateral meniscus, 161–3
lawnmower scanning technique, 121, 121
lawnmower technique, 69–71
left atrial pressure, 62

left atrium (LA)
  A4C view, 33
  PSAX view, 30–2
left upper quadrant (LUQ), 105–8,
  182–3
left ventricle (LV)
  A2C view, 34
  A3C view, 34
  A4C view, 33
  echo assessment of function of, 38–9
  global dysfunction of, 42–6
  in hypovolaemia, 59–60
  ischaemic dysfunction of, 39–42
  PLAX view of, 29–30
  post-MI complications of, 39–43
  PSAX view, 30–2
  SC view, 34–5
  thrombus formation in, 42–3
left ventricle end diastolic pressure
  (LVEDP), 62
left ventricular assist system (LVAS),
  127–8
left ventricular hypertrophy (LVH),
  33–4, 45–8
left ventricular non-compaction
  cardiomyopathy (LVNCC), 48–9
left ventricular outflow tract (LVOT),
  33–4, 47–8
leg. See lower limb
leiomyoma, 185
ligament, US characteristics of, 141–3
Lindegaard Ratio, 177–8
linear probe, 9–10
  LUS using, 68
  soft tissue and musculoskeletal US
    using, 140–1
  vascular US using, 127
lipoma, 146
liver. See also hepatobiliary system
  abdominal US of, 117–18, 122–6
  abscess of, 123
  acoustic impedance of, 7
  acute hepatitis of, 123
  cirrhosis of, 123
  cysts of, 123–4
  FAST of, 105–7
  fatty disease of, 123
  masses of, 123
  measurements of, 123
  propagation velocity through, 4–5
  vasculature of, 123–6
lobar pneumonia, COVID-19 with,
  222–3
long axis, 12
long COVID, 226
long head of biceps tendon, 150–2
lower limb
  DVT assessment in, 128–33

MSKUS of, 159–67
  vascular anatomy of, 129–31
lumbar puncture, US guided, 170–4
lung cancer, 89–90
lung hepatisation, 77–8, 87
lung point, 75, 81–3
lung pulse, 75, 81
lung sliding
  in BLUE protocol, 72
  endotracheal intubation
    confirmation using, 202
  LUS sign of, 73–4, 219–20
  pneumothorax absence of, 75, 80–3,
    201–2
  sea-shore sign of, 74
lung ultrasound (LUS), 96
  A lines on, 18, 74–5, 219–20, 225–6
  alveolar syndrome on, 85–8
  anatomy seen on, 69–70
  asthma and COPD on, 95
  B lines and comet tails as lung sign
    on, 76
  basic views of, 68–9
  BLUE Protocol, 1–2, 69, 71–3
  consolidation on, 76–8, 84–8, 91–2,
    95, 220–1, 224–5
  COVID-19 compared with
    pulmonary oedema on, 229–30
  COVID-19 hospital experiences
    with, 221–2
  COVID-19 progression on, 84–5,
    217, 219–26
  COVID-19 role of, 201, 217, 221–5
  diaphragm on, 79–81
  heart block on, 193
  indications for, 68
  interstitial syndrome on, 76, 82–5,
    191–3, 229–30
  lung point on, 75, 81–3
  normal lung on, 219–20
  pleural effusion on, 78–9, 83–4,
    87–94, 221–2
  pleural fluid on, 78–9
  pleural line thickening and
    irregularity on, 79–80, 84–5,
    219–20
  pneumothorax on, 75, 80–3, 201–2
  prehospital, 201–2
  probe selection for, 68
  pulmonary embolism on, 95
  quad sign on, 78–9
  remote, wilderness and austere
    medicine use of, 203–4
  rib shadows/bat wing sign on, 72–3
  scanning methods for, 69–73,
    218–20
  sea-shore sign on, 74
  shred and tissue signs on, 76–8, 86–7

signs interpreted in, 68–9
sinusoid sign on, 78–9
sliding sign on, 73–4, 219–20
spine sign on, 78–9
stratosphere sign/bar code sign on,
  75
thoracocentesis guidance by, 95
LUQ. See left upper quadrant
LUS. See lung ultrasound
LV. See left ventricle
LVAS. See left ventricular assist system
LVEDP. See left ventricle end diastolic
  pressure
LVH. See left ventricular hypertrophy
LVNCC. See left ventricular non-
  compaction cardiomyopathy
LVOT. See left ventricular outflow tract
lymph nodes, US appearance of, 145–6
lymphoedema, 196–7

M mode, 13
  lung sliding in, 74
  PLAX view, 30
  PSAX view, 32
  sinusoid sign in, 78–9
  stratosphere sign/bar code sign in, 75
machine. See ultrasound machine
Malaysia, training and accreditation
  pathways in, 237–44
MAPSE. See mitral annular plane of
  systolic excursion
marker, probe and display, 11–12
MCA. See middle cerebral artery
McConnell's sign, 57
measurements, image, 24
mechanical ventilation, for COVID-19,
  224–5
medial collateral ligament, 161–2
medial meniscus, 161–2
median nerve, 156
medium
  acoustic impedance of, 5–7
  propagation velocity through, 4–5
metacarpophalangeal joints, 157–8
metastatic lymph nodes, 145
metatarsal phalangeal joints, 166–7
MI. See myocardial infarction
Mickey Mouse sign, 120, 129
middle cerebral artery (MCA), 176–7
  infarct of, 205
  vasospasm of, 177–8
military medicine, 200, 212–13,
  216
mirror image artefact, 19
mitral annular plane of systolic
  excursion (MAPSE), 38–9
mitral regurgitation (MR), 41–2, 49–51
mitral stenosis (MS), 50–1

mitral valve (MV)
  A4C view, 33
  exaggerated inflow variability of, 54–5
  PLAX view of, 29–30
  PSAX view, 30–2
  rheumatic heart disease of, 215
  SC view, 34–5
  systolic anterior motion of, 47–8
modes, imaging, 12–17
modified parasternal windows, 30–1
moisture, equipment maintenance and considerations in, 212
molar pregnancy, 185
Morison's pouch, 105–7, 184–5, 201
MR. *See* mitral regurgitation
MS. *See* mitral stenosis
MSKUS. *See* musculoskeletal ultrasound
Murphy's sign, 118–19
muscle
  acoustic impedance of, 7
  propagation velocity through, 4–5
  US characteristics of, 141–3
musculoskeletal ultrasound (MSKUS), 140, 149–50, 167
  beginner's approach to, 150
  of elbow, 154–6
  of foot and ankle, 162–7
  of hand and wrist, 156–8
  of hip, 159–61
  interventions using, 150
  of knee, 160–3
  normal anatomical structures on, 141–3
  probe selection for, 140–1
  remote, wilderness and austere medicine use of, 206
  scanning methods for, 140–2
  of shoulder, 150–4
MV. *See* mitral valve
myocardial infarction (MI)
  acute MR after, 41–2
  ischaemic LV dysfunction and RWMAs after, 39–42
  thrombus formation after, 42–3
  ventricular septal rupture after, 41–3
myocarditis
  COVID-19, 225–7
  global LV dysfunction in, 42–6
myometrium, 180–1

necrotising fasciitis (NF), 145
nephrotoxicity, 190–2
nerves, US characteristics of, 141–3
neurology, 168, 178–9. *See also* transcranial Doppler
  GCA, 174–6
  lumbar puncture, 170–4

papilloedema, 168–71, 173–4
remote, wilderness and austere medicine, 204–5
scanning methods in, 169–73
New Zealand, training and accreditation pathways in, 237–44
NF. *See* necrotising fasciitis
non-cardiogenic pulmonary oedema, 84–5

obstetric and gynaecological (O&G) ultrasound, 180, 189
  ectopic pregnancy, 110, 184–5
  free fluid in pelvic cavity, 181–5, 188–9
  hydrosalpinx on, 188
  intrauterine pregnancy confirmation, 182–4
  IUD malposition or displacement on, 186
  molar pregnancy, 185
  ovarian cysts on, 186–7
  ovarian torsion, 187–8
  ovarian tumours on, 186–7
  pelvic anatomy on, 180–2
  PHUS in early pregnancy complications, 203
  PID on, 188–9
  scanning method for, 180–2
  tubo-ovarian abscess on, 188
  uterine fibroids (leiomyomas) on, 185
obstructive airway disease, 95
O&G ultrasound. *See* obstetric and gynaecological ultrasound
ONSD. *See* optic nerve sheath diameter
optic disc elevation, 169–71
optic nerve sheath diameter (ONSD)
  in AMS and HACE, 204–5
  in papilloedema, 168–71
organ rupture, 110–11
orientation
  imaging planes, 12
  of probe and display markers, 11–12
ovarian abscess, 188
ovarian cysts, 186–7
ovarian torsion, 187–8
ovarian tumours, 186–7
ovary, transabdominal pelvic US of, 180–2

PA. *See* pulmonary artery
paediatric multisystem inflammatory syndrome temporarily associated with COVID-19 (PIMS-TS), 229
palliative and end of life care, 195, 199
  abdominal paracentesis, 195–6
  heart failure management, 196–8
  lymphoedema diagnosis, 196–7
  withdrawal of medical care, 197–8

pandemic. *See* Coronavirus disease 2019
papilloedema, 168–71, 173–4
paracentesis, US guided, 110–11, 195–6
parapneumonic effusions, 90–3
parasternal long axis (PLAX) view, 29–30
  of pleural and pericardial fluid, 29–30, 52–3, 78
  of pulmonary embolism, 56–7
parasternal short axis (PSAX) view, 30–2
  of pericardial effusion, 52–3
  of septal flattening, 57–8
patella tendinopathy, 161–2
patient details, 8
PCA. *See* posterior cerebral artery
PD. *See* power Doppler
PE. *See* pulmonary embolism
pectoralis major tendon, 150–1
pelvic cavity
  free fluid in, 181–5, 188–9
  masses in, 186–7
  normal anatomy of, 180–2
pelvic inflammatory disease (PID), 188–9
pelvic views, FAST, 105–9
pendulum peristalsis, 121, 195–6
penetration, 7
pericardial effusion
  echo of, 50–5, 227
  post COVID-19, 227
pericardial fluid, 29–30, 52–3, 78
pericardial tamponade. *See* cardiac tamponade
period, 4–5
peripheral nerve blockade, 206
peripheral venous access, US guided, 136–9
peroneus longus and brevis tendons, 164–5
PG. *See* porcelain gallbladder
phased array probe, 9–11
  echo using, 27
PHUS. *See* prehospital ultrasound
physics of ultrasound, 4
  production and characteristics of sound waves, 4–5
  tissue interactions with sound waves, 5–7
PI. *See* pulsatility index
PID. *See* pelvic inflammatory disease
piezoelectric crystals, 4
PIMS-TS. *See* paediatric multisystem inflammatory syndrome temporarily associated with COVID-19
plankton sign, 91, 93–4
plantar fasciopathy, 164–5

PLAPS. *See* posterolateral alveolar and/or pleural syndromes

PLAX view. *See* parasternal long axis view

pleural effusion
  echo of, 52–3
  haemothorax, 93–4
  hydropneumothorax, 94
  LUS of, 78–9, 83–4, 87–94, 221–2
  parapneumonic effusions, complex effusions and empyema, 90–3
  size of, 88–90

pleural fluid
  echo of, 29–30, 52–3, 78
  LUS of, 78–9

pleural line thickening, 79–80, 84–5, 219–20

pleural sliding. *See* lung sliding

pneumonia. *See also* parapneumonic effusions
  COVID-19 with, 222–3
  LUS of, 77–8, 85–8
  South Pole diagnosis of, 207–9

pneumonitis, COVID-19, 229–30

pneumothorax. *See also* hydropneumothorax
  e-FAST of, 201
  LUS of, 75, 80–3, 201–2
  stratosphere sign/bar code sign in, 75

POCUS. *See* point of care ultrasound

POD. *See* Pouch of Douglas

point of care ultrasound (POCUS), 1, 3. *See also specific topics* benefits of, 1
  COVID-19 role of, 201, 217, 221–5
  ease of training in, 2
  evidence base for, 1–2
  as mandatory skill for generalists, 2–3
  momentum behind, 2

polycystic kidney disease, 115–16

polycystic liver disease, 123–4

popliteal vein, DVT assessment in, 129–33

porcelain gallbladder (PG), 118–19

portable ultrasound machines, 1–2, 11, 200, 203, 213–14

portal hypertension, 124–5

portal veins
  abdominal US of, 117–18, 120, 123–6
  echo assessment of, 62–3
  flow within, 124–6

post disaster medicine. *See* humanitarian and disaster relief medicine

posterior cerebral artery (PCA), 176–7

posterior interosseous nerve, 154

posterolateral alveolar and/or pleural syndromes (PLAPS), 72–3

post-partum DCM, 43–5

Pouch of Douglas (POD), 108–9, 180–2, 184–5

power button, US machine, 8

power Doppler (PD), 15–16, 141–2

pregnancy
  ectopic, 110, 184–5
  intrauterine, 182–4
  molar, 185
  of unknown location, 184

prehospital ultrasound (PHUS), 200, 216
  early pregnancy complications, 203
  echocardiography in cardiac arrest, 202
  e-FAST for trauma, 201
  endotracheal intubation confirmation using, 202
  LUS, 201–2
  vascular and procedural, 202–3

presets, selection of, 11

probe
  abdominal US, 97–8
  all-in-one hand-held, 2, 11, 200
  angle of incidence of, 7
  care for, 24
  curvilinear, 9–10
  echo, 27
  FAST, 105
  governance and quality assurance policy for, 231
  high frequency compared with low frequency, 7
  key elements of, 4–5
  linear, 9–10
  LUS, 68
  movements and manipulation of, 13–14
  phased array, 9–11
  selection of, 9–12
  soft tissue and musculoskeletal US, 140–1
  vascular US, 127

probe marker, 11–12

Project Morpho, 213

propagation velocity, 4–5

proximal septal hypertrophy, 46–7

PSAX view. *See* parasternal short axis view

pseudogestational sac, 182–3

pulmonary artery (PA), 30–1

pulmonary embolism (PE)
  COVID-19 and, 227–8
  echo of, 56–9, 205–6
  LUS of, 95

pulmonary fibrosis, 85

pulmonary hypertension, high altitude, 204

pulmonary oedema
  COVID-19 differentiation from, 229–30
  high altitude, 204
  LUS of, 76, 82–5, 204

pulmonary valve (PV), 30–2

pulsatility index (PI), 178

pulse wave (PW) Doppler, 16. *See also* transcranial Doppler
  of hepatic vein flow, 124–5
  of portal vein flow, 124–6

pulsus paradoxus, 51, 54–5

PV. *See* pulmonary valve

PW Doppler. *See* pulse wave Doppler

pyelonephritis, 116

QA. *See* quality assurance

quad sign, 78–9

quadriceps muscles, 159–60

quadriceps tendon, 160–1

quality assurance (QA), 231–2, 235
  education, training and continual professional development, 234–5
  image optimisation, 232–3
  in remote, wilderness and austere medicine, 212
  reports, 233–4

RA. *See* right atrium

radial vein, 133–5

rarefaction, sound, 4–5

record, image, 24, 231–2

reflection, 7

refraction artefact, 19–20

regional wall motion abnormalities (RWMA), 39–42

remote, wilderness and austere medicine, 200, 203, 216
  equipment maintenance and considerations in, 211–12
  foreign body removal in, 206, 209–11
  hip fracture diagnosis and management at South Pole, 208–10
  LUS use in, 203–4
  musculoskeletal injury and peripheral nerve blockade in, 206
  neurology US use in, 204–5
  pneumonia differential diagnosis at South Pole, 207–9
  research conducted in, 212
  teleultrasound in, 212
  training and quality assurance in, 212
  tropical diseases in, 206–7
  vascular US use in, 205–6

renal tract
  abdominal US of, 112–17
  anatomy of, 112–13
  bladder residual volume, 116, 190–2
  calculi in, 114–15
  cancer of, 116
  CKD of, 116
  cysts of, 115–16
  Hospital at Home care for,
    190, 191, 191, 192
  hydronephrosis of, 112–15
  pyelonephritis of, 116
  scanning methods for, 113
reports, 233–4
resolution, 5, 7
respiratory failure, BLUE Protocol for,
    1–2, 69, 71–3
respiratory phasicity, 131, 133
return of spontaneous circulation
    (ROSC), 37–8
reverberation artefact, 18, 74–5, 86
rheumatic heart disease (RHD), 214–15
rib shadows, 72–3
right atrial pressure
  echo assessment of, 35–6, 62
  IVC collapsibility as marker of,
    104–5
right atrium (RA)
  A4C view, 33
  diastolic collapse of, 52–4
  PSAX view, 30–2
  RV inflow view of, 30–1
right upper quadrant (RUQ), 105–7,
    182–3
right ventricle (RV)
  A4C view, 33
  diastolic collapse of, 52–4
  dilatation of, 56–7, 59
  echo assessment of function of, 55–6
  hypertrophy of, 57–8
  inflow and outflow view of, 30–1
  McConnell's sign in, 57
  PLAX view of, 29
  pressure and volume overload of,
    57–8
  SC view, 34–5
ring down artefact, 18–19
ring of fire sign, 184
rocking, probe, 14
ROSC. See return of spontaneous
    circulation
rotation, probe, 14
rotator cuff interval, 150, 152
ruptured ovarian cysts, 187
RUQ. See right upper quadrant
RV. See right ventricle
RWMA. See regional wall motion
    abnormalities

SAM. See systolic anterior motion
saphenofemoral junction (SFJ),
    129–30
SARS-CoV-2. See Severe Acute
    Respiratory Syndrome
    Coronavirus
SBO. See small bowel obstruction
SC view. See subcostal view
scanning method, 36.120. See also
    specific US techniques
  image acquisition, 12–21
  image optimisation, 21–4, 232–3
  image saving, 24, 231–2
  machine knobology, 8–9
  orientation and imaging planes, 12
  probe and preset selection, 9–12
scapholunate ligament, 157–8
SCUF. See Society of Clinical
    Ultrasound Fellowships
sea-shore sign, 74
sebaceous cysts, 146
sector width, 21–2
septal bulge, 46–7
septal flattening, 57–8
septic shock, 197–8
Severe Acute Respiratory Syndrome
    Coronavirus 2 (SARS-CoV-2),
    217. See also Coronavirus disease
    2019
SFJ. See saphenofemoral junction
SFV. See superficial femoral vein
shock
  echo assessment of, 59–63
  septic, 197–8
short axis, 12
shortness of breath. See dyspnoea
shoulder, MSKUS of, 150–4
shred sign, 76–8, 86
side lobe artefact, 20–1
silent hypoxia, 223–4
simple ovarian cysts, 186
Singapore, training and accreditation
    pathways in, 237–44
sinusoid sign, 78–9
60-60 sign, 57–8
sliding, probe, 13
sliding sign, 73–4, 219–20
  endotracheal intubation
    confirmation using, 202
  pneumothorax absence of, 75, 80–3,
    201–2
small bowel, 121
small bowel obstruction (SBO), 121,
    195–6
snow storm appearance, molar
    pregnancy, 185
Society of Clinical Ultrasound
    Fellowships (SCUF), 236

soft tissue ultrasound, 140, 143, 167.
    See also musculoskeletal
    ultrasound
  abscess on, 143–5
  Baker's cyst on, 148–9, 162
  cellulitis on, 143–4
  foreign bodies on, 148–9
  fractures on, 147
  ganglion cysts on, 146
  haematoma on, 147–8
  lipoma on, 146
  lymph nodes on, 145–6
  necrotising fasciitis on, 145
  normal anatomical structures on,
    141–3
  probe selection for, 140–1
  scanning methods for, 140–2
  sebaceous cysts on, 146
  tendonitis and tenosynovitis on, 148
sonographic Murphy's sign, 118–19
sound waves
  production and characteristics of,
    4–5
  tissue interactions with, 5–7
South Africa, training and
    accreditation pathways in, 237–44
South Pole
  equipment maintenance and
    considerations in, 211
  hip fracture diagnosis and
    management at, 208–10
  pneumonia differential diagnosis at,
    207–9
spectral Doppler, 16
specular reflection, 7
spine sign, 78–9
spleen
  acoustic impedance of, 7
  FAST of, 106–7
  propagation velocity through, 4–5
splenic rupture, 111
splenomegaly, 124–5
spongy myocardium. See left
    ventricular non-compaction
    cardiomyopathy
SSN view. See suprasternal view
sternal fracture, 147
sternoclavicular joint, 153–4
stratosphere sign, 75
string of pearls sign, 187–8
stroke, ischaemic, 177, 205
stroke volume (SV), 33–4, 60–1
subacromial bursa, 152
subclavian vein, 133–5
subcostal (SC) view, 34–5, 52, 54
subpleural consolidation, 76–7, 84–6,
    220–1
subscapularis, 150, 152

superficial femoral vein (SFV), 129–30, 132–3
supraspinatus, 150, 152–3
suprasternal (SSN) view, 35–6
SV. *See* stroke volume
swirl sign, 143–4
systolic anterior motion (SAM), 47–8

Tanga sign, 121
TAPSE. *See* tricuspid annular plane of systole excursion
target sign, 122
TAUS. *See* temporal artery ultrasound
TB. *See* tuberculosis
TCD. *See* transcranial Doppler
TDI. *See* tissue Doppler imaging
teleultrasound, 212
temporal artery ultrasound (TAUS), 174–6
tendinopathy, 141–2, 148
tendon, US characteristics of, 141–3
tendonitis, 148
tenosynovitis, 148
TGC. *See* time gain compensation
THI. *See* tissue harmonic imaging
thoracic ultrasound. *See* lung ultrasound
thoracocentesis, LUS guided, 95
thrombus. *See also* deep vein thrombosis; venous thromboembolism
    in acute pulmonary embolism, 59
    echo of, 63–4
    post-MI LV, 42–3
tilting, probe, 14
time gain compensation (TGC), 22–3
tissue Doppler imaging (TDI), 17
tissue harmonic imaging (THI), 23–4, 140–1
tissue sign, 76–8, 87
tissues. *See also specific tissues*
    propagation velocity through, 4–5
    sound wave interactions with, 5–7
TR. *See* tricuspid regurgitation
training and accreditation
    ease of, 2
    governance and quality assurance, 234–5
    pathways, 236–44
    in remote, wilderness and austere medicine, 212
transabdominal pelvic ultrasound
    confirmation of intrauterine pregnancy using, 182–4
    free fluid on, 181–5, 188–9
    scanning method for, 180–2
transcranial Doppler (TCD), 176

intracranial vasospasm on, 177–8
ischaemic stroke on, 177, 205
pulsatility index and ICP estimation, 178
remote, wilderness and austere medicine use of, 205
scanning method for, 176–7
transducer. *See* probe
transfer medicine. *See* prehospital ultrasound
transthoracic echocardiography (TTE), 213
trauma. *See* focused assessment with sonography in trauma
triceps tendon, 156
tricuspid annular plane of systole excursion (TAPSE), 55–6
tricuspid regurgitation (TR), 57–8
tricuspid valve (TV)
    A4C view, 33
    exaggerated inflow variability of, 54–5
    PSAX view, 30–2
    RV inflow view of, 30–1
    SC view, 34–5
trochanteric bursitis, 159–60
tropical disease, 206–7
TTE. *See* transthoracic echocardiography
tubal ring sign, 184
tuberculosis (TB), 92–3, 207
tubo-ovarian abscess, 188
tumours. *See also specific cancers*
    cardiac, 64
    ovarian, 186–7
TV. *See* tricuspid valve
twinkle artefact, 114
2D mode, 13

UGRA. *See* ultrasound guided regional anaesthesia
ulnar collateral ligament, 156–8
ulnar nerve, 156–7
ulnar vein, 133–5
ultrasound (US), 24.30. *See also specific topics*
    physics of, 4–7
ultrasound guided regional anaesthesia (UGRA), 206
ultrasound (US) machine. *See also* probe
    care for, 24
    governance and quality assurance policy for, 231
    imaging modes, 12–17
    knowledge and understanding of, 8–9
    portable, 1–2, 11, 200, 203, 213–14

presets of, 11
United Kingdom, training and accreditation pathways in, 237–44
United States of America, training and accreditation pathways in, 237–44
UPJ. *See* ureteropelvic junction
upper limb
    DVT assessment in, 133–6
    MSKUS of, 150–8
    vascular anatomy of, 133–4
ureter, 113–14
ureteropelvic junction (UPJ), 113–14
urinary retention, 116, 190–2
US. *See* ultrasound
uterus
    fibroids (leiomyomas) of, 185
    transabdominal pelvic US of, 180–1

vaginal stripe, 180–1
valvular heart disease
    A4C view, 33
    echo assessment of, 49–51
    infective endocarditis, 64–5
    PLAX view of, 29–30
    rheumatic, 215
vascular ultrasound, 127, 139
    in COVID-19, 227–8
    general principles and scanning methods for, 127–8
    lower limb DVT assessment using, 128–33
    prehospital, 202–3
    probe selection for, 127
    remote, wilderness and austere medicine use of, 205–6
    upper limb DVT assessment using, 133–6
    venous and arterial vascular access guidance by, 136–9, 225
vasospasm, TCD of, 177–8
veins, 127–8. *See also* vascular ultrasound
velocity. *See* propagation velocity
venous access, US guided, 136–9, 225
venous excess ultrasound (VEXUS), 62–3
venous gas emboli (VGE), 206
venous thromboembolism (VTE), 227–8. *See also* deep vein thrombosis
ventilation, for COVID-19, 224–5
ventricular septal defect (VSD), 41–3
vesicoureteric junctions (VUJ), 113–14
VEXUS. *See* venous excess ultrasound
VGE. *See* venous gas emboli
viruses. *See also* Coronavirus disease 2019

viruses. (cont.)
   LUS changes caused by, 226
volume assessment. *See*
   haemodynamics
VSD. *See* ventricular septal defect
VTE. *See* venous thromboembolism
VUJ. *See* vesicoureteric junctions

wall echo shadow (WES), 118–19

water
   acoustic impedance of, 5–7
   propagation velocity through, 4–5
water bath, soft tissue and
   musculoskeletal US using, 141–2
waterfall sign, 76, 220–1
wavelength, 4–5
WES. *See* wall echo shadow
whirlpool sign, 187

wilderness medicine. *See* remote,
   wilderness and austere
   medicine
withdrawal of medical care, 197–8
wrist, MSKUS of, 156–8

yolk sac, 183

zoom, image optimisation with, 21–2